Disorders of Nutrition and Metabolism in Clinical Surgery

To Bartha, Andrew, Philip and Douglas

For Churchill Livingstone

Publisher: Georgina Bentliff
Project Editor: Lucy Gardner
Editorial Co-ordination: Editorial Resources Unit
Copy Editor: Susan Beasley
Production Controller: Nancy Henry
Design: Design Resources Unit
Sales Promotion Executive: Hilary Brown

Disorders of Nutrition and Metabolism in Clinical Surgery

Understanding and Management

Graham L. Hill MD ChM FRACS FRCS FACS
Professor of Surgery, University of Auckland, New Zealand

Foreword by
J. C. Goligher ChM(Edin) FRCS(Edin & Eng) HonDSc(Leeds) HonMD(Mult) HonFRCS(I) HonFRACS HonFACS
Emeritus Professor of Surgery, University of Leeds; Consulting Surgeon, St Mark's Hospital for Diseases of the Rectum and Colon, London

CHURCHILL LIVINGSTONE
EDINBURGH LONDON MADRID MELBOURNE NEW YORK AND TOKYO 1992

CHURCHILL LIVINGSTONE
Medical Division of Longman Group UK Limited

Distributed in the United States of America by Churchill Livingstone Inc., 650 Avenue of the Americas, New York, N.Y. 10011, and by associated companies, branches and representatives throughout the world.

First published 1992

ISBN 0-443-04457-0

British Library Cataloguing in Publication Data
A catalogue record for this book is available from the British Library.

Library of Congress Cataloging in Publication Data
Hill, Graham L.
Disorders of nutrition and metabolism in clinical surgery: understanding and management / Graham L. Hill; foreword by J. C. Goligher.
p. cm.
Includes bibliographical references and index.
ISBN 0-443-04457-0
1. Surgery — Nutritional aspects. 2. Alimentary canal — Surgery. I. Title.
[DNLM: 1. Metabolic Diseases — therapy. 2. Nutrition Disorders — therapy. 3. Surgery, Operative. WO 500 H646d]
RD52.N88H55 1992
617′.919 — dc20
DNLM/DLC
for Library of Congress 91–46102

Produced by Longman Singapore Publishers (Pte) Ltd.
Printed in Singapore

Foreword

It was in 1925 that my most famous predecessor in Leeds, Berkeley Moynihan — who was not only a great abdominal surgeon but also a superb orator of quite Churchillian calibre — was responsible for the arresting and oft-quoted remark: 'Now that we have learnt Lister's lesson on how to avoid surgical sepsis, surgery is safe for the patient; what remains for us to do is to make the patient safe for surgery.' Well, despite its obvious oversimplification, this statement embodies a substantial truth. Since it was made, much has happened to assist progress towards the target set by Moynihan. Assuredly three of the most important aids to that end, which immediately spring to mind, are the general availability of blood transfusion, the introduction of antibiotic therapy and the better understanding of metabolic and nutritional disorders in surgical patients. Indeed, these advances have become such an integral part of modern surgical management it is now difficult to contemplate surgery without them and undeniable that many patients, who in earlier years would have succumbed after major surgical interventions, now owe their recovery from such operations largely to the beneficial effect of one or more of these therapeutic measures.

Of course, readily available blood transfusion and antibiotic therapy came on the scene in response to urgent wartime needs in 1939 and 1942/43 respectively. That lent their arrival a certain dramatic impact, which, together with the relative simplicity of their underlying rationales, ensured for both of them an immediate wide acceptance. By contrast, the evolution during the last 55 or so years of knowledge relating to disturbances of metabolism and nutrition in surgical patients and its incorporation in routine surgery has been a more gradual and fitful process. Most surgeons of my generation can recall in that period the successive bursts of enthusiasm displayed by different groups of researchers dealing with various specific issues within this large field — such as the understanding and control of fluid and electrolyte imbalance after surgical operations, the correction of protein deficiencies by intravenous administration of amino-acid solutions, the pros and cons of intravenous lipid emulsions as a specially rich source of energy, the perfecting of the technique of central venous cannulation via the subclavian vein (which did so much to popularize prolonged parenteral feeding), and the development of enteral tube feeding, to mention but some of the more important topics. All this work aroused much interest, but initially its ultimate great potential for ordinary surgical practice was perhaps not as widely appreciated as it should have been. However, during the past 20 or so years, awareness on this point has grown sharply and it is now generally accepted that the prevention and treatment of metabolic and nutritional disorders, certainly in major cases, is an essential item of first-rate contemporary surgical care. Much of this special attention can often be provided by the regular surgeon in charge of the patient, but, when faced with a highly complex situation, he or she should unquestionably secure the collaboration of an acknowledged expert.

This work on metabolic and nutritional disturbances has naturally generated an abundant and rapidly expanding literature, with many papers being published in different sorts of journals. It would obviously be a considerable convenience for the average clinical surgeon to have available a comprehensive treatise summarizing these numerous contributions and indicating their relevance to practical management. The provision of such a work has been the task Graham Hill has set himself in writing his new book on *Disorders of Nutrition and Metabolism in Clinical Surgery — Understanding and Management*, which also reflects strongly the findings of his own extensive personal experience and researches. To be asked to contribute a Foreword affords me immense pleasure, not least because it provides the opportunity to acknowledge publically how indebted I am to him for enlightening me on the modern management of these disorders. That happened in 1975, when, after working for 2 years with Stanley Dudrick in Texas, he rejoined me as my deputy in Leeds. The great emphasis in my department on advanced gastrointestinal and colorectal surgery meant that we had an abundance of patients particularly liable to experience metabolic problems, thus providing him with ideal opportunities to demonstrate how they should be investigated and treated. I have always felt extremely grateful to him and have followed with keen interest the progress of his career after he moved to the Chair of Surgery in Auckland, New Zealand, where his department has rightly become celebrated for its many important contributions to knowledge in this field.

It has indeed been a delight to browse through the pages of this splendid volume. Of course, I have approached it, not as someone specially versed in metabolic matters, but as an ordinary practising surgeon — and, moreover, one now virtually at the end of his active professional life! It is hardly surprising therefore that some of the more abstruse sections of the text should have proved rather difficult for me to master, but perhaps even more remarkable that, thanks to the great clarity of the writing and illustrations, I was able to understand far more of the biochemical data than I might have expected. However, I have no doubt that to those younger, more physiologically orientated surgeons who may wish to remain responsible themselves to the limit of their abilities for the metabolic care of their patients, this book will prove eminently readable and entirely comprehensible, and should provide them and their staff with good guidance to keep them on the right lines in their efforts. As regards the use metabolic specialists may make of this book, admittedly they will already be familiar with most or all that is mentioned in it, but they may find it convenient to have this information fully recorded in this compact well-referenced form, and also be interested to compare their own views with those of the author on various controversial issues.

I believe that surgeons should feel extremely grateful to Graham Hill for having gone to the trouble to produce this magnificent work, which provides such sound practical advice and also affords occasional fascinating glimpses of possible exciting developments in the future. I am convinced that it will be widely consulted and cannot fail to become an outstanding success.

J. C. Goligher

Preface

Just when we thought that nutrition and metabolism had settled into a comfortable place in surgical care the revolution in cell biology has come along. Now, in clinical practice and looming on the horizon, we have the ability to modify the patient's response to serious sepsis at a molecular level, provide nutrients which act as pharmacological agents and manufacture growth factors which have the potential to reduce or eliminate protein catabolism, improve response to nutritional therapy and enhance wound healing. All this is heady stuff and it would be easy to lose perspective and forget the vital impact high quality nutrition and metabolic care have in the daily care of the surgical patient. It is for this reason that this book is presented. It is a guidebook for the general surgeon and his or her team which seeks to be authoritative and practical and focused on patient care. It is based on an understanding of the fundamentals of nutrition and metabolism within the context of high standards of surgical care. It also seeks to place the exciting new advances in molecular biology in context even though balanced perspectives are difficult to attain at this time of rapid change.

This book has been put together by a busy general surgeon who has been fortunate to have had a wide clinical experience in several areas including Australasia, the United Kingdom, the United States, and South East Asia. It is this broad practical base combined with an active interest in clinical and scientific research in the area of nutrition and metabolism that has led to the belief that a book from such a background might have a place in the vast array of surgical literature.

More than 20 years ago, as a lecturer in surgery in Professor Alan Clarke's Department of Surgery in Dunedin, New Zealand, I met Dr Stanley Dudrick, who was on a James IV Travelling Fellowship to that part of the world. His new practical developments and clinical research caught my imagination and I resolved then that this type of work would be worthy of life-long study. Later, in Professor John Goligher's great Department of Surgery in Leeds, England, I was introduced to the serious nutritional and metabolic problems of patients undergoing very major and complex gastrointestinal surgery. Professor Goligher encouraged me to take up an offer to work in Dr Stanley Dudrick's Department of Surgery at the University of Texas at Houston, where I was further able to develop my interests and experience first hand the work of that growing and active department.

Later, rejoining John Goligher at the Leeds General Infirmary, I was able to join forces with Dr Lewis Burkinshaw's Medical Physics group who were starting work in the area of in vivo neutron activation analysis. We were able to develop these new physics systems into clinical facilities which enabled us to make direct body composition measurements, and study the effect of various nutritional regimens on the composition of the body. The lessons learnt in Leeds formed the basis for the development of the clinical interests and the laboratories at the Department of Surgery at the University of Auckland, New Zealand, where I moved in 1980. There, from ideas born overseas, we set up a nutritional assessment/body composition laboratory alongside our surgical wards where a wide variety of general surgery was being performed in a tertiary care setting. Not only were patients with complex diseases of the alimentary tract available for study but patients with major trauma and critically ill intensive care patients also were able to be measured in a body composition facility specially designed for that purpose.

Background and scope of the book

This book is based mainly on studies of patients from our surgical wards studied in the University Department of Surgery at Auckland Hospital. More than 600 surgical patients covering most of the commonly encountered metabolic problems have been entered in various protocols and studies over the past 10 years. Not discussed here are those problems and diseases of which we have no personal experience. In particular, burns have not been covered, nor have the special nutritional and metabolic problems of children.

The book is organised into four parts and covers those areas which are everyday occurrences in busy surgical clinics. The first part of the book deals with fundamental principles underlying metabolic care, the compositional and physiological changes that occur in normal convalescence after major surgery and then some of the more difficult problems encountered in metabolic care in the perioperative period. A fairly formal account of water and salt and acid base therapy is then given. The second part of the book is a comprehensive account of nutritional care. Modern ideas of the classification of adult protein energy malnutrition and new discoveries of the effect of nutritional therapy in treating it are then covered. Practical aspects of nutritional assessment are explained as are the therapeutic modes of enteral and parenteral feeding. This section finishes with four case management problems, a learning technique used most successfully by Dr George Blackburn of Boston. The next section of the book, Part 3, covers the particular nutritional and metabolic problems encountered in the practice of the surgeon who deals with complex problems of the alimentary tract. We present here much of our own practical approach in this area together with research that has been centred around these types of patients. Finally the book finishes with an insight for the general surgeon into serious surgical illness, including in particular those patients with organ failure. This is not meant to be a comprehensive account of intensive care. It is specifically designed for those members of general surgical teams who find this area somewhat confusing and baffling and this section is aimed to introduce them to the terminology used in critical care, the type of treatments given and the role that they may be expected to play if they are working in a team situation with critical care specialists alongside. This section is not designed for those who are experts in critical care and manage this side of patient care entirely themselves.

There has been no attempt to cover the extensive literature on the subject but an up-to-date and representative bibliography is provided which will enable the reader to explore certain topics in more depth.

Acknowledgements

This book would never have been possible without the dedication, enthusiasm and education of the author by a series of assistants and research fellows, both here in Auckland and formerly in Leeds. Their names appear as the various studies are presented and each one has a share in whatever worth this book may prove to have.

I am particularly indebted to members of the Department of Surgery in Auckland, who worked closely in the development of the techniques used and helped to plan the experiments presented here. Dr Stephen Streat not only worked in the Department as a research fellow but also provided direct assistance by reviewing the sections on trauma and serious sepsis. Dr J. Shaw, while working in the Department, performed a vast array of isotopic studies in general surgical patients and I have drawn from his various publications to explain some aspects of glucose, fatty acid and protein kinetics in surgical disease.

The development of the surgical research laboratory at the University of Auckland, which is a unique facility, would not have been possible without Dr Alan Beddoe, Mr Herman Zuidmeer, Dr Grant Knight, Dr Sudeep Mitra, Dr John Sutcliffe and Dr Lindsay Plank. Dr Lewis Burkinshaw from Leeds has also given a guiding hand to our work over the years.

This book was put together during a sabbatical at Green College, Oxford University whilst the author was a guest in Professor Peter Morris' Department of Surgery. Sir Crispin Tickell, Warden of Green College, kindly provided for me a superb office environment in a small astronomical observatory in the College grounds. Dr Julian Britton and his wife, Mona, made every effort to make our stay at Green College and in Oxford a most profitable and happy one. At Oxford University, away from the busy clinical life, I was able to concentrate undisturbed and bring together the various threads of our many clinical studies. Many others, however, worked hard and long to make this book possible. Most of the laboratory measurements mentioned in the case reports and the various studies were done in the Auckland Hospital Department of Surgery laboratories by Dr Grant Knight and more recently, Mrs Mary White. Mrs Bartha Hill processed the manuscript and produced all the computer graphics for the book.

The support of the Medical Research Council of New Zealand is acknowledged with gratitude. The University of Auckland has done all in its power to ensure the work has been encouraged and developed. We are grateful also to the Auckland Medical Research Foundation and the Royal Australasian College of Surgeons for being of assistance. The help of Baxter Healthcare Ltd (New Zealand Ltd) and managers, Mr Ned Lipes and Mr Con Crighton, is again gratefully acknowledged.

This book is based on hundreds of clinical measurements of our sick surgical patients and we are grateful for their cheerful and willing contributions which have led to the better understanding and overall nutritional and metabolic care of surgical patients.

Auckland, New Zealand 1992 Graham L. Hill

Contents

PART 1

Metabolic Care

PART 1

Metabolic Care

Part 1 Contents

1. Understanding metabolic care

INTRODUCTION

Many surgeons feel that surgical metabolism is a complex topic which is particularly difficult to grasp and hence they shrink away from learning about it. It is true that some textbooks and some experts present metabolic principles in unnecessary detail and this, quite understandably, can be daunting to the surgical mind. There are, however, a number of basic concepts which the surgeon needs to grasp in order to be in a position to manage the many complex metabolic problems that present in modern surgical practice.

In this chapter, we will present these basic concepts. A broad overview of the chemical composition of the body will be given and a description of how the body reacts to simple starvation will be compared to a description of the integrated metabolic response of the body to trauma and serious sepsis. This is bedrock knowledge and it is difficult to proceed to an understanding of metabolic care without it.

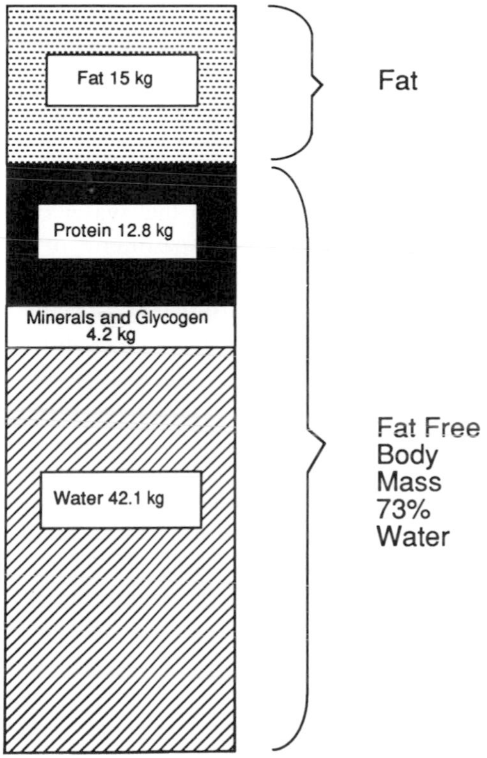

Fig. 1.1 The components of body mass in a healthy 40-year-old male subject. An in vivo neutron activation technique and measurements of body water and body weight were used to measure these body compartments. (Data from Beddoe et al 1984.)

SECTION I
THE CHEMICAL COMPOSITION OF THE BODY

Figure 1.1 shows the chemical composition of a normal 40-year-old male.

BODY FAT

It can be seen that this normal 40-year-old man is composed of 15 kg of fat. The majority, about 12 kg, is *storage fat*, that is, fat in subcutaneous, intermuscular, intraabdominal and intrathoracic locations. The remaining 3 kg is termed *essential fat*, that is, lipids of bone marrow and lipids in the central nervous system and other organs.

Storage fat is in the form of triglyceride which is chemically and physically like olive oil. It is stored mainly in specialised cells called adipocytes where it is stored without accompanying water. When fat is required as a fuel for the heart, skeletal muscle, liver or kidney, it is hydrolysed to three fatty acids and glycerol (a carbohydrate). Tightly bound to albumin the fatty acids are transported to these organs where on combustion they yield 9.4 kcal for every gram of fatty acid burned.

THE FAT FREE BODY MASS

Figure 1.1 shows that the fat free body mass is composed of water, glycogen, protein and minerals.

Body water

From Figure 1.1 it can be seen that water comprises by far the biggest compartment of the body. Clinically this is important for it means that appreciable gains or losses from body weight in the short term are due largely to changes in body water. The hydration of the fat free body is remarkably constant. In man, together with all other animal species measured, 73% of the fat free body mass is water. We shall see later that an almost universal accompaniment of surgical illness is an expanding hydration of the fat free body. In some particularly sick patients the hydration coefficient may reach 80% or more.

Carbohydrate

Carbohydrate stores in the body are very small, (600–700 g). It is stored in the form of glycogen; 500 g are in muscle and 200 g in the liver. Glycogen is made up of large branching-chain molecules of glucose which form a gel with potassium rich water between the chains. As cells build up glycogen 2–4 g of water are stored for each gram of glycogen. These small stores of carbohydrate in the body quantitatively are not important as energy reserves but they are vitally important in situations of stress where they provide the first extra glucose when glucose is needed urgently. Repletion of body glycogen results in an increase in total body potassium and total body water.

Body protein

Not all of the 12 or 13 kg of protein in the body is available for metabolic interchange. About 45% forms the scaffold of the body — it is the structural proteins of collagen, fascia, ligaments, dermis and of the walls of blood vessels. When body tissues are consumed in wasting diseases these structures are maintained intact while lean cellular tissues are oxidised. The remaining 55% of body protein is in cells or circulating proteins and here lies the engine room of the body. Each protein molecule has an important function: as an enzyme, as a contractile unit or structural unit, or in one or more other proteins performing a physiological function. *The important point is that if cellular protein is consumed as a fuel, as it always is in surgical illness, there will, as a consequence, be a loss of some body function.* We will see later (Ch. 5) that by the time 20% of body protein stores have been burnt there is objective evidence of physiological dysfunction in most organ systems of the body. When the normal quantity of protein in the body is present any extra protein taken in is broken down, the nitrogen is excreted as urea and the carbon skeletons of the amino acids are used as energy or stored as fat.

Minerals

By weight, most of the minerals in the body are in the skeleton. Though the rest of the minerals weigh less than half a kilogram, they are of crucial importance in determining water distribution. We will discuss the physiology of this in more detail in Chapter 4.

SECTION II
ENERGY DEMANDS

THE RESTING STATE

Of all the organs of the body the brain has the most constant demand for energy. Whether the subject is asleep, sitting an examination or watching television the demand is constant. It uses about 20% of the resting energy expenditure. The liver and viscera together use 30% of resting energy expenditure, the heart 5%, the kidneys 10%, and the remainder is used by muscle. In exercise, muscle may take up to 90% of the total energy expenditure.

THE STRESSED STATE

In stress situations, catecholamines and glucagon rise and, as a consequence, liver and muscle glycogen break down with an outpouring of glucose into the circulation. Glycogen is a limited source of glucose however, and hepatic glucose production is increased shortly after, being also initiated by catecholamines and glucagon. The raw material for this newly manufactured glucose comes mainly from amino acids, principally from two muscle amino acids, alanine and glutamine. The energy for the manufacturing process comes not from glucose but from the breakdown of body fat.

These basic changes seen in physiologic stress extend to surgical illness where in trauma and sepsis increased glucose requirements are met by increased hepatic manufacture of glucose from amino acids produced from the breakdown of muscle protein. We shall see how in prolonged starvation the body adapts its fuel requirements to spare muscle protein but in serious surgical illness this adaptive process does not occur and muscle is cannibalised to provide alanine and glutamine which are the raw materials for glucose production. The increased glucose is produced to meet the energy demands of the brain, the wound and the infected or traumatised site.

SECTION III
METABOLIC INTERCHANGES IN PROGRESSIVE STARVATION

THE NORMAL SUBJECT JUST AFTER A MEAL

The glucose from the *carbohydrate* consumed in a meal is absorbed and its first priority is to provide fuel for the brain which requires 100–125 g of glucose per day. The next priority is to replenish liver glycogen and once this is replete the extra glucose is siphoned off and stored as fat.

Food protein is broken down into amino acids which after absorption replenish protein in the liver and muscle and replace protein broken down since the previous meal. Amino acids not required for protein synthesis are stripped of their amino group to form urea and the remaining carbohydrate residues are used by the liver for energy or for fat synthesis or for the formation of new glucose. Three amino acids (leucine, isoleucine and valine) which are together called the branched-chain amino acids (BCAAs) are metabolised in the periphery by adipocytes for fat synthesis and in muscle cells for energy. This is why it has been thought that the provision of amino acid solutions enriched with branched-chain amino acids might help to preserve protein in serious surgical illness where, as we have seen, muscle is being cannibalised to provide branched-chain amino acids which then form alanine and glutamine, the substrates for hepatic glucose production.

Fat from food is absorbed as triglyceride and when combined with lipoproteins forms chylomicrons. In the fasting state these are used by muscle as fuel although after a meal they are removed primarily by adipose tissue for incorporation into fat droplets and stored for energy.

THE NORMAL SUBJECT AFTER AN OVERNIGHT FAST

After an overnight fast, when all the food from the previous meal has been absorbed, the brain is consuming the majority of the body's glucose although skeletal muscle derives about a third of its energy from glucose. Free fatty acids are beginning to be mobilised from adipose tissue to provide the rest of the fuel requirements of muscle (Layzer 1991). Liver glucose production is being maintained both from glycogen and from the formation of new glucose (gluconeogenesis). Insulin levels are low and this initiates muscle protein breakdown with the release of amino acids, mainly alanine and glutamine. These are the optimal substrates for the production of new glucose in the liver and, to a lesser extent, in the kidney.

EARLY STARVATION

Figure 1.2 shows the fuel metabolism in a normal man who has been fasted for 1–2 days. The brain is now living primarily off new glucose produced by the liver. By the second day of starvation about 75 g of muscle protein is being broken down daily. This is not enough to supply all the substrate for the manufacture of glucose for the brain, and glycerol (from fat) and lactate (from glucose utilisation in the haemopoietic tissues) are the other sources of fuel. This shunting of lactate back to the liver for recycling into glucose is called the Cori cycle. The gluconeogenic precursors coming from the periphery are pushed into gluconeogenesis with almost 100% efficiency and for this reason, the liver derives its own energy directly from fatty acids. Figure 1.2 also shows that about 160 g of triglyceride is broken down daily to supply energy needs.

LATER STARVATION

Figure 1.3 shows the picture of fuel metabolism in prolonged fasting. A major adaptive change has now occurred, the prime purpose of which is to reduce the loss of muscle protein. Blood levels of acetoacetate and beta hydroxybutyrate (ketones) which have gradually built up over the first week of starvation are now high and sufficient to be consumed by the brain as its primary fuel. Glucose oxidation by the brain is diminished accordingly. With less and less need for brain glucose hepatic gluconeogenesis is needed less and muscle proteolysis is much diminished. Therefore, instead of 75 g of muscle protein per day, only 20 g of muscle protein a day is being consumed and urinary nitrogen which is around 11–15 g per day in normal subjects falls to 4 or 5 g per day. This is due to the marked diminution in urinary urea (Fig. 1.4). This adaptation enables the preservation of a large proportion of body muscle and allows starvation to continue as long as there is some triglyceride to produce free fatty acids and glycerol.

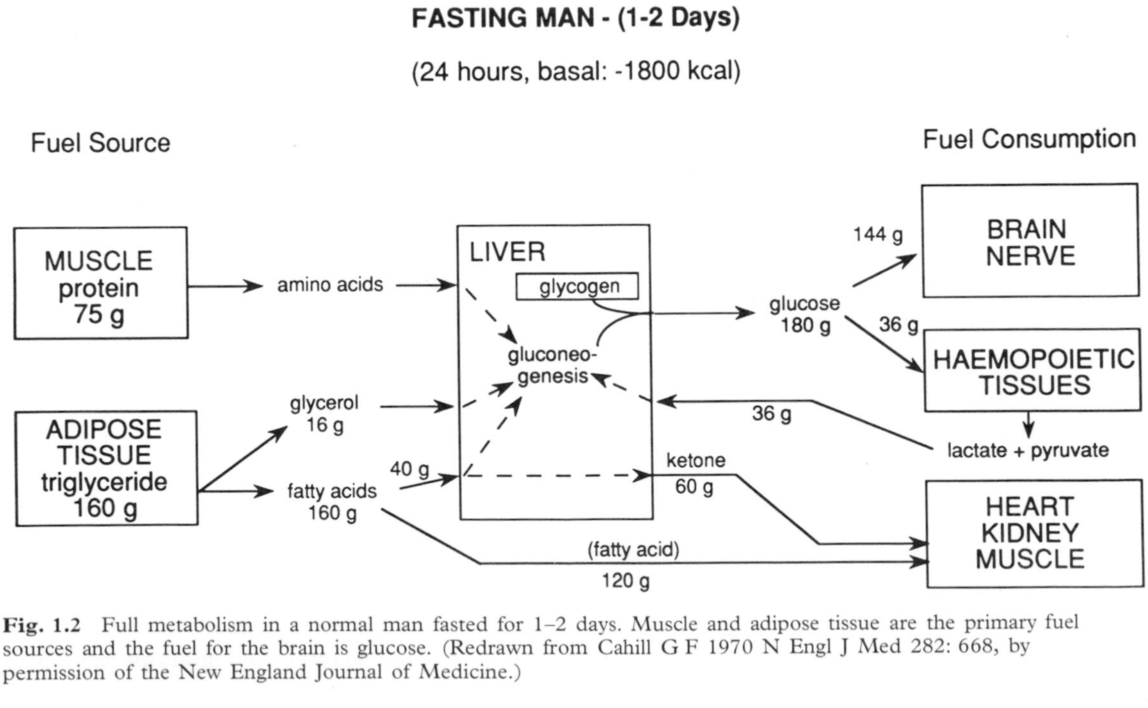

Fig. 1.2 Full metabolism in a normal man fasted for 1–2 days. Muscle and adipose tissue are the primary fuel sources and the fuel for the brain is glucose. (Redrawn from Cahill G F 1970 N Engl J Med 282: 668, by permission of the New England Journal of Medicine.)

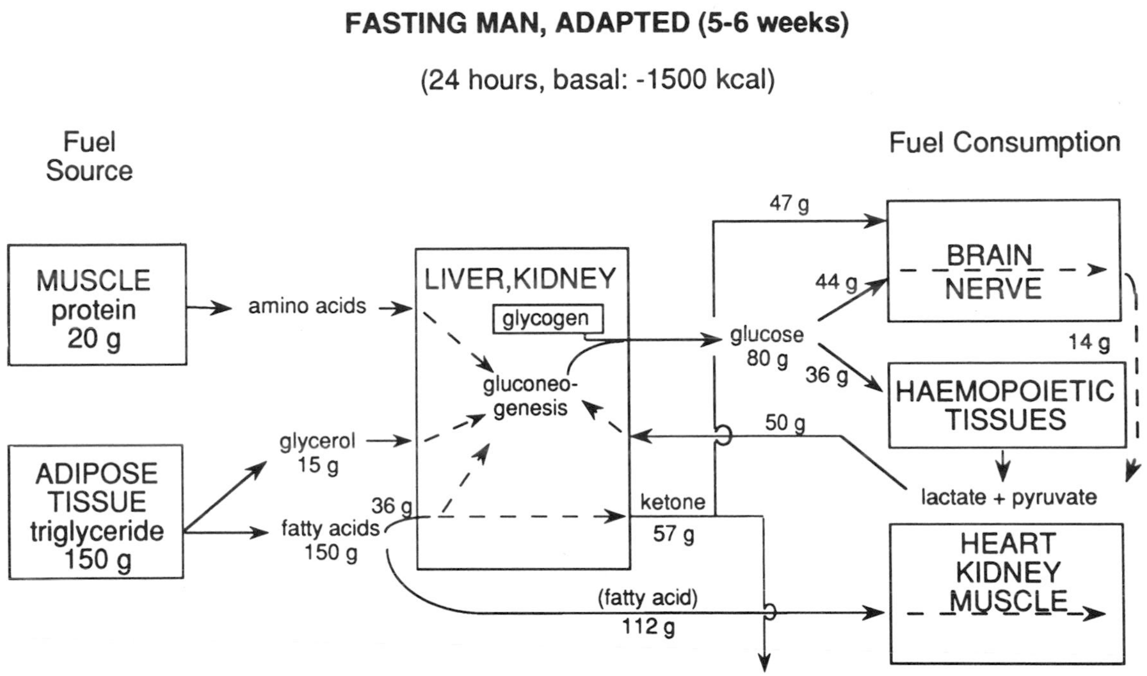

Fig. 1.3 Fuel metabolism in prolonged fasting (5–6 weeks). The fuel for the brain is mainly ketones. The subject has adapted by burning less muscle protein. (Redrawn from Cahill G F 1970 N Engl J Med 282: 668, by permission of the New England Journal of Medicine.)

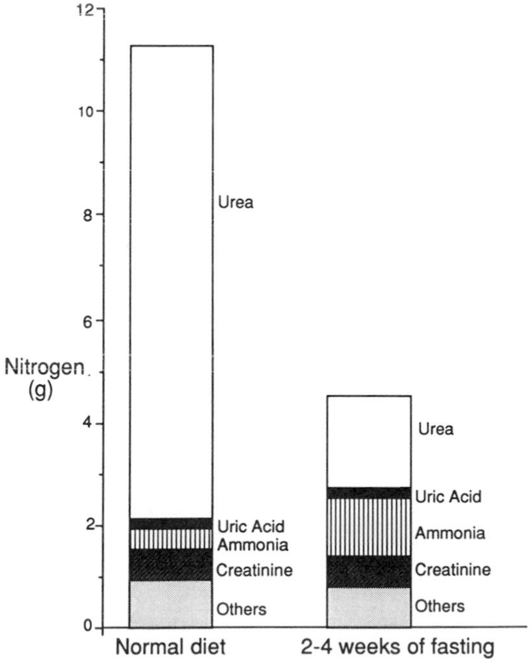

Fig. 1.4 The urinary constituents in the fed state (left column) and after 2–4 weeks of starvation (right column). The extremely small amount of urea excreted by the starving subject is apparent.

ENDOCRINE RESPONSES TO FASTING

Figure 1.5 describes the hormonal response to fasting. There is a decline in circulating insulin, an increase in glucagon and a fall in triiodothyronine. The primary signal early in fasting is the lower insulin level which in the presence of elevated levels of glucagon provokes not only hepatic breakdown of glycogen but also the initiation of gluconeogenesis. The low insulin level also initiates proteolysis in skeletal muscle with release of amino acids. As the liver enters a gluconeogenic mode, in the presence of low insulin levels and in the permissive presence of glucagon, glucocorticoids and thyroid hormone it begins to produce ketone bodies. Fasting decreases the conversion of thyroxine to triiodothyronine resulting in a modest form of hypometabolism with the result that there is a decrease in overall caloric expenditure due to a decreased oxygen consumption. There is also a small decrease in catecholamine levels.

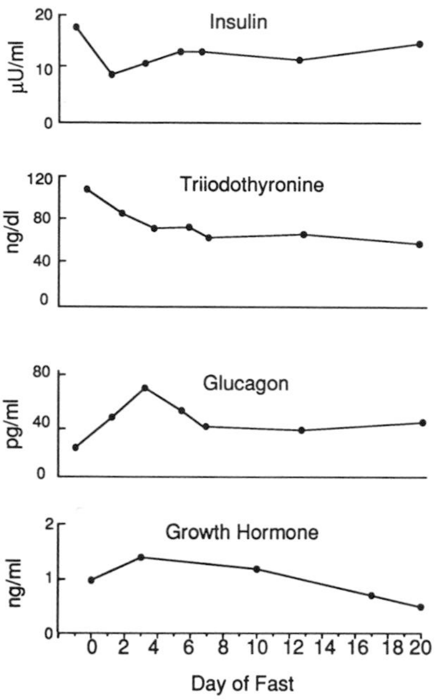

Fig. 1.5 Hormonal response to fasting. Insulin and triiodothyronine concentrations decline and glucagon concentration increases. Growth hormone does not change. (Redrawn from Aoki & Finlay 1986 The metabolic response to fasting. In: Rombeau J L, Caldwell M D (eds) Clinical nutrition, W B Saunders, Philadelphia, vol 2: 11, with permission of W B Saunders.)

SECTION IV
METABOLIC INTERCHANGES IN TRAUMA

Trauma produces a neuroendocrine response which results in changes in hormone concentrations which are quite different to those we have observed in prolonged starvation. Cortisol, glucagon, and the catecholamines, epinephrine and norepinephrine, are increased in proportion to the severity of the trauma. They produce muscle proteolysis (cortisol), glycogenolysis and enhanced gluconeogenesis (cortisol and glucagon), and oxidation of fat (epinephrine, cortisol and thyroid hormone). Insulin action is antagonised by raised levels of growth hormone and epinephrine. The net result on fuel metabolism is seen in Figure 1.6.

The fundamental change is a requirement of the wound or damaged tissue for glucose and a loss of the adaptive decrease in proteolysis that is seen in prolonged starvation. Muscle proteolysis produces branched-chain amino acids which are converted to alanine and glutamine as precursors for new glucose formation by the liver. Glucose is the fuel used by the wound and haemopoietic tissues. Lactate from the wound and glycerol from fat oxidation are also substrates for new glucose. In the plasma there are marked rises in free fatty acids, glycerol, glucose, lactate, and amino acids, particularly alanine and glutamine. Alanine is the main gluconeogenic precursor. Glutamine is the fuel for the gut, kidney and cells of the immune system (Fig. 1.7).

The neuroendocrine response to trauma will be described more completely in Chapter 4 but it should be noted here that interruption of the normal neural pathways up the mid brain can abolish it altogether (Hume & Egdahl 1959). When injury is limited, as in straightforward elective surgery, the response is slight and short lived. In major accidental trauma the neuroendocrine response is marked and the metabolic effects are substantial. When trauma is very severe, and particularly when infection supervenes, more profound haemodynamic alterations together with hypermetabolism and marked proteolysis occur. The neuroendocrine responses are necessary for this hypermetabolic response but are not completely responsible for it. In the next section we will see how peptide regulatory factors are the key factors in initiating and propagating the metabolic response in severe trauma and serious sepsis.

SECTION V
METABOLIC INTERCHANGES IN SERIOUS SEPSIS

Patients with serious sepsis have a dimension of hypermetabolism, proteolysis and extracellular water expansion that cannot be explained by the neuroendocrine responses that are seen after major surgery or moderate trauma.

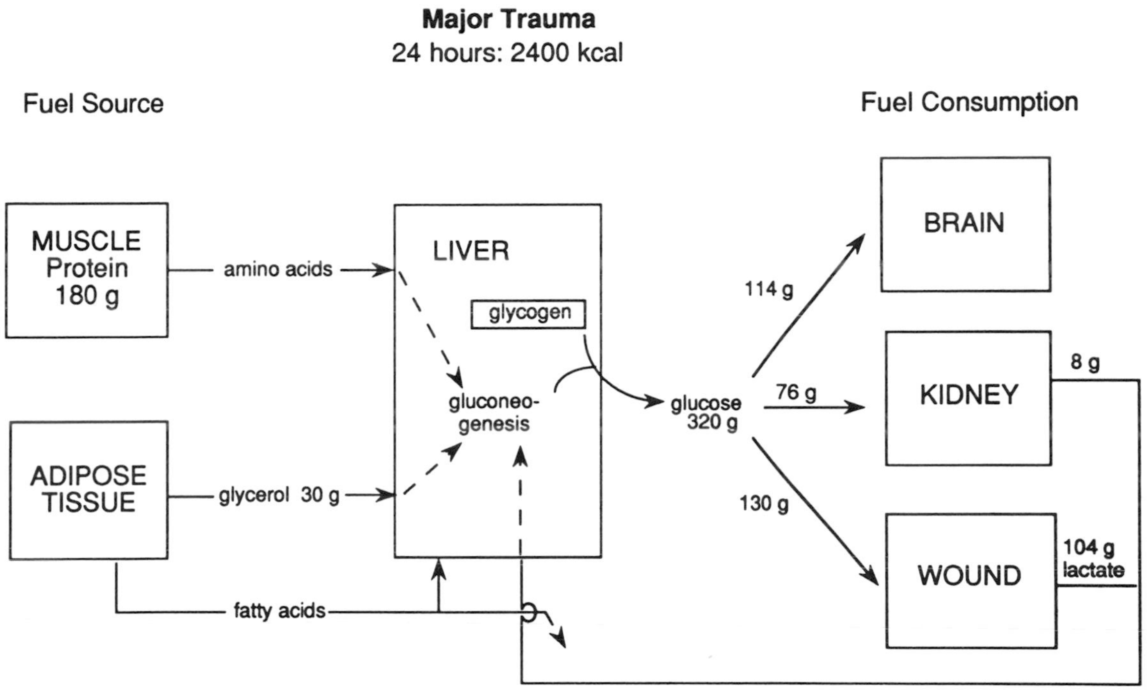

Fig. 1.6 Fuel metabolism in a patient with major trauma (simplified schema). Shown is the substantial glucose requirement of the injured tissue. Lactate is produced from wound anaerobic metabolism and is returned to the liver for recycling into glucose (Cori cycle). Muscle is cannibalised to produce amino acids (particularly alanine and glutamine) which are precursors of new glucose. Fatty acids supply the energy necessary for gluconeogenesis.

Although infusion of the catabolic hormones, cortisol, glucagon and the catecholamines can reproduce many of the clinical and metabolic changes seen in patients with serious sepsis, they cannot reproduce the massive proteolysis that is seen in these patients. Up to 250 g of muscle protein per day may be broken down in patients

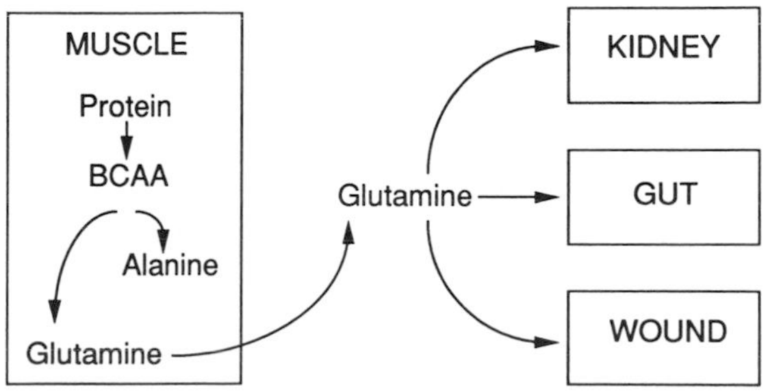

Fig. 1.7 Proteolysis provides branched chain amino acids (BCAA) within muscle which donate nitrogen to form alanine and glutamine. Glutamine is essential for functioning of cells in the healing wound, as fuel for the gut and for ammonia formation in the kidney.

with serious sepsis. It is now realised that peptide regulatory factors, in particular cytokines produced from inflammatory cells at the site of the infection itself are the links between the wound or inflammatory mass and the metabolic and immunologic responses that are occurring (Fong & Lowry 1990). The interleukins 1, 2 and 6 (IL-1, IL-2, IL-6), tumour necrosis factor (TNF) and interferon γ may have important roles in this regard. At least two of these cytokines, TNF and IL-2, are postinflammatory, circulating signals that can initiate and propagate the metabolic response in serious sepsis. Endotoxin is a potent stimulus for the production of TNF. Recent research suggests that cytokines potentiate the release of other cytokines and mediators as well as the classic hormones, catecholamines, glucagon and cortisol (Michie & Wilmore 1990). The effects of circulating cytokines are profound (Welbourn et al 1990). For instance, TNF has been shown to produce hypotension, shock, increased capillary permeability, fever and profound effects on the immune system. It has metabolic effects including muscle proteolysis, increased amino acid uptake by the liver, the production of acute phase proteins and increased lipolysis. IL-1 has been called proteolysis inducing factor and also is a principal inducer of acute phase protein synthesis. IL-2 and IL-6 serve predominantly as immune stimulants though both have metabolic effects.

The net result of cytokine release into the circulation is to induce hypermetabolism with increased whole body oxygen consumption, massive proteolysis and a general exaggeration of the changes in fuel metabolism that occur in trauma. Figure 1.8 shows the characteristic alterations in the exchange of substrates between organs that occur; it is the hyperdynamic circulation which develops in serious sepsis that enables these exchanges to take place. The inflammatory cells in the wound require glucose (probably also glutamine) as their primary fuel. Here glucose releases its energy through the glycolytic pathway with CO_2, water and lactate as the end products. This lactate is transported back to the liver for recycling into glucose. The whole gluconeogenic process requires energy which is supplied by free fatty acids. Most of the glucose required for the healing wound or inflammatory mass is produced by the liver not only from lactate but from alanine released from muscle and to a lesser extent from other gluconeogenic amino acids. Muscle is the major supplier of amino acids, the most abundant amino acids released from muscle being alanine and glutamine. Glutamine serves as a primary fuel for the enterocyte, producing ammonia and other products such as alanine which are shuttled back to the liver. Glutamine also helps to buffer the increased acid load in the kidney by the formation of ammonia (see Ch. 19).

In Chapter 19 we will learn more about the hyperdynamic state that occurs in critically ill surgical patients. The important thing to grasp here is the substantial need for glucose by the inflammatory mass with the substrates for this coming from the breakdown of muscle protein. To support these interchanges and particularly to

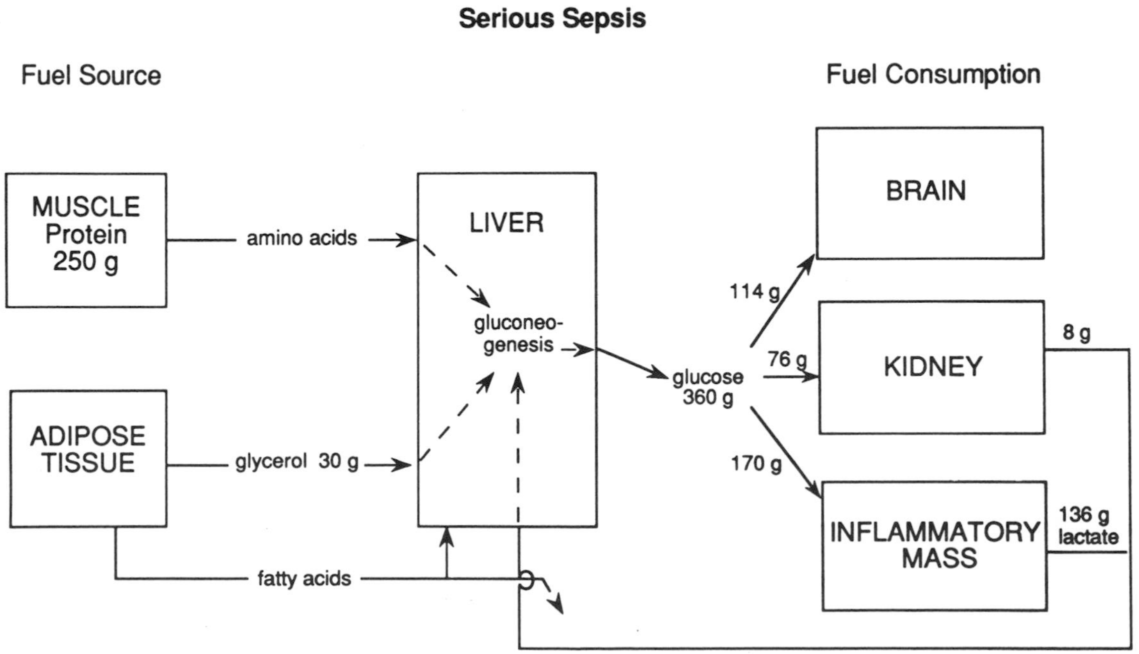

Fig. 1.8 Fuel metabolism in a patient with serious sepsis. The substantial daily loss of muscle protein is shown. The inflammatory mass is using glucose as fuel. This comes from gluconeogenesis in the liver. The substrates used for new glucose production are amino acids (particularly alanine and glutamine) from muscle, glycerol from fat, and lactate from the metabolising inflammatory cells.

support the increased glucose requirement for the cells in the inflammatory mass there is a whole body need for more energy; more oxygen is consumed and the metabolic rate is raised. To allow these interchanges to occur there is increased cardiac output and a hyperdynamic circulation.

The practical surgical lesson is that until the septic focus is controlled cytokines will continue to be produced and hypermetabolism with autocannibalism will continue unabated. Surgeons have known for centuries the dramatic and beneficial effect of draining pus, removing necrotic debris and preventing continuing contamination. The realisation that peptide regulatory factors are released from inflammatory cells in the septic focus has now taught us why this effect is so dramatic. The solution to the problem of continuing hypermetabolism is often in the hands of the surgeon and it cannot be emphasised too greatly that until the continuing production of cytokines from inflammatory cells is stopped the best that can be done at present is to partially stem the tide of cellular protein loss and support the hypermetabolic state. Recombinant technology, by providing monoclonal antibodies to endotoxin and various cytokines, has opened up a new era in the treatment of serious sepsis.

SECTION VI
IMPACT OF RECENT ADVANCES IN BIOTECHNOLOGY AND THE TREATMENT OF SERIOUS SEPSIS

Many of the systemic responses to Gram negative bacteraemia can be triggered by endotoxin. Endotoxin is the lipopolysaccharide component of the bacterial cell wall. A human monoclonal antibody that binds to the active component of endotoxin-lipid A has been produced and its administration has been shown to halve the mortality of patients with the sepsis syndrome (Ziegler et al 1991). Other monoclonal antibodies have been raised against tumour necrosis factor and other components of the inflammatory cascade. Immunotherapy has the potential to influence the outcome of serious surgical illness in the same way that antibiotics did in earlier times (Dunn 1988, Shimamoto et al 1988, Khazaeli et al 1990).

SECTION VII
METABOLIC TERMS — SOME DEFINITIONS AND EXPLANATIONS

NITROGEN BALANCE

The average western diet contains around 80 g of protein. Since 16% of this protein is nitrogen (i.e. there is 1 g of N in 6.25 g of protein), that means about 13 g of nitrogen per day is ingested. A normal subject who is maintaining a constant weight excretes an amount of nitrogen equal to his or her intake — he or she is therefore referred to as being in zero nitrogen balance. Of the 13 g a day intake of nitrogen around 11 g are excreted in the urine (≈70% in the form of urea) and the remainder in the faeces (1 g) and from exfoliation of the skin (1 g).

Nitrogen balance can give an overall picture of whether total body protein is being built up (anabolism) or broken down (catabolism). Where nitrogen balance is positive more is being taken in than is being excreted and body protein is being synthesised; when nitrogen balance is negative there is net catabolism of body protein.

Nitrogen balance data are frequently shown in metabolic charts. The convention usually used is that of Moore and Ball (1952) in which intake is charted upward from zero, output downward from the top of the intake line. The resultant lower line is the balance.

PROTEIN TURNOVER

Protein and indeed other processes in metabolism are in a dynamic state, i.e. protein is constantly being broken down and constantly being synthesised. Protein is thought of as being in a compartment or a pool and the total volume of the pool is influenced by the rate at which protein is added to or removed from it. These rates can be determined by infusing a small amount of isotopically labelled protein (usually an amino acid). At steady state, the tracer appears in the pool and, providing the pool size is constant, the rate of the appearance of the labelled protein is equal both to the rate of disappearance from the pool and the total rate of movement through the pool. The process is referred to as the flux or turnover of protein.

PROTEIN SYNTHESIS AND PROTEIN CATABOLISM

Total body protein is thought of as a single metabolic pool from which protein is withdrawn in two directions — namely for protein synthesis or for protein catabolism (breakdown). If synthesis exceeds breakdown there is a net gain of total body protein (net protein synthesis) and if breakdown exceeds synthesis there is a net loss of total body protein (net protein catabolism).

AMINO ACIDS

Essential amino acids

Isoleucine, leucine, valine, lysine, methionine, phenylalanine, threonine and tryptophan are essential dietary components. The lack of any one of these in the diet results in an inability to retain protein. The subject will therefore go into negative nitrogen balance. In the adult at least 20% of dietary protein should be in the form of essential amino acids.

Branched-chain amino acids (BCAAs)

Three of the essential amino acids, isoleucine, leucine and valine are called BCAAs. While most amino acids are taken up and metabolised by the liver to a large extent, branched-chain amino acids are utilised by skeletal muscle. In muscle, BCAAs provide the nitrogen and glucose provides the carbon for the formation of alanine and glutamine. Alanine is a precursor for gluconeogenesis in the liver, glutamine is utilised in the kidney, intestine and cells of the immune system.

Aromatic amino acids

Phenylalanine, tyrosine and tryptophan are the aromatic amino acids for which metabolism is normally regulated in the liver. In liver failure their plasma levels rise and they are more available for entry into the brain. Synthesis of brain serotonin may in this way become uncontrolled.

Amino acid pool

This is an amino acid pool in the body which is localised in the plasma, interstitial fluid and in the cell sap and is in dynamic equilibrium with the total body protein pool. It comprises free amino acids, amounting to about 100 g, primarily made up of non-essential amino acids.

COUNTER-REGULATORY HORMONES

These are the so-called catabolic or stress hormones namely cortisol, catecholamines, glucagon and growth hormone which are secreted as part of the neuroendocrine response to injury or sepsis.

BODY CELL MASS, FAT FREE MASS AND LEAN BODY MASS

Body cell mass is the total mass of cells in the body. It therefore represents that part of the body in which all energy exchange occurs, where oxygen is consumed and CO_2 is produced. It is estimated by multiplying the total body potassium by a factor which may vary according to the state of sickness or health of the patient. *Fat free mass* is the mass of the body that remains after all the ether extractable fat has been removed. Although often used interchangeably with lean body mass, in the strictest terms it is different. *Lean body mass* has been defined as that part of the body which is totally devoid of fat except for a small amount of essential lipid, probably 2%. Others, erroneously, define lean body mass as the difference between the body mass and adipose tissue.

CHANGES IN BODY WEIGHT

To properly understand surgical metabolism body weight should be thought of in terms of its components. The latter comprises total body water, total body protein, minerals and glycogen. It is helpful to further subdivide both the body water, into plasma, interstitial water and intracellular water, and the body protein, into muscle protein, visceral protein and structural protein. From Figure 1.1 it can be seen that much of body weight comprises water, so this means that in clinical practice appreciable gains in weight over a short term (anything less than 48 hours) are largely due to increases in body water. The synthesis of new lean tissue, about one fifth of which is protein and four fifths water proceeds so slowly that it is a cause of weight change that is discernible only over a period of a week or so. The synthesis of lean tissue rarely proceeds at a faster rate than 150 g per day. Fat and protein can be lost at rates as rapid as 200–300 g per day, but rapid loss of water as from an enterocutaneous fistula, may produce weight loss approximately ten times faster. Thus short term rapid weight loss generally signifies loss of salt and water. Continuing severe tissue trauma which, for example, accompanies invasive sepsis, may account for about 500–600 g per day. Weight loss over and above this is water loss.

TRANSFER OF ENERGY

Because of their high degree of structural order, the complex molecules contained in fat, proteins and carbohydrates contain much chemical energy and during catabolism this is set free and conserved as the chemical energy inherent in the covalent bonding structure of the terminal phosphate groups in the ATP molecule. The ATP so formed is free to diffuse to those sites in the cell where transport work, mechanical work or biosynthetic work is required. The hydrolysis of ATP or other high energy phosphate compounds releases energy which can be captured by other reactions which need energy to proceed. Thus ATP provides energy for fat or protein anabolism, muscular contraction and membrane transport. ATP is formed from the oxidation of nutrients such as carbohydrates and fats which yield, on full combustion, CO_2 and water.

ENERGY BALANCE

The first law of thermodynamics states that energy can be neither created nor destroyed. Therefore the total amount of energy which is taken in by the body (oral or intravenous) must be accounted for by the energy put out by the body according to the equation:

Energy input = Energy output
Chemical energy of food = Heat energy + work energy ± stored chemical energy

If intake of food energy is greater than the energy put out as heat and work the body stores energy and the patient gains weight as fat. If, on the other hand, the caloric content of the food eaten is less than the energy output, there is a negative energy balance and the body stores of protein and fat are utilised and the patient loses weight. The weight loss that occurs after a major surgical operation is almost entirely accounted for by a lack of energy intake for there is very little increase in energy output after an uncomplicated surgical operation (Ch. 2).

Although this physical law must apply in surgical patients the time scale for the regulation between energy intake and output is in weeks rather than days and there is little direct relationship between food intake and energy output on any one day. The energy requirements of surgical patients in hospital are assessed poorly by means of appetite and it has been shown that patients recovering in hospital after a major operation rarely eat more than was eaten prior to coming to hospital even if their energy output is considerably increased. However, it is a well attested fact that energy intake rises markedly when the patient is convalescing in his or her own home environment and it is at this time that positive energy balance is achieved and body weight and composition return towards normal.

ENERGY VALUE

Energy is stored in three substances in the body: protein, fat and carbohydrate (glycogen). The metabolisable energy values of these substances have recently been determined. Protein on combustion yields 4.70 kcal/g, fat yields 9.44 kcal/g and glycogen 4.18 kcal/g (Livesey & Elia 1988). In this book and for clinical work in general these figures are rounded off to 4, 9, and 4 respectively. Protein is taken as 4 kcal/g because protein composition is variable. Taking these values and the data from Figure 1.1 the energy values of the different compartments of the body can be calculated (Table 1.1).

RESPIRATORY QUOTIENT (RQ)

Measurement of oxygen consumption and carbon dioxide production can give the surgeon some idea as to what fuel the patient is consuming. The oxidation of carbohydrate and fat to CO_2 and water in the body is complete. The ratio of the CO_2 produced to the O_2 consumption is the RQ.

For carbohydrates the RQ is 1, for mixed fat the RQ is 0.7. The RQ for protein oxidation is not as clear cut because protein composition is variable and complete oxidation does not always occur. The RQ of protein oxidation is normally taken as 0.8. The process of lipogenesis in which fatty acids are derived from glucose has an RQ greater than 1.

Table 1.1 Energy stores in a 40-year-old normal man — 74.1 kg

	kg	kcal
Adipose tissue triglyceride	12	113 280
Protein		
cellular	7	32 900
structural	5	23 500
Carbohydrate		
muscle glycogen	0.5	2 090
liver glycogen	0.2	836
free glucose	0.02	80

FAT CANNOT BE CONVERTED TO CARBOHYDRATE

Inter-relationships of the three major energy sources within the body are complex but the important clinical point is that carbohydrate can readily be converted to fat and can be aminated to form protein but there is no conversion of fat to carbohydrate and little conversion to protein.

2. Metabolic management of patients undergoing major surgery

INTRODUCTION

Over many years surgeons have been interested in the early metabolic responses in patients undergoing major surgery particularly whilst they are still in hospital, but it is only recently that long term changes in metabolism, body composition, physiology and psychological function have been studied over the weeks and months following surgery. In this chapter we will look at what is known about the metabolic changes brought about by the surgical procedure and show how they may persist for weeks and in some cases months before the patient is restored to full health. On this basis we will set out a management programme for the metabolic care of patients undergoing uncomplicated major elective surgery.

SECTION I
THE METABOLIC RESPONSE TO SURGERY

Dr David Cuthbertson (1932) divided the metabolic response to injury into an early *ebb phase* characterised by hypovolaemia and subsequent sympathetic and adrenal response, and a later *flow phase* during which the injured patient loses protein at an accelerated rate. The duration of the flow phase depends on the severity of the injury, and it is gradually replaced by a convalescent *anabolic phase* during which the protein and energy stores lost in the early post-injury period are repleted (Table 2.1).

Table 2.1 Metabolic response to injury — the ebb and flow phases of Cuthbertson

Ebb phase	Flow phase
Hypometabolic	Hypermetabolic
Decreased energy expenditure	Increased energy expenditure
Extremities cold and clammy	Extremities warm
Cardiac output below normal	Cardiac output increased
Core temperature low	Core temperature elevated
Normal glucose production	Increased glucose production
Blood glucose elevated	Blood glucose normal or slightly elevated
Catecholamines elevated	Catecholamines high normal or elevated
Glucagon elevated	Glucagon elevated
Insulin concentration low	Insulin concentration low or elevated
Mediated by central nervous system	Mediated by central nervous system and cytokines

THE EBB PHASE

The ebb phase is largely a result of hypovolaemia, and it lasts until circulating blood volume is restored. The pale, clammy and tachycardic patient visited by the surgeon soon after surgery is in the ebb phase. Hume & Egdahl (1959) demonstrated the importance of the brain in the early endocrine response to injury. They disconnected a limb from the body of an anaesthetised animal, leaving only the sciatic nerve and femoral vessels. When they measured the level of corticosteroids in adrenal venous blood in response to a burn to the isolated limb they found an immediate rise; when the sciatic nerve was divided this response did not occur. These same workers showed subsequently that the early hormone response to injury did not occur unless the central nervous system was intact. Thus pain, hypovolaemia, acidosis and hypoxia initiate the neural afferent signals to the brain, this is processed by the hypothalamus, leading to increased activity of the sympatho-adrenal system which is accompanied by release of adrenocorticotrophic hormone (ACTH) and growth hormone (GH) from the anterior pituitary, and anti-diuretic hormone (ADH) from the posterior pituitary. Plasma cortisol levels rise as a consequence of the release of ACTH and the renin-angiotensin system is activated. These vasoconstrictor influences decrease renal blood flow, glomerular filtration rate, sodium excretion and urine flow. Volume retention extends beyond the ebb phase but diuresis occurs within the first 72 hours in most patients. Plasma insulin levels are variable during the ebb phase, however they are low relative to the prevailing high glucose concentration. This is probably a result of sympathetic inhibition of insulin release from the pancreas and glucocorticoid induced insulin resistance in peripheral tissues.

The ebb phase may be prolonged if the patient suffers from postoperative haemorrhage, or barely occur at all if the the operative procedure involved little blood loss or tissue damage. Once normovolaemia has been restored this acute ebb phase is replaced by the flow phase.

THE FLOW PHASE

The flow phase is characterised by oxidation of muscle protein to supply glucose which is essential fuel for the brain and healing tissues in particular. The accelerated loss of protein results from an increase in the rate of breakdown of muscle protein rather than a reduction in the rate of protein synthesis. In Chapter 1 we saw how in severely injured patients, such as those who have suffered major trauma or serious sepsis, this phase is associated with an accelerated metabolic rate, although as we shall see the resting metabolic expenditure of patients who have undergone elective surgical procedures is only slightly increased. The patient's energy requirements during this phase are mostly met by fat oxidation. The plasma concentrations of the counter-regulatory stress hormones fall during this phase although the plasma insulin level increases during the flow phase to reach a maximum level paradoxically at the time of the greatest rate of loss of body protein. The reason for the inappropriate rise in the plasma concentration of insulin is little understood, as is the apparent resistance to its usual anabolic effects.

Given that the plasma concentrations of the catecholamines, glucagon and cortisol are falling during the flow phase, it is difficult to attribute the increased loss of protein observed over this period to their catabolic actions. Although there is little doubt that the central nervous system and neuroendocrine response to surgical injury explains most of the metabolic changes observed during the flow phase after major surgery the stress hormones are not completely responsible for all of them. Much recent research has been focussed on the possible role of *cytokines* released from cells at the site of the wound. Many different cell types release cytokines which have not only local effects but systemic effects as well. Interleukin-1, Interleukin-6 tumour necrosis factor (TNF) and interferon gamma are important mediators of the integrated metabolic response but with the exception of Interleukin-6 these cytokines have yet to be detected in the plasma of postoperative patients (Cruickshank et al 1990). Infusion of TNF replicates many of the clinical and metabolic features of sepsis, including fever, hypotension, anorexia, hyperglycaemia and a negative nitrogen balance (Tracey et al 1986, Michie et al 1988, Flores et al 1989). Many of the features of the endocrine and metabolic reaction to sepsis, such as insulin resistance and protein loss, are present in injured patients and it is surprising that to date TNF has not been detected in the serum of patients after major surgery.

SECTION II
PERIOPERATIVE ENERGETICS

Over the first 2 weeks following a major operation the patient accrues a substantial energy deficit.

Only half of the energy requirement is met from intravenous dextrose and food and in order to achieve energy balance, body fat stores and, to a lesser extent, glycogen and protein stores are burned. In 1968 Kinney and his collegues conducted a study of energy balance in 10 patients undergoing major surgery. This remarkable and detailed study of energy intake and energy expenditure showed that resting energy expenditure, in health around 22 kcal/kg/day, increases very slightly early after surgery but from then on, unless there is a complication, remains at normal values (Fig. 2.1).

Energy expended during physical activity falls to very low levels (about 1 kcal/kg/day) over the first 4 postoperative days and hence during this period total energy requirements are substantially reduced; from normal 26 kcal/kg/day to 22 kcal/kg/day. By the end of the first postoperative week, activity energy expenditure has doubled and by the end of the second week total energy requirements are near normal values (25 kcal/kg/day) and the patient is eating sufficient to approach energy balance (Fig. 2.2). Once home, appetite improves and positive energy balance is achieved with accumulation of fat and protein and restoration of normal values for fat, protein and body weight.

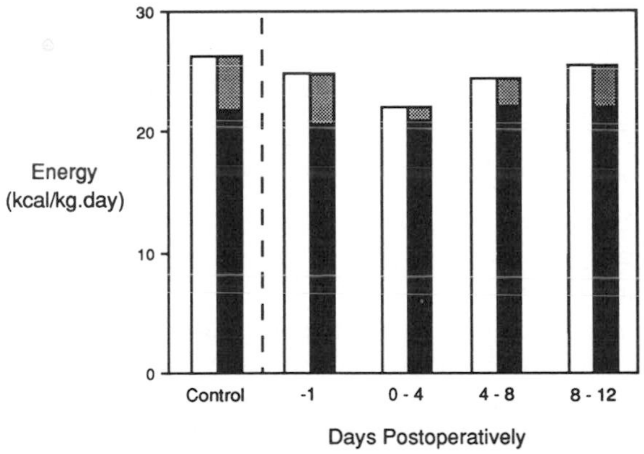

Fig. 2.1 Components of total energy expenditure in 10 patients undergoing uncomplicated major surgery. It can be seen that resting energy expenditure rises slightly postoperatively. The reduction in total energy expenditure occurred during the period of reduced physical activity. Key: □ = total energy expenditure; ■ = resting energy expenditure; □ = activity energy expenditure. (Reprinted from Hill G L, Douglas R G, Schroeder D S 1992. World J Surg (in press), with permission of the World Journal of Surgery.)

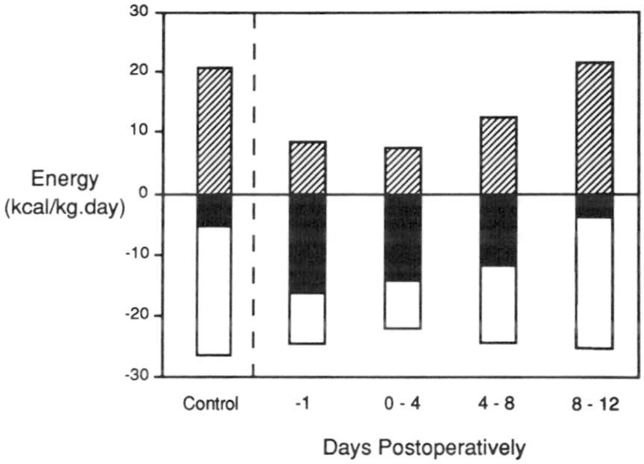

Fig. 2.2 Energy balance in 10 patients after uncomplicated major surgery. Energy intake is plotted above the base line and energy output below it. It can be seen that energy balance ■ was in all cases negative although at 8–12 days just before discharge from hospital energy intake was almost sufficient to achieve energy balance. (Reprinted from Hill G L, Douglas R G, Schroeder D S 1992 World J Surg (in press), with permission of the World Journal of Surgery.)

SECTION III
CHANGES IN BODY COMPOSITION AFTER SURGERY

We measured the changes in body composition that occurred after major uncomplicated gastrointestinal surgery in 46 patients (23 male, 23 female, average age 47 years). Just before surgery each had measurements of body weight, total body fat, protein and water by the methods set out in Appendix 1. The measurements were repeated at 7, 14, 28, 90, 180 and 360 days later. Only 16 patients had measurements beyond 90 days. None of the patients in the study received nutritional support perioperatively. Postoperatively they received 2–3 L 4.3% dextrose and 1/5 N saline until they were able to take sufficient fluids orally.

BODY WEIGHT

After uncomplicated surgery 3 kg of body weight were lost. The maximum weight loss had occurred by the end of the second postoperative week. From then on weight was gained slowly and steadily (Fig. 2.3). At 3 months the weight

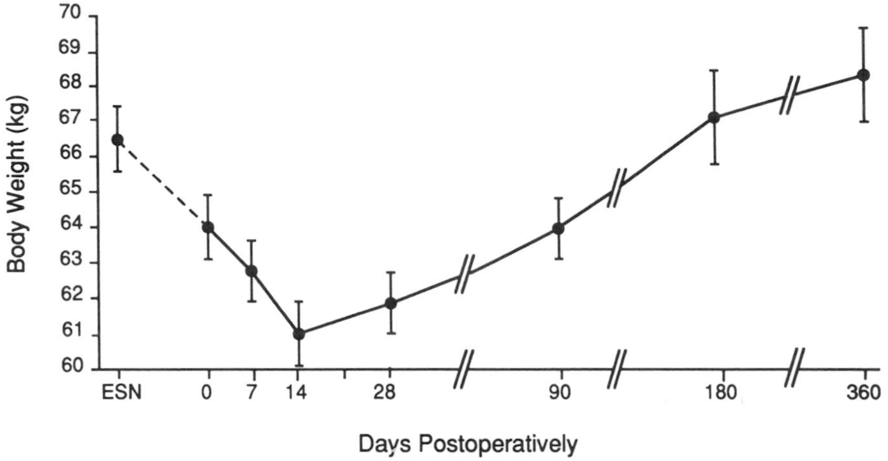

Fig. 2.3 A study of the postoperative changes in body weight in 46 patients undergoing major surgery of the alimentary tract. ESN = Estimated normal weight, mean ± s. e. m. (Reprinted from Hill G L, Douglas R G, Schroeder D S 1992 World J Surg (in press), with permission of the World Journal of Surgery.)

loss over the postoperative period had been restored but, in those who had had preoperative deficits, weight gain continued until normal values were achieved — usually taking about 6 months but sometimes as long as 1 year. Many patients overshot their preillness or well weight and were as much as 2–3 kg overweight at 1 year. The excess weight gain was due to accumulation of fat and the condition is aptly named — post-traumatic obesity.

TISSUE COMPOSITION OF WEIGHT CHANGES

The postoperative weight loss resulted from oxidation of fat and breakdown of protein to provide energy and amino acids during the first 2 postoperative weeks. Figures 2.4, 2.5 and 2.6 show how 3000 g of body weight lost over the first 2 weeks postoperatively was composed of 1400 g fat, 600 g protein, and 1000 g of water.

Fat

Most of the fat loss occurred in the first few days postoperatively when the energy deficit was greatest — a kilogram or more was lost in the first week (Fig. 2.4).

After 2 or 3 months, when the patients were well and protein stores had been repleted fat gain was at its maximum. Post-traumatic obesity occurs when this fat gain continues; the result of a continuing positive energy balance. The surgeon should alert his patients to this common problem and encourage more physical activity and a tighter control on appetite.

Protein

Protein catabolism occurred over the first 2 postoperative weeks with losses of total body protein of 600 g or so (6% of body protein) (Fig. 2.5).

Hereafter, with the resumption of normal food intake, protein was slowly and surely accreted to reach preoperative levels at 3 months and normal values at 6 months to 1 year. The protein was lost mainly from muscle but our studies of the loss of potassium and nitrogen in these 46 patients suggest that some non-cellular protein was lost as well. There are about 3 mmol of potassium to each gram of nitrogen in muscle; a K:N ratio of 3. Over the first 7 postoperative days the ratio of the loss of K:N was much higher than this (about 10), showing that potassium was lost from cells in excess of protein; either because glycogen was being mobilised and with it bound potassium-rich water, or an intracellular potassium

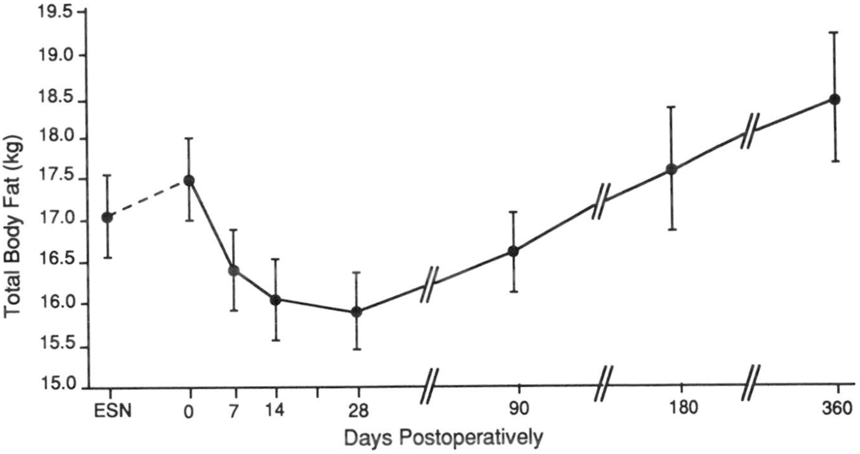

Fig. 2.4 A study of the postoperative changes in total body fat in 46 patients undergoing major surgery of the alimentary tract. ESN = estimated normal body fat, mean ± s. e. m. (Reprinted from Hill G L, Douglas R G, Schroeder D S 1992 World J Surg (in press), with permission of the World Journal of Surgery.)

deficiency was developing. Probably both of these were occurring. After 2 weeks when the patients were in positive energy balance, potassium was replaced at a ratio of 6 : 1 suggesting that there had been an intracellular deficiency which was now being repaired. Late in convalescence, when protein gains were small, the K:N ratio of the tissue gained was less than 3 showing that body protein as a whole, not just cellular protein was being laid down. Kinetic studies have shown that the loss of total body protein in the early postoperative period is due to an increase in the rate of protein breakdown rather than a reduction in the rate of protein synthesis (Clague et al 1983). The duration and extent of this loss of body protein is a function of body stores of protein

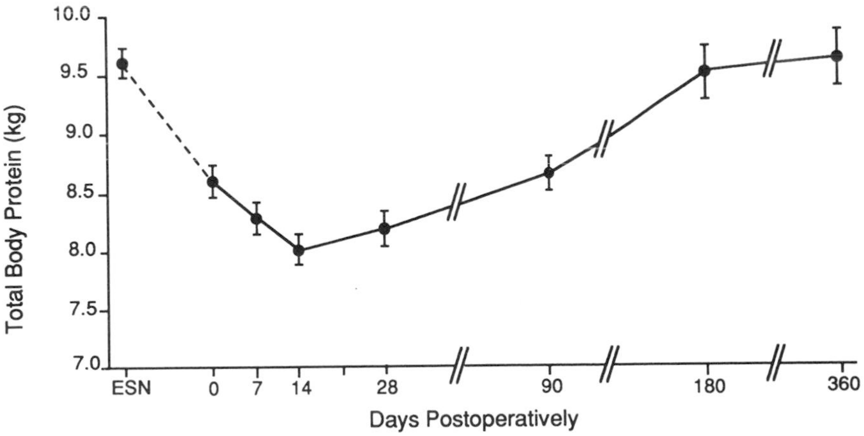

Fig. 2.5 A study of the postoperative changes in total body protein in 46 patients undergoing major surgery of the alimentary tract. ESN = estimated normal body protein, mean ± s. e. m. (Reprinted from Hill G L, Douglas R G, Schroeder D S 1992 World J Surg (in press), with permission of the World Journal of Surgery.)

(the larger the stores of protein, the greater the loss) and whether or not the patient is protein depleted prior to surgery (depleted patients suffer less loss of body protein).

The protein loss would have been greater in the early postoperative period if the fluid regimen used had not contained dextrose. The infusion of 130–150 g of dextrose per day results in a 40% reduction in urine nitrogen loss (Craig et al 1977, Swaminathan et al 1980).

Water

Over the first postoperative week when antidiuretic hormone levels were high, water was retained in spite of close attention to water balance by the attending surgeons (Fig. 2.6).

The patients experienced a fall in plasma sodium levels due to additional sodium-free water which arose from loss of cell substance and the oxidation of protein and fat. This can be understood by reference to Figures 2.4 and 2.5. Here it can be seen that 300 g of protein were oxidised during the first postoperative week. Since 1 kg of wet muscle contains about 200 g of protein, this loss of 300 g protein represents the loss of about 1500 g of wet muscle, comprising 300 g protein and 1200 ml of sodium-free potassium-rich water which is added to the extracellular space. Furthermore, the oxidised protein itself yields sodium-free water; 300 g protein upon full oxidation produces about 120 ml water.

Over the same period 1100 g of fat were oxidised. Since each 1000 g of fat that is completely oxidised yields 1000 ml of sodium-free water, the oxidation of 1100 g yields a further 1100 ml, making a total of nearly 2.5 L (1200 + 120 + 1100) of endogenous water added over this time period. Because antidiuretic hormone levels were high in the postoperative period this endogenous water was not excreted normally, resulting in early positive water balance, increased hydration of the fat free body and bodily hypotonicity. Normal tonicity had returned by the end of the first postoperative week and hydration of the fat free body had returned to normal within a month of operation. The oliguria and salt and water retention occurring over the first few days postoperatively were also related to high aldosterone activity and may have also been partly due to decreased atrial natriuretic peptide. Alterations in vascular tone that are associated with positive pressure ventilation decrease venous return to the right side of the heart and may as a consequence decrease secretion of this hormone.

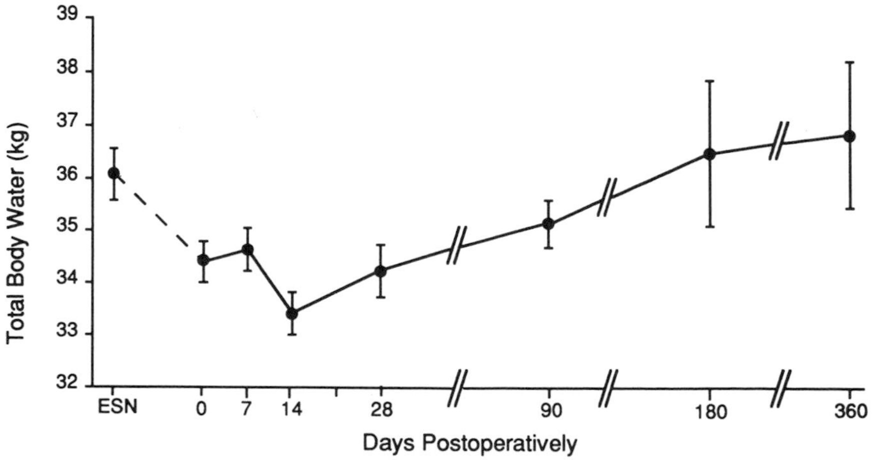

Fig. 2.6 A study of the postoperative changes in total body water in 46 patients undergoing major surgery of the alimentary tract. ESN = estimated normal total body water, mean ± s. e. m. (Reprinted from Hill G L, Douglas R G, Schroeder D S 1992 World J Surg (in press), with permission of the World Journal of Surgery.)

SECTION IV
POSTOPERATIVE FATIGUE AND SKELETAL MUSCLE FUNCTION

One of the most unpleasant effects of surgery is the long period of mental and physical tiredness that follows it. In a study of 84 patients (37 male, 47 female, average age 54 ± 18 years, s.d.) undergoing major surgery of the alimentary tract (Schroeder & Hill, 1992) we found that many of the patients, because of their illness, had a

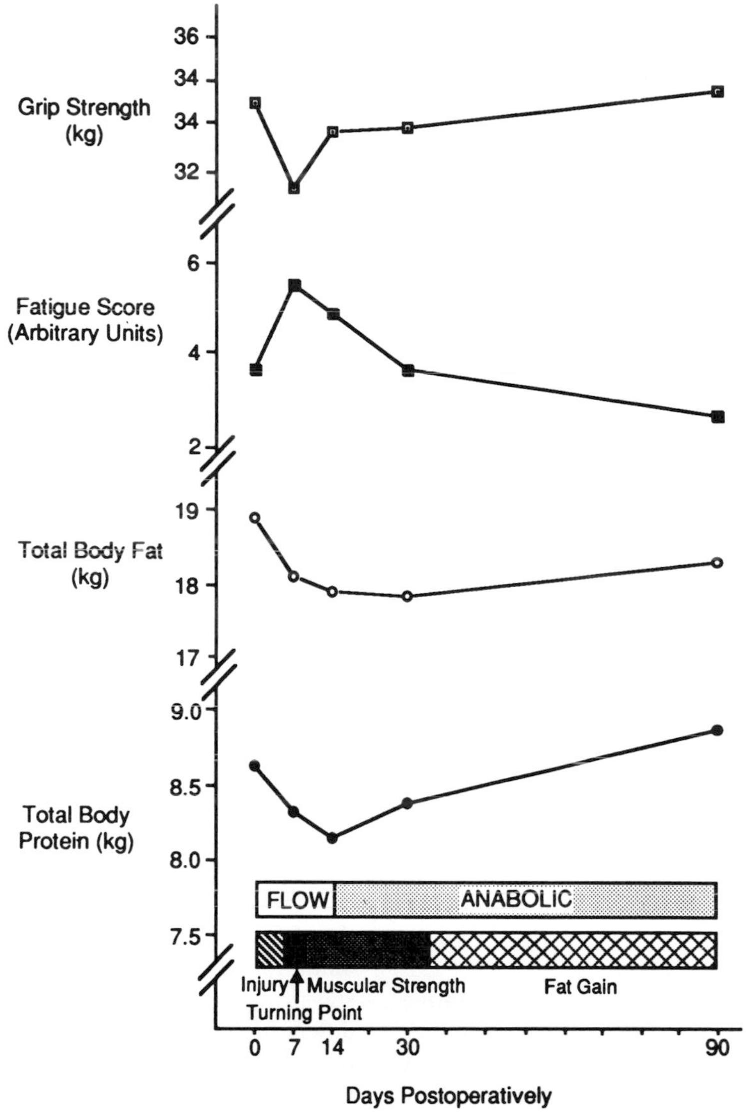

Fig. 2.7 The changes in total body protein and total body fat together with associated changes in postoperative fatigue and muscle function in 84 patients undergoing major surgery of the alimentary tract. In the lower part of the figure Cuthbertson's flow and anabolic phases are shown (the ebb phase was too short to show) together with F D Moore's phases of convalescence. (Reprinted from Hill G L, Douglas R G, Schroeder D S 1992 World J Surg (in press), with permission of the World Journal of Surgery.)

subjective feeling of fatigue prior to the operation itself and this became worse postoperatively, being greatest at the end of the first week (Fig. 2.7). 1 month postoperatively most patients were back to preoperative levels of fatigue and by 3 months it had all but disappeared. A few patients, however, particularly those in whom postoperative weight loss was most marked had more pronounced fatigue which was also much prolonged, a situation which has been previously described (Christiansen & Kehlet 1984). We found that fatigue was most troublesome in those patients who came to surgery already tired. There was evidence that patients who had few reserves of body protein (those with small muscle mass), the elderly, and those who knew they had cancer, even though a curative operative operation had been performed, suffered most from prolonged fatigue.

Voluntary muscle function also changes after surgery and we found that the pattern of deterioration that occurred was in some ways similar to that which occurs for fatigue (Fig. 2.7). It might be thought then that postoperative fatigue was a simple matter of loss of muscle protein affecting muscle function adversely and the whole effect therefore was that of physical tiredness. Unfortunately it is much more complicated than this. For instance, postoperative enteral nutrition, which preserves body protein stores postoperatively, does not prevent postoperative fatigue (Schroeder et al 1991). Also, involuntary skeletal muscle function unlike voluntary muscle function has been shown not to deteriorate postoperatively (Schroeder & Hill 1991). Thus postoperative fatigue which is an exclusively human problem (it does not occur in animals) has a psychological basis as well as a physiological one (Lancet 1979).

In summary then, whereas postoperative fatigue is experienced by all patients to a greater or lesser extent it is not much of a problem in patients who feel well prior to surgery or those who are physically robust. Those patients presenting for surgery already feeling tired, however, especially if elderly and with a diagnosis of cancer, are likely to suffer from prolonged fatigue. The cause of this debilitating condition is as yet unknown, but psychological factors are predominant. As yet no therapeutic manipulation has been found which prevents postoperative fatigue.

SECTION V
PHASES OF CONVALESCENCE

Dr Francis D Moore (Moore 1959a) described surgical convalescence in terms of four sequential phases starting immediately with the operation itself, and stretching out for 3 or even 12 months until the patient was functionally rehabilitated and returned to normal activity.

Moore's four phases are the *injury phase*, the *turning point phase*, the *gain in muscular strength phase*, and the *phase of fat gain*.

In Figure 2.7 it can be seen how these four phases very adequately describe the process of operative injury and convalescence when they are considered in terms of body composition, physiologic function and of postoperative fatigue. In the same figure Cuthbertson's flow and anabolic phases are also shown. In major elective surgery the ebb phase is too short to be properly depicted in the figure.

THE INJURY PHASE

The patient

The injury phase of Moore comprises not only the ebb phase described earlier but also part of the flow phase. This phase extends over the first 4 postoperative days. It begins as a phase of high catecholamine and adrenocorticoid activity. It is the time of maximal energy deficit and maximal oxidation of fat and protein. Protein synthesis stays the same or is increased and protein breakdown increases. Potassium is lost in excess of nitrogen due to mobilisation of glycogen from liver and muscle. In the beginning the patient is cold and clammy, pale and tachycardic; throughout he or she is tired, takes little interest in food and visitors and likes to be left undisturbed. The duration of this phase depends on the magnitude of the operation and the disturbance in physiology brought about by it. Hypovolaemia, atelectasis and acid base imbalance all prolong it and the development of a postoperative complication such as sepsis, peritonitis, embolus or necrosis extends this relatively minor alteration in metabolism into another order of magnitude.

The wound

Soon after surgical closure of the wound the fibrinous coagulum between the two surfaces is infiltrated with neutrophils and macrophages. By the third day capillary buds spring from the wound edge and fibroblasts migrate into the area and, soon after, collagen formation commences. Collagen content of a wound closely parallels its tensile strength during these early days. There is considerable variation in the wound healing response during the injury phase. Enforced starvation prior to surgery (Windsor Knight & Hill 1988), hypoalbuminaemia (Dickhaut et al 1984), and deficiencies in vitamin C and zinc (Sanstead et al 1982) cause an impairment in the wound healing response as also do high steroid dosages (Orgill & Demling 1988). Thus the surgeon should take special precautions with wound closure of those who have been eating poorly in the days leading up to surgery. Although zinc deficiency sufficient to cause wound healing difficulties is uncommon in patients undergoing elective surgery, vitamin C deficiency is more common. It may be present to some extent in up to 25% of patients undergoing elective surgery (Hill et al 1977). The effect can be considerable; although granulation tissue is formed at the wound site the fibroblasts lack orientation and, due to a deficiency in phosphatase, collagen formation does not occur.

When high dose steroids are given experimentally little granulation tissue is formed, fibroblasts remain small and collagen formation is reduced. These steroid doses are far in excess of those which are used clinically. Nevertheless clinical evidence suggests that the wound healing response is poor in patients chronically on steroids and the surgeon needs to ensure that the fascial closure is thorough and that skin sutures or clips remain longer in the patients on high dose steroids.

Generally speaking the wound healing response occurs in an area of high metabolic activity even though the rest of the body is catabolic. The inflammatory cells in the wound have a marked capacity for glycolytic metabolism and glucose is the preferred fuel for the healing wound. The liver produces this glucose by recycling carbon from lactate but it also comes from amino acids derived from skeletal muscle protein. It is remarkable how the wound is anabolic while the rest of the body is catabolic in the vast majority of patients during the injury phase. The wound is synthesising new collagen, gaining strength and healing in spite of an overall consumption of body fat and protein which are being oxidised to provide for the energy economy of the body. *This priority of the wound is a feature of the injury phase.* Later on, this high priority is lost and if the patient remains catabolic over a prolonged period the wound stops healing and contributes like any other part of the body to the consumption of tissues required to sustain life.

THE TURNING POINT PHASE

The patient

Around the middle to the end of the first postoperative week the patient starts to take an interest in his surroundings and wonders at his dishevelled appearance. He wants to get up, and shave and comb his hair, and women patients may be seen to be looking in the mirror and applying lipstick. This phase normally lasts only 1 or 2 days but if a septic complication is present or developing the change is incomplete and prolonged.

It is this time that the desire to get up and get moving is tempered by extraordinary tiredness, and the patient quickly returns to bed. Most patients now take an interest in food and a few sips of water are soon regarded as insufficient and a soft diet is begun (Fig. 2.8). The stage of maximum fatigue and loss of skeletal muscle strength is finishing. Endocrine function has returned towards normal although protein catabolism is continuing. Because endocrine activity has now decreased, somewhere between 3 and 5 days, a diuresis occurs. Potassium loss in the urine is less as intracellular deficits in potassium are made up. The transient

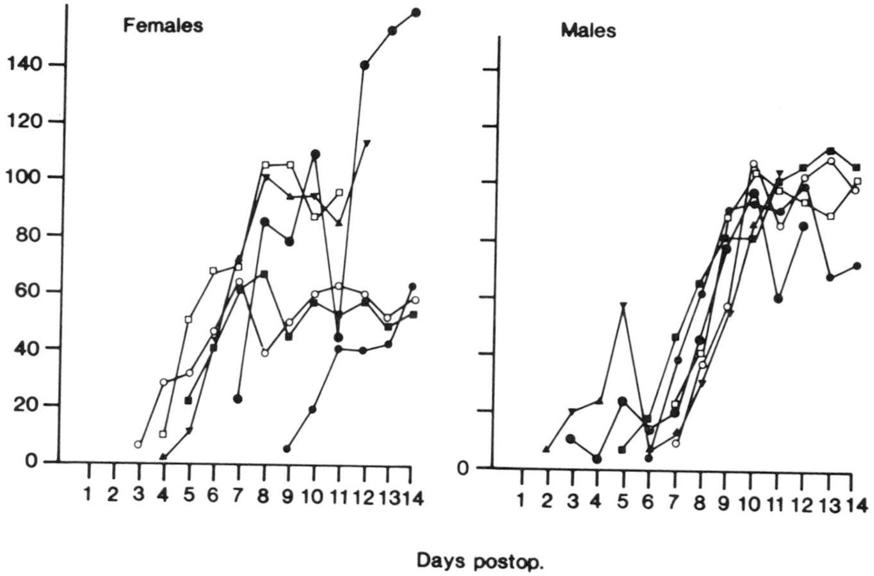

Fig. 2.8 Daily voluntary food intake (energy) that occurred over the first 2 postoperative weeks in 12 patients after colorectal surgery. On the vertical axis the results are expressed as a percentage of the estimated previous home voluntary food intake. (Redrawn from Hackett A F, Yeung C K, Hill G L 1979 Br J Surg 66: 415, by permission of the publishers.)

hypotonicity (from hyponatraemia) returns to normal and the expanded extracellular fluid volume returns towards normal. Activity energy expenditure is increased during the turning point phase but because energy intake is still substantially less than normal (Fig. 2.8) an energy deficit persists which is balanced by catabolism of fat and protein. The key to success at this stage is the increasing provision of a good diet.

The wound

The wound in normal circumstances is very tender though not red. It is firmly apposed but can be disrupted by strong traction. Microscopically, fibroblastic activity is vigorous and collagen fibrils are forming. By the seventh postoperative day sutures can be removed because of this increased tensile strength. Bowel anastomoses at this stage start functioning but disruptions of these or other wounds indicate failure to gain this expected tensile strength.

THE MUSCULAR STRENGTH PHASE

The patient

The patient now passes into a period of 2 to 8 weeks where there is rapid psychological and physiological improvement. The excitement and reality of going home is experienced, voluntary food intake is now near normal and the wound is less painful. This together with normal bowel function and diminishing fatigue leads to encouragement. At the end of 8 weeks body composition, physiologic function and the feeling of tiredness all have been restored to near the state that they were just prior to the operation.

The wound

The wound is now reaching its maximum collagen content. On palpation it feels thickened and heaped up and the fine thin line observed soon after operation is now red and coarse. Tensile strength continues to be increased, however, by crosslinking of collagen and by remodelling of new collagen by lysis and resynthesis.

THE FAT GAIN PHASE

The patient

The final period of convalescence is a gain in body weight due to accumulation of body fat and its supporting structure. This happens because there is continuing positive energy balance with intake of energy being greater than that used for work and heat. The protein that is gained together with this fat is thought to be that of the supporting structure in adipose tissue for there is little change in total body water even up to 1 year postoperatively. Somewhere during the fat gain phase the patient returns to normal daily activity.

The wound

The wound continues to gain in tensile strength by continuing development of crosslinks with collagen fibrils and also by a process of remodelling new collagen by collagenolysis and resynthesis. All elements of the scar become less vascular and it now becomes pale and less heaped up both at the skin surface and in the subcutaneous tissues. Maximal tensile strength probably occurs around 100 days and the gain in strength levels off at approximately 80% of normal. Scar tissue shrinks during wound maturation and this continues over a period of 3 to 12 months. During this time it may undergo a period of stretching as well as contraction. Vitamin C deficiency at this stage has a profound effect on collagen formation and the scar may open again if the deficiency is profound.

SECTION VI
METABOLIC MANAGEMENT OF THE PATIENT UNDERGOING MAJOR SURGERY

Our management recommendations are based on the measured changes in metabolism, body composition, physiology and psychology. They begin before the patient enters the operating room and end when the patient is functioning again in his/her normal environment.

PREOPERATIVE MANAGEMENT

If the surgeon takes time to give a careful and relevant description of what is going to take place in hospital and describes the sensations that will be experienced and how these are to be coped with then there is evidence that hospital stay will be shorter (Egbert et al 1964). He may choose to explain to those who are likely to experience excessive postoperative fatigue that it will be a long convalescence so that disappointment and discouragement can be prevented (Schroeder & Hill 1991). The physiotherapist may help also by teaching the patient exercises that will be used postoperatively and how to turn in bed and move so that pain is minimal. If investigations have gone on for several days and particularly if little food has been consumed over the previous week then the wound healing response will be impaired and special care needs to be taken (Windsor Knight & Hill 1988). If there is any question of deficiency vitamin C is given. The prescription of prophylactic antibiotics and taking proper precautions against venous thrombosis both add to a smooth postoperative course.

AT THE TIME OF SURGERY

The surgeon

That the magnitude of cell injury, the amount of necrotic tissue created and the presence or absence of infection influence the release of cytokines helps the surgeon set goals and plan strategies for the operative task. *The goal is to keep cytokines out of the circulation!* The least damaging, least contaminating and the most expeditious procedure is the way to do it. The strategies include excellent exposure, sharp dissection along anatomical planes, careful haemostasis, accurate apposition of tissues and careful suturing without strangulation. These strategies, so essential to a smooth postoperative course, are the result of a mind set and ideas developed some days or hours before the procedure. The wise surgeon, no matter how familiar the procedure, will go through it all in his mind step by step, particularly in relation to the particular patient. It is the sort of approach that characterises those surgeons whose patients 'seem to fly through'.

At the conclusion of the operation thorough peritoneal toilet minimises the risk of leaving necrotic debris or clot behind and careful haemostasis throughout ensures that large haematomas do not interfere with postoperative recovery.

The anaesthetist

Although spinal or epidural anaesthesia prevent the greater part of the classical endocrine response to surgery the effect is maximal in pelvic surgery, e.g. prostate, gynaecological procedures, and lower limb orthopaedic procedures, but is much less in abdominal and chest procedures probably because of insufficient afferent neural blockade (Kehlet 1987). In any event most major surgical procedures require general anaesthesia, but the haemodynamic effects induced by it as well as by the operative procedure can be minimised by the anaesthetist. Hypovolaemia must be prevented, fluid deficits from radiological procedures or mechanical bowel preparation should be replaced soon after sleep is induced. During the operation, blood pressure should be manipulated to within 10–20% of the preoperation level and urine output within the range of 0.5–1 ml/kg/h by the addition of a balanced salt solution given in amounts over and above maintenance requirements. The amount of this extra 'third space requirement' is dependent on the nature, extent and duration of the operation and it may also extend for 12 hours or so into the postoperative period. Proper attention to fluid volume and control of blood pressure, pulse rate and urine output will lessen the endocrine response to the operation (Roberts et al 1985), reduce the time of the injury phase and lead to a reduction of hospital stay.

Blood requirements (mainly given as packed red blood cells) during operation are a controversial topic and a decision to transfuse requires expert clinical judgment (NIH 1988). The combination of hypovolaemia and anaemia though may lead to severe morbidity and possible mortality. There is a minimum haemoglobin value for each patient below which inadequate oxygen delivery is likely to occur. The decision to transfuse takes into account the presence or absence of perioperative anaemia, the intravascular volume, the extent of the operation, the probability of continuing massive blood loss and the presence of coexisting conditions such as impaired pulmonary function, inadequate cardiac output, myocardial ischaemia, or cerebrovascular or peripheral arterial disease.

MANAGEMENT DURING THE POSTOPERATIVE PHASE

Pain relief

Postoperative pain serves no useful function and if inadequately controlled may adversely affect respiratory function and intracardiac demands, decrease intestinal motility, and induce skeletal muscle spasm which in itself impairs mobilisation. If regional anaesthesia has been used it should carry through the operation and probably go on for 24–48 hours.

Systemic administration of opioids, either given according to a fixed administration regimen or according to a demand based regimen, has unfortunately no important modifying effect on the endocrine response to the operation. Nevertheless its effect is vital in reducing or eliminating postoperative pain, improving respiratory function, decreasing cardiac demands and controlling muscle spasm.

Intravenous fluids

If on return to the ward the patient is tachycardic and peripherally shut down (ebb phase) more crystalloid is required. In most situations this is provided by isotonic crystalloid solutions (Ringer's lactate) in sufficient quantities to keep blood pressure and pulse rate near normal preoperative levels and urine output at 0.5–1 ml/kg/h. In many patients losses will continue from the intravascular compartment for 12 hours or so and during this time isotonic fluid replacement will be required.

After some hours the capillary leak will close and fluid will be slowly mobilised from the periphery into the vascular space, and increased urine output results. At this point fluids should change to maintenance rates or lower and from isotonic saline to hypotonic saline.

In adequately hydrated patients who have undergone a straightforward procedure with minimal blood loss maintenance fluid alone is all that is required. Maintenance requirements for a 70 kg patient are normally 100 ml/h of dextrose/saline to which 20 mmol of potassium per litre has been added. The provision of 130–150 g of dextrose in the postoperative fluid regimen has, by suppressing endogenous glucose production, a modest protein sparing effect. The urinary urea nitrogen is about 40% less when dextrose is given in this way (Swaminathan et al 1980). Because of the dissolution of cells which floods the extracellular water with potassium it is advisable to refrain from giving potassium for the first 24–48 hours postoperatively.

Energy and protein supplied either by the enteral or parenteral route can prevent completely the loss of protein after uncomplicated major surgery. Unfortunately there is no obvious clinical benefit either early or late from preventing protein loss although some suggest that specially formulated enteral diets may have a place in reducing postoperative complications (Bower 1990a, Yeung et al 1979b). It has been shown, however, that the wound healing response is enhanced by postoperative nutrition and in large granulating wounds this may be of some clinical benefit (see Ch. 10, Fig. 10.3). The whole topic of perioperative nutrition is discussed in more detail in Chapter 18. Hormonal manipulation has also been tried. Insulin added to TPN regimens and intramuscular growth hormone administration result in reduced postoperative protein loss, preservation of body composition and increased hand grip strength (Jiang et al 1989, Inculet et al 1986). Much more work will be required, however, before this can be used routinely in major surgery (Ziegler et al 1990).

Role of nurse, physiotherapist and dietitian

The best metabolic care as the patient passes into the 'turning point phase' and beyond is encouragement of positive attitudes by the nursing staff, insistence upon increasing mobilisation by the physiotherapist and the provision of attractive and nourishing food by the dietitian. Indeed the key of success is the resumption of eating as the anabolic phase commences. Early on, the patient prefers carbohydrates to protein but by the middle of the second week a balanced diet, equivalent in energy and protein content to that being consumed at home just prior to admission, should be being consumed (Fig. 2.8). Some patients with artificial dentures experience some gum shrinkage after surgery and the discomfort of chewing in these circumstances limits protein intake. Provision of special dietary supplements in patients who are slow to reach energy and protein balance appears to be beneficial (Isaksson et al 1959).

Can anything be done to limit postoperative fatigue?

Although careful preoperative counselling can limit the toll of surgery by shortening hospital stay it has not been shown that this has any effect on the magnitude or duration of postoperative fatigue. Postoperative nutrition, sufficient to abolish net protein loss, similarly has not been shown to limit postoperative fatigue. On the other hand, it appears that subjects who are extremely fit prior to surgery of modest magnitude experience little if any fatigue postoperatively.

SECTION VII
MINIMALLY INVASIVE SURGERY AND THE METABOLIC RESPONSE

Minimally invasive surgery, in particular laparascopic cholecystectomy, in which the gallbladder is removed through tiny abdominal incisions, is of particular practical and scientific interest. Even though a general anaesthetic is required and the procedure may be prolonged, it seems to be associated with shortened convalescence and minimal postoperative fatigue (Neugebauer et al 1991). Although preliminary investigations suggest that the neuroendocrine responses are the same as those that occur after open operations (Cuschieri 1991) full scientific evaluation of the metabolic effects of these procedures and the postoperative physiological and psychological effects is awaited (Paterson-Brown et al 1991).

Acknowledgements

We are grateful to the World Journal of Surgery for permission to reproduce here some of the material contained in our paper: Hill G L, Douglas R G, Schroeder D S 1992 Metabolic basis of management of patients undergoing uncomplicated surgery. World J Surg (in press).

3. Metabolic management of special problems in perioperative care

In the previous chapter the metabolic changes associated with uncomplicated elective major surgery were described. Perioperative management was arranged on a solid understanding of the endocrine, body composition, physiological and psychological changes that were shown to occur. Not all patients, however, come to surgery with 'all systems normal', apart of course from their primary surgical disease, and not all escape major postoperative complications. In this chapter some of the special problems encountered in perioperative metabolic care will be discussed and, based on understandings of disordered metabolism and physiology, a management programme is set down.

SECTION I
THE PATIENT WHO DEVELOPS SEPSIS IN THE EARLY POSTOPERATIVE PERIOD

The normal metabolic response to a major operation and the well ordered convalescence described in the previous chapter is interrupted catastrophically if the patient develops a septic complication in the early postoperative period.

Example

A man of 55 years of age who underwent a curative low anterior resection of the rectum for carcinoma without a defunctioning colostomy is a typical example. The operation went smoothly and the postoperative course was entirely as predicted until the fifth day when after passing a loose bowel movement extreme pain developed in the lower abdomen, he became faint, and retired to bed quickly. Within an hour he was clearly critically ill with tachypnoea, low systolic blood pressure, high pulse rate and was peripherally shut down; he was clearly in the ebb phase of septic shock. This patient illustrates the type of major postoperative septic complication that can occur in general surgery and threaten the patient's life.

DISORDERED METABOLISM ACCOMPANYING POSTOPERATIVE SEPSIS

Endocrines and cytokines

The patient had just passed through the turning point, taking a new interest in life and beginning to eat food without discomfort. He was passing bowel movements, he had a soft abdomen and normal bowel sounds. He was walking gingerly around the ward although this was a real effort and he was pleased to get back to bed after a short time. Stress hormones would be expected to be near normal levels. He had been afebrile but with the onset of this acute episode his body temperature shot up and he became shocked as a result of an outpouring into the circulation of catecholamines, cortisol and glucagon initiated by the release of mediators within the pelvis where a massive faecal leak had occurred. In the pelvic tissues surrounding the faecal leak Gram negative organisms and endotoxin were in high concentration and soon after there was a gram negative bacteraemia. Tumour necrosis factor and other cytokine production was increased and could be detected in the circulation. These peptides regulate the acute phase response, and potentiate the release of other cytokines and classical hormones in a self propagating cascade (Long & Lowry 1990) — see Figure 4.5. The result is cardiovascular collapse, leaky capillaries and shock. If the situation is not rapidly controlled the circulatory disturbance can be so profound that multiorgan failure occurs. Accompanying the stress hormone release aldosterone and ADH were again at high levels, causing antidiuresis with salt and water retention, a situation which could not be relieved until sepsis was controlled and eliminated.

Protein, fat and water metabolism

In a patient such as this there would be a marked increase in protein catabolism with increased amino acid loss from muscle, increased amino acid uptake in the liver and increased synthesis of acute phase proteins although albumin synthesis would be decreased markedly. There would be increased lipolysis, decreased fatty acid synthesis and rapid expansion of extracellular fluid from leaky capillaries. The massive loss of body protein, lipolysis and fluid expansion can be reduced but not prevented by any known pharmacological agent or treatment including maximum nutritional therapy, hormonal manipulation and (probably) monoclonal antibodies to endotoxin and TNF. The only thing that returns these changes towards normal is elimination of the sepsis.

Body composition

Table 3.1 shows the body composition changes that would be expected in our patient.

It can be seen that the normal postoperative changes in body weight, fat, protein and water have been considerably altered by the pelvic sepsis. Table 3.1 shows there was lipolysis and proteolysis at a markedly increased rate and a 5 L expansion of extracellular water associated with resuscitation. Resting metabolic expenditure was raised about 40%. Protein losses of this magnitude have implications for all postoperative patients but particularly for those who are already depleted prior to surgery and who can ill afford to sustain further losses with their accompanying physiological impairments.

Energetics

Surprisingly, total energy expenditure is not increased. Resting metabolic expenditure, however, is raised 38% above normal levels but because the patient is prostrate and physical activity is severely curtailed total energy expenditure is not raised.

Table 3.1 Changes in body composition and metabolic expenditure that would be expected over a 10 day period in a 55-year-old man who had a leak from a low anterior resection on postoperative day 5.

	Est. value when well	Preop.	4 days postop.	6 days postop.	10 days postop.
Body weight (kg)	64.0	61.0	63.0	68.5	63.5
Total body fat (kg)	15.0	14.0	13.4	13.0	12.5
Total body protein (kg)	10.0	9.5	9.25	8.9	8.5
Total body water (L)	35.0	33.8	36.6	42.6	36.8
Extracellular water (L)	17.0	16.5	19.0	23.9	19.9
ECW/FFM	0.35	0.35	0.38	0.43	0.39
RME_m	1250	1225	1202	1535	1293
RME_p	1216	1189	1155	1112	1096
RME_m/RME_p	1.02	1.03	1.04	1.38	1.18

Key: ECW = extracellular water; FFM = fat free body mass; RME_m = resting metabolic expenditure–measured; RME_p = resting metabolic expenditure–predicted

Organ function

Organ function in terms of skeletal muscle function and respiratory muscle function is affected early because of alterations in cellular chemistry and a decrease in resting membrane potential, and later as a result of the loss of cellular protein. In patients who have large stores of protein and in whom the septic episode is quickly brought under control this loss of cellular protein may be of little clinical significance but it can prove to be a major difficulty in those who are on the edge of significant physiological impairments because of prior protein depletion.

METABOLIC MANAGEMENT

The goal for the surgeon is to resuscitate the patient and eliminate the sepsis as quickly as possible. Antibiotics are given and the sepsis is definitively controlled by drainage or defunctioning or both as soon as the circulation is stabilised. The place of immunotherapy in sepsis is fully discussed in Chapter 19 but a single dose of a human monoclonal antibody that binds to lipid A is indicated if rapid surgical resolution of the septic state is not anticipated. Those patients with lingering sepsis may need, in addition, intensive haemodynamic monitoring, cardiorespiratory support and therapeutic nutrition (see Ch. 19).

Defence of the circulation

Physical examination revealed a patient in considerable pain. His face was ashen and his extremities were pale, cold and clammy. He had a rapid pulse rate (130/min) and his blood pressure was 90/60. Only a small amount of concentrated urine was present in his urine bag. He was given a bolus of 2 L of Ringer's lactate solution and broad spectrum antibiotics intravenously. Over the next 2 hours he received 3.5 L of Ringer's lactate to maintain urine output at 30 ml/h and blood pressure at 110/80. It was clear that a major intraabdominal catastrophe had occurred and after a rectal examination revealed a defect in the anastomosis a decision was made to reexplore his abdomen without further investigations. Prior to induction of anaesthesia a nasogastric tube was passed to ensure the stomach was empty of fluid.

Drainage

At surgery the old incision was reopened, and a pelvis full of feculent pus was found. After drainage a hole the size of a postage stamp was seen on the anterior surface of the anastomosis deep in the pelvis. The colorectal anastomosis was taken apart by pinching through the staple line with the fingers and the colon was brought up in the left iliac fossa and an end colostomy made. The pelvis was washed out with an antiseptic solution and no attempt was made to oversew the open rectal stump. Two vacuum suction drains were placed in the pelvis and the abdomen was closed.

During the procedure, because the patient's urine volume had fallen below 0.5 ml per kg per hour, another 3 L of crystalloid were given. The anaesthetist chose not to give colloid at this stage, for albumin administered to patients with disrupted endothelial membranes merely passes out into the interstitium. The added fluid resulted in a urine output of 1 ml per kg per hour and the circulation continued to be stable.

On returning to the ward the patient continued on antibiotics maintenance fluids together with a litre of crystalloid every 4 hours sufficient to keep urine output at 0.5–1 ml/kg/h.

Postoperative care

The next day the patient was sitting up out of bed, looking much improved. He was afebrile, with a normal blood pressure and pulse, a good urine output and well perfused extremities. A day later a spontaneous diuresis developed, the colostomy began to function and he commenced on oral fluids. Plasma albumin was 25 g/L and salt-poor albumin was given to bring it up to 35 g/L. This was given to restore osmotic pressure, aid gastric emptying and decrease swelling of the intestine as manifest by the swollen oedematous colostomy.

The response to treatment of postoperative sepsis does not always go as smoothly as this and *indecision or lack of effective drainage to control the sepsis in the pelvis results in continuing circulatory instability, the possibility of organ failure and further massive loss of protein.* This may lead to a period of time in the critical care unit for intensive therapy. The management of this situation will be discussed in Chapter 22.

Our patient who had his normal postoperative course interrupted has sustained a further protein and energy deficit and it could be argued that he should have been started on nutritional support as soon as he was haemodynamically stable. Reference to Table 3.1 shows that without nutritional support he continued to lose body fat and protein and by the tenth postoperative day he had sustained a total loss (from well values) of 2.5 kg of fat and 1.5 kg (15%) of protein. The normal stepwise increase in voluntary food intake (Fig. 2.8) had been interrupted and delayed for a further 4–5 days and it would be expected that further losses of body fat and protein would continue to occur. A course of total parenteral nutrition commenced on day 6 would have prevented this tissue loss. As a general rule, patients who develop major intraabdominal catastrophies in the early postoperative period should be commenced on TPN as soon as they are haemodynamically stable. In Chapters 5 and 6 of this book it will be explained how nutritional supplementation is indicated when protein stores are, or are expected to become, depleted to the extent that physiological impairments occur. Clinically this usually occurs when total weight loss is greater than 15%.

SECTION II
THE ELDERLY PATIENT UNDERGOING MAJOR SURGERY

There are fundamental differences in the early response to surgery and the subsequent convalescence in elderly patients from that set out in Chapter 2. Although there is an increasing mortality from surgery with advancing age, physiological status is the fundamental determinant, not age alone (Boyd et al 1980, Warner et al 1988). It is for this reason that there is an enormous range of abilities to withstand and benefit from the same surgical procedure in elderly patients.

The reason elderly patients are more at risk from major surgery is that in virtually every organ system there is a decline in physiologic reserve. The surgeon should think of it as *a decreasing ability to maintain homeostasis with advancing age.* Fundamental to correct metabolic management then is an understanding of the alteration that age brings about in body composition and fluid and electrolyte and acid base homeostatic mechanisms.

SURGICAL METABOLISM

Body composition changes with advancing years

Patients in their 70s and 80s have only half the muscle mass they had when they were young (Cohn et al 1976). Proportionately there is more extracellular water and less intracellular water in the elderly, making intolerance of excessive sodium loads an ever present problem. The elderly patient may well have had a constant body weight for years, for an increasing body fat mass hides the shrinkage in body muscle and other protein stores. The deficit in muscle mass is accompanied by proportional decreases in bodily functions in particular skeletal muscle strength and endurance (Larsson et al 1979) and most aspects of respiratory muscle function (Wahba 1983). The patient therefore has little reserve should the usual protein losses after surgery be exceeded. This is graphically highlighted by the well known fact that elderly patients withstand major postoperative complications poorly.

Fluid and electrolyte homeostasis — changes with advancing years

Elderly patients are less able to defend the extracellular space when challenged because of:

- *a diminished ability to excrete salt and waterloads*, predisposing to expansion of extracellular fluid volume and bodily hypotonicity if inappropriate hypotonic solutions are given (Crane & Harris 1976)

- *a diminished ability to concentrate urine and conserve water* which taken with an impairment in thirst response and baroreceptor sensitivity predisposes to dehydration and hypernatraemia particularly when fluid intake is limited and insensible losses are high (Helderman et al 1978)
- *impaired cardiac and peripheral vascular responses* which are so often present in the elderly making compensation for these diminished abilities slow and inefficient.

Acid base balance is less efficient in the elderly

Although the pH of body fluids is normally only slightly affected by age, the efficiency of acid base homeostasis is decreased in the elderly. Elimination of an acid load is prolonged in the elderly not only because buffering systems are limited in capacity but also because effective renal mass is diminished and the capacity of renal regulation of acid base status is smaller (Rowe 1980).

The metabolic response to surgery in the elderly

The endocrine and cytokine release in response to pain and the surgical trauma itself appear to be the same as in younger subjects (Watters et al 1990) but their effect on protein catabolism and the kidney is changed. Because of the smaller muscle mass the net amount of protein catabolised is proportionately less in the elderly and is usually of little clinical significance. The situation radically changes, however, if postoperative complications accompanied by large protein losses occur. Because of the diminished skeletal muscle protein reserve this results in rapid deterioration in physiological functions with profound implications for recovery.

METABOLIC MANAGEMENT OF ELDERLY SURGICAL PATIENTS

Based on the broad view that major organ systems have reduced physiological reserve as age advances a general programme for the metabolic management of elderly patients undergoing major surgery can be arranged in three stages; preoperative management, postoperative management and management of the phases of injury and recovery.

Metabolic management prior to surgery

More than the usual attention is paid to preoperative evaluation of the elderly patient undergoing major surgery. Occult cardiac disease is looked for closely. This includes a history, a physical examination, electrocardiography and chest X-rays. The risk of postoperative cardiac complications appears to be substantially greater when congestive heart failure is not properly controlled (Gerson et al 1985). Patients with symptomatic peripheral vascular disease also are liable to have perioperative difficulties. Elderly patients are particularly at risk of postoperative respiratory complications, and simple spirometry is the most useful pulmonary function test (Tisi 1979). Elderly patients with weight loss and hypoalbuminaemia are likely to have an expanded extracellular space and sodium-containing fluids should be used sparingly. When impairments are found which are secondary to diminished protein reserves, nutritional supplementation will be of value in restoring function prior to surgery (see Ch. 6). The progressive decline in renal function which occurs with advancing age is a consistent finding. The serum creatinine concentration may well be normal despite substantial concurrent decreases in glomerular filtration rate; this is because of the decreased muscle mass in the elderly and glomerular filtration rate is as a consequence better assessed by the determination of creatinine clearance.

Intraoperative metabolic management

Intraoperative physiological monitoring is of importance in the geriatric population because of limitations in cardiovascular and pulmonary function and a diminished ability to maintain fluid and electrolyte, acid base and temperature homeostasis. Continuous measurement of blood pressure and electrocardiographic monitoring for rate and rhythm, and monitoring of respiratory rate, peripheral tissue oxygenation, end tidal carbon dioxide tension and body temperature should be considered in all elderly patients (Charlson et al 1990). An indwelling urinary catheter to monitor urine output is needed in all major surgery in which significant fluid administration is anticipated.

Some argue that invasive haemodynamic monitoring should be used in nearly all elderly patients undergoing major abdominal or thoracic surgery (Del Guercio & Cohn 1980). This is because abnormalities of cardiac, pulmonary and oxygen transport which are not easily identified by usual methods may be detected and dealt with earlier.

The key guideline for the anaesthetist in metabolic care is the prevention of major alterations of blood pressure and heart rate and the avoidance of perturbations of fluid, electrolyte and acid base status. Again, the inseparable dependence of reducing change in vascular volume and fluid and electrolyte and acid base homeostasis on gentle clean non-damaging surgery cannot be overestimated. The relationship between the impairments brought about by the anaesthetist and the surgeon and postoperative recovery and convalescence is close and of fundamental importance to the care of the elderly.

Postoperative management

The efforts of the surgical team are directed at limiting postoperative stresses which arise from hypoxaemia, hypothermia and pain.

Postoperative respiratory complications are common in elderly patients with respiratory failure and resultant inadequate oxygen transport being more common than in younger patients. They are an important cause of death in this population. Resting arterial oxygen tension and content decrease progressively with advancing age and the further decrease associated with operation that occurs after major surgery is particularly prominent in the elderly. In addition, the ventilatory responses to both hypoxia and hypercapnia are blunted in older people. Postoperative hypothermia is more prominent in the elderly and oxygen demand is markedly increased by postoperative shivering. Abdominal procedures with general anaesthesia induce decreases in vital capacity that may persist for up to 2 weeks postoperatively. The result is increased closure of small airways, ventilation–perfusion mismatch and increased alveolar–arterial oxygen gradient.

Tactics employed to increase oxygenation include the use of epidural or subarachnoid anaesthesia, local anaesthetics and the encouragement of the early resumption of physical activity to get the patient sitting and moving. Incentive spirometers, breathing exercises and intermittent positive pressure breathing are also of some benefit in reducing pulmonary complications after surgery and may help shorten hospital stay (Celli et al 1984). Supplemental oxygen via a mask or nasal prongs should be routinely provided to elderly patients who have undergone major abdominal or thoracic procedures, for a period of several days or until physical mobility is restored.

Falls in core temperatures are common in elderly patients undergoing surgery and the extent increases with advancing age. Hypothermia should be minimised or prevented in the operating room by controlling room temperature, minimising exposure of body surfaces, warming intravenous fluids and ventilator gases and using a warming blanket. Some of these techniques can also be used postoperatively.

Analgesia plays a critical role in allowing early resumption of physical activity, increasing residual lung volume and improving respiratory gas exchange. Postoperative pain is itself a stimulus to the elaboration of stress hormones and for all these reasons postoperative pain should be managed as detailed in Chapter 2, but of particular note in elderly patients is the respiratory depression brought about by opiates which should be used very sparingly (if at all) in the elderly.

Postoperative fluid therapy

Mention has been made of the blunted ability of the elderly patient to deal with a water and a salt load and also the deficient ability to conserve salt and water when that is required. Reduced glomerular filtration rate accounts for the decreased ability of the kidneys to excrete an acute load of salt or water and this predisposes the patient to extracellular fluid volume overload. Hyponatraemia coupled with water intoxication is a serious disorder in the elderly presenting with anorexia, weakness, lethargy, confusion and maybe coma. The elderly are prone to excessive secretion of antidiuretic hormone particularly during the stress of surgery. This excess of antidiuretic hormone secretion is accompanied by extracellular fluid expansion, hyponatraemia and inappropriately concentrated urine (Rowe 1980). There is no substitute to the very accurate titration of water and salt requirements for the elderly patient recovering from major surgery.

SECTION III
THE JAUNDICED PATIENT REQUIRING MAJOR SURGERY

Metabolic management of the patient with obstructive jaundice revolves round the following facts:

- There is an energy deficit due to the malabsorption of fat and if the jaundice has persisted for more than 2 weeks or so malnutrition to a greater or lesser extent is always present.
- Vitamin K deficiency occurs and blood clotting is not normal.
- The bile is infected and surgery causes bacteraemia with the possibility of invasive sepsis as a consequence.
- Renal failure is a possibility in jaundiced patients undergoing surgery.
- The wound healing response may be impaired in patients with obstructive jaundice.

PREOPERATIVE METABOLIC PREPARATION

Decompression with nutritional therapy

If the obstruction has extended over several weeks malabsorption of fat and the fat soluble vitamins results not only in protein energy malnutrition but also in vitamin K deficiency with reduced prothrombin levels. There is some evidence that preoperative decompression either endoscopically or transhepatically may improve outcome but only if nutritional therapy is given as well (Foschi et al 1986). Thus, where protein energy malnutrition is of sufficient intensity to impair physiological performance (see Ch. 5), a combination of decompression and a short course of either total parenteral nutrition or, if practical, enteral feeding should be given. 5 days or so of good quality nutrition will result in improvements in grip strength, respiratory function and restoration of the levels of the short half life plasma proteins, prealbumin and retinol binding protein (see Ch. 6).

Prevention of renal failure

If care to preserve urine output is not taken patients who are operated on with unrelieved jaundice may develop postoperative acute renal failure. The renal damage appears to arise mainly from the nephrotoxic effects of bacterial endotoxin. If the patient has undergone potentially dehydrating investigations or procedures (such as mechanical bowel preparation) an intravenous infusion should be started the evening before operation and 2 litres of dextrose and saline administered overnight. Because all obstructed biliary tracts are for all intents and purposes contaminated, antibiotics are given for 24 hours preoperatively and if the operation has been particularly large or contaminating these should be continued for 5 days after.

Normalise blood clotting

Vitamin K, 10 mg each day for 5 days, is recommended but larger doses than this may depress prothrombin levels (Cohn 1975). Usually this therapy will correct Vitamin K deficiency due to straightforward biliary tract obstruction.

INTRAOPERATIVE CARE

The surgeon again has a primary role in ensuring that haemostasis is accurate, surgery is gentle and not damaging, and contamination is kept to a minimum. Particular attention is given to the technique of wound closure. The anaesthetist's prime role is to prevent hypovolaemia and to ensure that during the procedure urine output is kept at 1 ml per kg per hour.

POSTOPERATIVE CARE

Postoperatively relatively larger amounts than usual of crystalloids are given in the hope of preventing postoperative renal failure. After relief of the obstructive jaundice the bile output may be more than 3 litres per day and salt depletion may quickly develop if close attention is not paid to sodium balance. If drainage is high it is therefore wise to collect the bile and have it analysed for sodium content, for in some instances the concentration of sodium in it can be greater than that of plasma.

If preoperative parenteral nutrition has been given then it should be continued postoperatively until the patient is taking 1000 kcal per day orally. Vitamin K should continue until this time as well. Generally, after this sort of surgery the patient finds difficulty reaching a satisfactory level of oral intake and it may be necessary to encourage the family to bring in favourite foods to stimulate appetite. Sip feeding of dietary supplements may be particularly helpful. It is worthwhile noting the adverse effects of hypoalbuminaemia in postoperative patients. Not only is gastric emptying slowed but intestinal absorption is impaired from the oedematous gut which develops in patients with low levels of plasma albumin.

SECTION IV
MANAGEMENT OF PATIENTS WITH ADRENAL INSUFFICIENCY UNDERGOING MAJOR SURGERY

It is not unusual in modern practice to perform surgery on patients who are on steroids. Classically the general surgeon encounters this in patients with inflammatory bowel disease or in those who are on steroids for asthma or another chronic condition. In such patients adrenocorticol secretion is inhibited and this inhibition may persist long after cessation of steroid therapy, up to one year or more (Br Med J Editorial 1980) This results from suppression of hypothalamic release of corticotrophin releasing factor or inhibition of pituitary release of ACTH. The problem of inhibition is less when therapeutic steroids have been given every other day but in any event the surgeon is wise to adopt a standard regimen in all patients who have been on steroids for a long time and who are to undergo a major operation (Harris & Kendall-Taylor 1989).

MANAGEMENT

Evening before operation

Give hydrocortisone hemisuccinate 100 mg by the intramuscular route (prednisone is four times more potent than hydrocortisone).

Day of operation

100 mg hydrocortisone hemisuccinate i.m. morning and evening. During operation hydrocortisone is continued 100–300 mg i.v.

First postoperative day

100 mg hydrocortisone i.m. every 12 hours.

Next 3 days

50 mg hydrocortisone i.m. every 12 hours.

Next 3 days and thereafter

25 mg hydrocortisone every 12 hours. Halve dose every 3 days with an aim to discontinue steroid 3 or 4 weeks from surgery.

If a postoperative complication develops the dose should be at least 100 mg i.m. daily until recovery. Blood pressure readings are probably the best early check on inadequate steroid dosage. They should be made every hour for the first 48 hours, thereafter every 6 hours till the patient is stable.

In exceptional circumstances and particularly when the hydrocortisone dose is lower than 100 mg per day the patient may become salt depleted. Usually this occurs in those who have had surgery for inflammatory bowel disease with greater than usual losses from an ileostomy and the correct treatment is to slow ileostomy output by the administration of constipating drugs and to replace losses litre for litre with Ringer's lactate solution.

Some, these days, suggest that the steroid regimen outlined above provides far more corticosteroid than is needed (Kehlet 1975). This conclusion is based on animal experiments and on human studies in which surgery is of lesser magnitude and prone to fewer complications than that usually required by the types of patients encountered in general surgery such as those with inflammatory bowel disease (Kehlet & Binder 1973). It is our view that it is dangerous to adopt a lesser regimen and there is general agreement that treatment with hydrocortisone at the high doses outlined above for several days followed by rapid tapering appears to provide protection, is not associated with observable detrimental consequences and is the proper treatment in patients who have received long term high dose steroid therapy within 1 year before operation.

THE SPECIAL SURGICAL PROBLEMS OF PATIENTS ON STEROIDS

In patients on high dose steroids there is a fundamental impact on systemic immunity with a decrease in white cell accumulation at sites of damage and healing. The whole cascade of events resulting in healing and control of inflammation is interfered with and slowed in patients on steroids. In practice the wound healing response is slow, the ability of the peritoneal cavity to localise sepsis is reduced and serious infections present late because of diminished physical signs (Fauci et al 1976). The surgeon must ensure then that suturing is non-strangulating, accurate and secure, that fascial closures are done with permanent materials and skin stitches stay in several days longer than usual. In emergency settings anastomoses performed within contaminated areas are avoided and defunctioning and exteriorisation are to be used more frequently than usual.

SECTION V
THE MANAGEMENT OF PATIENTS WITH MASSIVE WEIGHT LOSS WHO PRESENT FOR MAJOR SURGERY

Although the patient presenting for major surgery with massive weight loss will be discussed in detail later (Ch. 18) a few general principles will be outlined here.

Weight loss of itself is probably not important and if physiological impairments are not present postoperative complications do not seem to be higher than in patients without weight loss at all. On the other hand when weight loss is accompanied by clinically obvious impairments of organ function which include respiratory function, skeletal muscle function, psychological function, wound healing and hypoalbuminaemia, then postoperative complications are more common and postoperative stay is prolonged. Patients presenting with weight loss greater than 20% almost always have physiological impairments and are at increased risk of postoperative complications. Those with weight loss less than 10% are most unlikely to have physiological impairments and postoperative complications occur in these patients with the same frequency as in patients without any weight loss at all. It is those patients with weight losses somewhere between 10 and 20% who must be examined carefully for evidence of physiological impairments and if these are present consideration should be given to perioperative nutritional therapy. It is now clear, however, that preoperative TPN does more harm than good in patients with marginal malnutrition but in those with severe malnutrition (and this should be quite obvious on clinical examination) a short course of 7 days or so of nutritional support is both clinically effective and cost effective (Ch. 18).

SECTION VI
MANAGEMENT OF THE CANCER PATIENT PRESENTING FOR MAJOR SURGERY

There is a huge literature on the metabolic effects of cancer (see review of Douglas & Shaw 1990) and the surgeon could be excused for being confused as to whether any special precautions should be taken for the cancer patient over the perioperative period. The problem can be simplified by considering the following three clinical situations.

THE PATIENT WITH A LOCALISED MALIGNANCY UNDERGOING EXCISIONAL SURGERY

A patient with an adenocarcinoma of the colon, stomach, pancreas or hepatobiliary tract without a very large tumour or evidence of dissemination should be regarded as being metabolically identical to a similar patient with benign disease (Shaw & Wolfe 1988b). Preoperative weight loss, due to alterations in taste sensation, anorexia, or local effects of the tumour may occasionally be massive (Theologides 1979) but this is not often a problem. If physiological dysfunctions are considerable then preoperative nutritional replenishment is indicated and it can be expected that protein will be accreted at the same rate and to the same extent as in a patient with similar deficits who has benign disease (Hill et al 1991). Postoperatively, in a similar manner to a patient without cancer, dextrose infusion results in protein sparing and if TPN is required protein loss can be prevented (Shaw & Wolfe 1988b). The only difference these patients have from those with benign disease is that postoperative fatigue is likely to be prolonged. In a study of preoperative factors likely to be associated with postoperative fatigue we found that patients with a diagnosis of cancer, whether or not it was subjected to curative surgery, had a significantly prolonged period of postoperative fatigue (Schroeder & Hill 1992).

THE PATIENT WITH A LARGE TUMOUR OR DISSEMINATED MALIGNANCY

Patients with sarcoma (Shaw & Humberstone 1988), lymphoma (Humberstone & Shaw 1988), bulky tumours (Shaw & Wolfe 1988b) and those who have tumours that have spread to the liver and beyond (MacFie et al 1982) are hypermetabolic. It is unlikely that the tumour itself is totally responsible and it appears that peptide regulatory factors are at least partially involved (Douglas & Shaw 1990). These patients suffer from alterations in metabolism and interorgan substrate interchanges (Fig. 3.1) that are not dissimilar to those we have seen in sepsis (Brennan 1977, Douglas & Shaw 1990, Chen et al 1991).

If major surgery is required in very malnourished patients with advanced cancer it therefore cannot be expected that nutritional support will result in repletion of body stores of protein (Shaw & Wolfe 1988b). A few days of nutritional repletion will, however, restore some aspects of physiological function and the plasma levels of the short half life plasma proteins (see Ch. 6). Postoperative care should include special attention to fluid balance (avoiding excess sodium because of the expanded extracellular water) and nutritional support to prevent further loss of body protein.

PATIENTS WITH GASTROINTESTINAL MALIGNANCY PRESENTING FOR VERY MAJOR EXTIRPATIVE SURGERY

Typical examples of this type of patient include those with oesophageal or oesophagogastric tumours. These patients may present with considerable weight loss and require a difficult and prolonged operative procedure in which the risks of postoperative complications are high. Table 3.2 describes the measurements of body composition, plasma proteins and metabolic expenditure we made on 17 patients presenting for total gastrectomy and distal oesophagectomy for adenocarcinoma of the proximal stomach/lower oesophagus (Hill 1988). Preoperatively every effort was made to exclude metastases and none of these patients had hepatic, lung or peritoneal

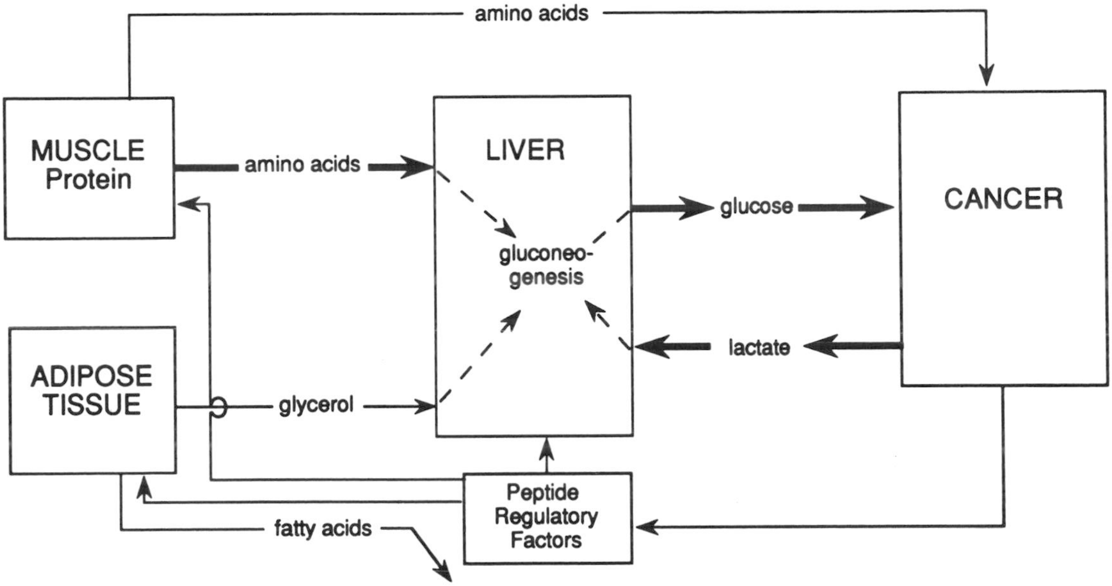

Fig. 3.1 A summary of the metabolic changes associated with advanced cancer. The interorgan substrate transfers are like those that occur in sepsis.

Table 3.2 Nutritional assessment profile of 17 patients with adenocarcinoma of the gastrointestinal junction. Although widespread metastases (liver, lung, peritoneal) were not present and resection was possible in each case none survived longer than 3 years. (Mean ± s.d.)

	Estimated value when well	Measured value	% change
Body composition			
Body weight (kg)	70.5 ± 13.2	59.4 ± 13.6	−15.8
Total body fat	16.5 ± 3.8	11.1 ± 5.5	−32.3
Total body protein (kg)	10.3 ± 1.9	8.5 ± 2.7	−18.1
Total body water (L)	39.7 ± 4.6	36.1 ± 8.6	−9.0
TBW: FFM	0.73	0.75	+2.5
Plasma proteins			
Plasma albumin (g/L)	35 – 48	36.3 ± 4.5	—
Plasma transferrin (g/dl)	220 – 330	177 ± 61	—
Plasma prealbumin (g/dl)	18 – 39	16.3 ± 8.1	—
Resting metabolic expenditure (kcal/24h)	1216 ± 152	1340 ± 326	+9%

metastases. Each underwent the planned procedure but there were no long-term survivors (i.e. greater than 3 years) suggesting the primary tumour had already escaped local control at the time of surgery. From the table it can be seen that the changes in body composition caused by the neoplasm are quite similar to those brought about by simple starvation (see Ch. 5, Table 5.3). Apart from the slightly increased resting metabolic expenditure (RME) and modest fall in plasma albumin there is little here to suggest septic metabolism. If nutritional repair had been required before surgery one would expect a modest gain in total body protein to occur. Postoperative TPN was given to each of these 17 patients and it resulted in preservation of body protein stores, restoration of plasma proteins to normal and a slight(but insignificant) increase in total body fat stores.

We suggest that these data show that patients requiring very major surgery for quite large gastrointestinal tumours which have not clinically metastasised may be treated in exactly the same way as similar patients without malignancy.

DOES TOTAL PARENTERAL NUTRITION CAUSE THE CANCER TO GROW?

There are animal data which suggest that nutrients provided by parenteral nutrition are consumed preferentially by the tumour (Fried et al 1985, Grube et al 1985) although there is considerable debate about a similar effect in cancer patients (Fischer 1984, Heys et al 1991). Some experimental data (Mullen et al 1980) and clinical common sense (Copeland 1990) suggest that if tumour growth stimulation occurs to an appreciable extent it would have been noted to be a clinical problem by now.

4. Fluid and electrolyte therapy and disorders of acid base balance

INTRODUCTION

Most surgical illness and operative intervention profoundly alter the balance and distribution of body fluids and electrolytes. A good understanding of the metabolism of salt, water and electrolytes is therefore essential to the care of surgical patients. In this chapter, some basic concepts of body composition and surgical physiology will be outlined before discussing the changes in body fluids that occur in surgical illness and how each of them may be treated.

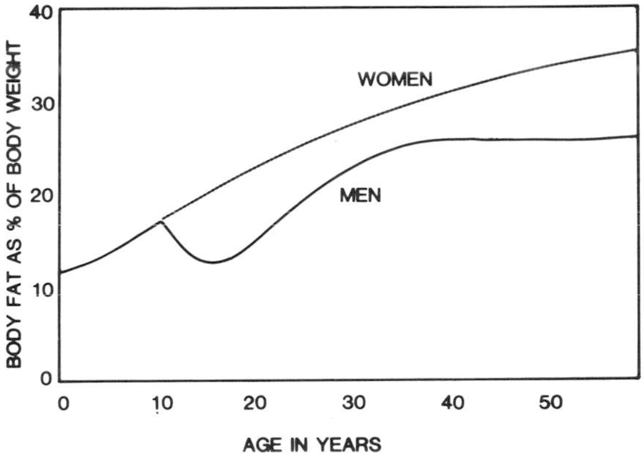

Fig. 4.1 This diagram shows that an increasing proportion of body weight is composed of fat as age increases. Note that after puberty the proportion of weight that is fat is always greater in females, i.e. if a female is the same weight as her male counterpart of the same age, her metabolic, fluid and electrolyte requirements will be less.

SECTION I
BODY MASS, BODY FAT, AND THE FAT FREE BODY MASS

The body mass may be thought of as being composed of two broad subdivisions, body fat and the fat free body mass.

In clinical practice it is usual to prescribe fluid, electrolyte, energy and protein requirements according to body mass. Since fluid and electrolyte exchanges in the body occur in its fat free portion, considerable errors may occur if no cognisance is taken of the varying proportion of body mass due to fat that occurs from patient to patient. Not only does body fat comprise a greater proportion of body weight in women but it increases in both sexes with increasing age (Fig. 4.1). It is important also to remember that not all the fat in the body is in subcutaneous tissue. Nearly half of it is in less visible sites, particularly the abdominal cavity. *A good clinical guide is the axiom: the more fat, the less lean. In other words, for two patients of equal weight the fatter patient has less fluid, electrolyte and metabolic requirements.*

SECTION II
ANATOMY OF BODY WATER AND ELECTROLYTES

BODY WATER CONTENT AND DISTRIBUTION

The total body water (about 42 L in a healthy 70 kg man) may be divided into two major compartments, the extracellular water (ECW or ECF) and the intracellular water (ICW or ICF) which are separated by the cell membranes. The ICW

(23 L) is the site of all the metabolic processes of the body and the ECW (19 L) is the compartment which provides a constant external environment for the cells. Edelman & Leibman (1959) have classified ECW into five phases (Fig. 4.2), namely:

- plasma (3 L)
- interstitial fluid-lymph (9 L)
- connective tissues and cartilage water (3 L)
- bone water (3 L)
- transcellular fluid (1 L).

Except for transcellular fluid each of these water phases corresponds to a well defined anatomical space. Transcellular fluid is that fraction of the ECW which is formed by the activity of the secretory cells but is not a transudate of plasma or lymph. The major component of the transcellular fluid is the intraluminal gastrointestinal water. Other transcellular fluids are found in the exocrine glands, liver, biliary tree, kidneys, eyes and the cerebrospinal fluid.

The emphasis from Figure 4.2 on subdivisions of body water helps understanding of fluid shifts that may occur in surgical patients. The most familiar example is that of the patient with distal intestinal obstruction in whom the total transcellular fluid content of the intestine may be 5 or 10 times that of normal and this is at the expense of other ECW. Major trauma or serious sepsis are other clinical examples in which large fluid translocations occur. In soft tissue injuries or after extensive dissection from a major surgical procedure extracellular fluid accumulates around the area of injury. In serious sepsis there is increased capillary permeability throughout the body and protein rich fluid passes out of the vascular space into the interstitium.

Almost all illness results in a redistribution of body water. ECW tends to be maintained as wasting proceeds. The ECW, including plasma and interstitial water, maintains volume while cell mass shrinks. The practical implication of this is that very wasted surgical patients who are not clinically sodium and water depleted are intolerant of excessive salt and water loads; there is a tendency to oedema, hypoproteinaemia and hypotonicity.

BODY SODIUM CONTENT AND DISTRIBUTION

Figure 4.3 shows the distribution of body sodium in the average normal adult male with a total body sodium of 4060 mmol. It gives a picture of how administered sodium will diffuse readily into

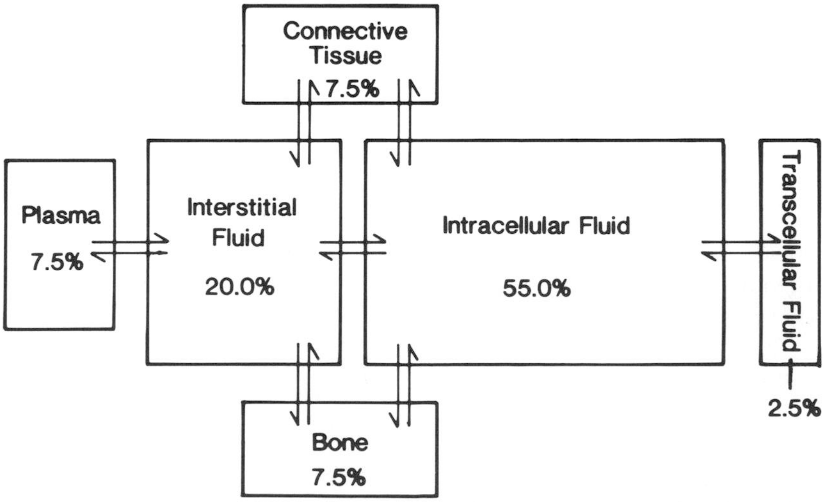

Fig. 4.2 Schematic diagram of the distribution of body water in a healthy young man. If labelled water is injected into the plasma of a patient it is distributed throughout these compartments within 2–4 hours. (Redrawn from Edelman I S, Leibman J 1959 Amer J Med 27: 256, with permission.)

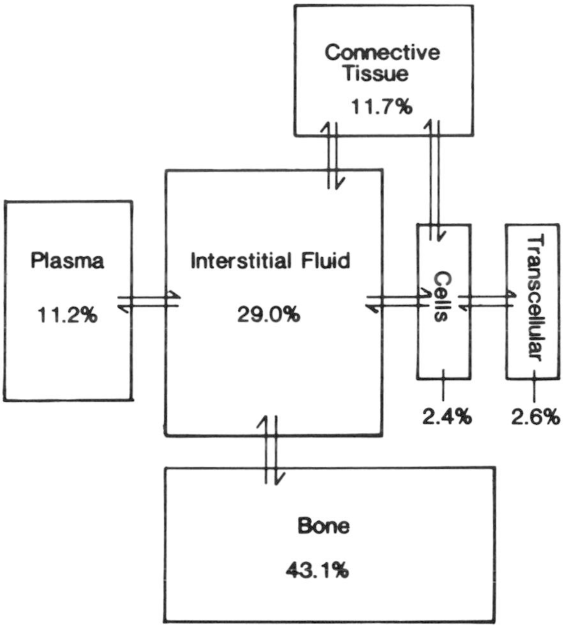

Fig. 4.3 Schematic diagram of the distribution of body sodium in a normal young adult man. (Redrawn from Edelman I S, Leibman J 1959 Amer J Med 27: 256, with permission.)

the different compartments of extracellular water. When radiolabelled sodium is administered it is found that there is a sizeable pool of rapidly exchangeable sodium, a slowly exchangeable pool of sodium and probably a non-exchangeable pool of sodium in bone. Bone contains more than 40% of the total body content of sodium; thus exchangeable sodium is significantly less than the total body quantity. All non-osseous sodium achieves exchange equilibrium with radiolabelled sodium in about 24 hours.

BODY POTASSIUM CONTENT AND DISTRIBUTION

Total body potassium content can be measured in a whole body counter and it can be demonstrated that almost all the potassium in the body is exchangeable in about 48 hours when the whole body counting method is compared with the radio-potassium-dilution technique. Almost all the potassium in the body is inside cells. Extracellular potassium is but a tiny fraction of the total body content. In a fit young male with 17 L of extracellular water only 65 mmol (out of a total body content of 3500 mmol) is effectively outside cells. The total plasma potassium may vary from as little as 7 mmol in a small woman to 21 mmol in a large man.

It is thought that most cells contain a constant concentration of potassium (150 mmol per L of ICW). Hence the total cell mass of the body (body cell mass) in a healthy man can be calculated from measurements of total body potassium. Unfortunately in some surgical illness and during recovery the concentration of intracellular potassium may vary considerably and in these situations body cell mass cannot then be estimated reliably. Body potassium depletion may occur when there is loss of cell substance but may also occur as a true intracellular depletion. Isolated pH changes invoke a change in the distribution of potassium between ICW and ECW. A certain amount of intracellular potassium (about 100–200 mmol) is associated with glycogen storage in liver and muscle cells. It can be rapidly lost or gained in early starvation or carbohydrate feeding.

BODY CHLORIDE CONTENT AND DISTRIBUTION

The 'ideal' 70 kg man contains about 2300 mmol of chloride. 70% of this is in plasma, interstitial fluid and lymph. It is thus predominantly an extracellular ion though some is present in intracellular fluid and specific chloride secreting cells such as the testes, ovary, intestinal and gastric mucosa and skin, and a significant part is localised in connective tissue. In clinical practice it is thought that since chloride is sufficiently restricted to the plasma and interstitial fluid it can be regarded as an index of extracellular fluid volume. Probably almost all the body chloride is exchangeable. Total plasma chloride content may change under pathophysiological circumstances independent of changes of plasma volume since hyperchloraemia may appear in some varieties of metabolic acidosis and hypochloraemia often is present in patients with metabolic alkalosis.

OTHER IONS OF CLINICAL IMPORTANCE

Magnesium

The total body content of magnesium in the average adult is about 1000 mmol, about half of which is incorporated in bone and is only slowly exchangeable. The distribution of magnesium is similar to that of potassium, the major proportion being intracellular. Plasma magnesium concentration normally ranges between 0.8–1.2 mmol/L. The kidneys show remarkable ability to conserve magnesium and this ion is essential for the function of most enzyme systems and depletion is characterised by neuromuscular and central nervous system hyperactivity. The normal daily intake of magnesium is about 10 mmol per day.

Calcium

Approximately 99% of the 1–1.2 kg of calcium in the body is concentrated in the skeleton. Thus a relatively small but profoundly important fraction of the total body calcium is in soft tissues and extracellular fluid. Calcium is an important mediator of neuromuscular function. The usual dietary intake of calcium is about 3 g a day, and most of this is excreted unabsorbed in the faeces. The normal serum calcium concentration is maintained by vitamin D, parathormone and calcitonin. Acidosis increases and alkalosis decreases the serum calcium concentration. Approximately half the serum calcium is bound to plasma proteins, mainly albumin, but it is the remaining ionised calcium (i.e. about 40% of the total serum calcium) which is the fraction responsible for the biological effect.

SECTION III
SURGICAL PHYSIOLOGY

OSMOLALITY AND TONICITY OF THE BODY FLUIDS

The chemical composition of the plasma, the interstitial fluid-lymph compartment and the intracellular fluid compartment of the body is shown in Table 4.1. It can be seen that the extracellular fluid has sodium as the principal cation and chloride and bicarbonate as the principal anions. There are minor differences in ionic composition between the plasma and interstitial fluid occasioned by the difference in protein concentration but for clinical purposes they may be considered equal.

The difference in ionic composition between the intracellular and extracellular fluid compartments is due to the selective permeability of the cell wall. Although water freely diffuses through this semipermeable membrane, the passage of sodium and its salts into cells is restricted, while that of potassium and its salts is promoted. This ability of water to diffuse freely across the cell membrane means that the total solute concentration (osmolality) of all body fluid compartments is identical (Flear et al 1980).

Apart from calcium, zinc, magnesium and other trace metals, nearly all the osmotically active cations in the body are represented by the exchangeable sodium and exchangeable potassium. In normal subjects it has been found that there is a high correlation between the sum of these cations and the total content of water in the body, demonstrating clearly the osmotic homogeneity of the body. In 1958 Edelman and his colleagues found in a variety of normal and pathologic subjects that there was a close relationship between the serum sodium concentration and the concentration of the total exchangeable cations in total body water (Fig. 4.4). Most clinical abnormalities of the serum sodium con-

Table 4.1 Electrolyte concentration of body fluids (mmol/L)

Electrolyte concentration	Plasma	Interstitial fluid	Intracellular fluid
Cations			
Na^+	142	144	10
K^+	4	4	150
Ca^{++}	2.5	1.5	2
Mg^{++}	1.5	0.5	20
Anions			
Cl^-	103	114	10
HCO_3^-	27	30	10
SO_4^{--}	1.5	1.5	70
PO_4^{---}	1	1	45

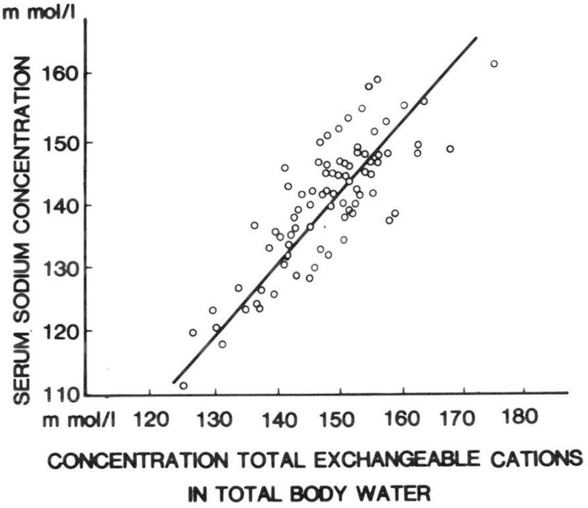

Fig. 4.4 This diagram shows the close relationship between serum sodium concentration and the concentration of the exchangeable cation ($Na_E + K_E$) in total body water for a wide variety of normal and sick subjects. F D Moore (1959) pointed out that this relationship is an expression of the osmotic homogeneity of the body and most clinical abnormalities of the serum sodium concentration can be explained by reference to it. (Redrawn from Edelman et al 1958 J Clin Invest 37: 1236, with permission.)

centration can be explained if this concept is understood. In surgical illness any condition that alters the effective osmotic pressure between the extracellular and intracellular compartments will result in redistribution of water between the compartments.

In surgical practice hypotonicity occurs quite commonly and is reflected by a low serum sodium concentration. The decrease in effective osmotic pressure in ECW will result in a transfer of water from the extracellular to the intracellular fluid compartments. It is important to understand that depletion or increases of the extracellular fluid compartment without a change in the concentration of ions (osmolality) will not result in transfer of water from the intracellular space. The intracellular fluid shares in losses or gains that involve a change in concentration or composition of the extracellular fluid but does not share in changes involving loss of isotonic volume only. It can be seen then that the distribution of water in the body is controlled by the osmolality of its fluid compartments. Dr F D Moore who wrote the classic *Metabolic Care of the Surgical Patient* teaches that the body as a whole acts as an osmometer in that an osmolality observed in any one part of the body must be present throughout the whole body.

In plasma about 98% of the osmolality consists of electrolyte: one half of this is sodium, i.e. the total plasma osmolality is numerically twice the sodium concentration in mmol/L plus a small increment (about 8 mOsmol/kg due to other particles). Clinically any plasma osmolality beyond 'twice the sodium' may be assumed to be due to abnormal accumulations of osmotically active particles, including glucose, urea, lactate, mannitol, alcohol and others in renal failure.

WATER GAIN AND LOSSES

Table 4.2 shows a water balance constructed for a normal 70 kg man living in a temperate climate. The normal subject drinks about 1500 ml of water a day and the rest of his water intake comes from water contained in solid food and from the food as it is oxidised in the body. Water is lost from the stool, urine, and also as insensible loss. Insensible losses are from the skin and the lungs and these increase when the patient is hypermetabolic, is over breathing or is febrile. Shown in this table are the minimal amounts of water that can be lost together with the maximum amounts that may be lost in extremes of surgical illness and stress.

SALT GAIN AND LOSSES

Normal man takes in about 100 mmol of sodium

Table 4.2 24-hours average intake and output of water in an adult

Intake		Output	
Oral liquids	1300 ml (0–1.5 L/h)	Urine	1500 ml (30 ml–1.4 L/h)
Water in food	900 ml (0–1500 ml)	Stool	200 ml (0–2.5 L/h)
Water of oxidation	300 ml (125–800 ml)	Insensible	
		Lungs	300 ml (200–1500 ml)
		Skin	500 ml (20 ml–1 L/h)
Total	2500 ml		2500 ml

and 100 mmol of chloride per day. Balance is maintained primarily by the kidneys which excrete salt that is taken in in excess of need. Under conditions of reduced intake or extrarenal losses of sodium the normal kidney can reduce sodium excretion to less than 1 mmol per day and sodium may disappear from the faeces and the sweat (Table 4.3). In clinical practice 1 mmol of sodium/kg body weight/day is a useful guideline for maintenance requirements.

POTASSIUM GAIN AND LOSSES

The normal subject takes in about 100 mmol of potassium per day and excretes about 60 mmol in the urine and the remainder in the faeces. Fluid from the small intestine contains much less potassium than that which is found in faeces. When potassium depletion occurs in patients with losses of small bowel content (e.g. enterocutaneous fistulas) it is because there has been renal conservation of sodium at the expense of potassium with consequent high output of urinary potassium.

COMPOSITION OF GASTROINTESTINAL SECRETIONS

To construct a proper balance sheet in a surgical patient who has abnormal losses from the gastrointestinal tract it is important to have a working knowledge of the volume and composition of the different types of gastrointestinal fluids (Table 4.4).

Gastrointestinal losses are usually isotonic or slightly hypotonic although there are considerable variations in their composition. In a patient with normal kidneys, though, these matter little. In clinical practice gastrointestinal losses are replaced by an isotonic salt solution. If the loss is from the stomach it is replaced litre for litre with 'normal saline' (0.9% saline) to which 15 mmol of K^+ have been added. Other losses from the gastrointestinal tract including that fluid which accumulates in the lumen of the intestine when it is obstructed can be replaced litre for litre with Ringer's lactate solution (Hartmann's). Villous tumours of the colon or rectum may secrete fluid with a high potassium concentration and clinical manifestations of hypokalaemia may be observed.

Table 4.3 Intake and output of sodium in an adult subject — shown are average values together with minimal and maximal values that are possible in sickness and health

Intake	Output	
Diet 50–100 mmol/day (0–100 mmol/h)	Urine	10–100 mmol/day (0–200 mmol/L)
	Stool	0–20 mmol/day (0–300 mmol/h)
	Skin	10–60 mmol/day (0–300 mmol/h)

ACID BASE FUNDAMENTALS

The meaning of pH

The pH notation is a useful means of expressing H^+ concentrations of the body, because the H^+ concentrations happen to be low, relative to those of other cations. Thus, the normal Na^+ concentration of arterial plasma that has been equilibrated with red blood cells is 145 mmol/L, whereas, the H^+ concentration is 0.00004 mmol/L (i.e. 0.00000004 mol/L). The pH (that is the negative logarithm of 0.00000004) is therefore 7.4. The enormous range encompassed by the logarithmic pH scale can be understood if it is thought of in linear terms. Thus, there is about twice as much H^+ in a solution of pH 7.1 (H^+ concentration is 0.000079 mmol/L) as there is at pH 7.4 (H^+ concentration is 0.000039 mmol/L). Body cells can function normally between pH 7.2 and pH 7.5, a range of 400% alteration in H^+ concentration.

The disposal of acid in the body

A variety of organic acids are produced during the metabolism of carbohydrate, fat and proteins. The body is constantly working to prevent a metabolic acidosis due to these metabolic processes and surgical illness may upset this balance. Appreciable quantities of lactic acid, pyruvic acid and other acids sometimes accumulate in the blood in surgical patients. Oxidation of sulphur-containing amino acids generates H^+ and SO_4^{2-} and metabolism of phosphorus-containing sub-

Table 4.4 Composition of gastrointestinal secretions

Intestinal tract locality	Volume (ml)	Na^+ (mmol/L)	K^+ (mmol/L)	Cl^- (mmol/L)	HCO_3^- (mmol/L)
Saliva	1500	10	25	10	30
Gastric juice (fasting)	1500	60	15	90	15
Pancreatic fistula	700	140	5	75	120
Biliary fistula	500	145	5	100	40
Jejunostomy	2–3000	110	5	100	30
Ileostomy	500	115	8	45	30
Proximal colostomy	300	80	20	45	30
Diarrhoeal stools	500–15 000	120	25	90	45

stances such as nucleoproteins generate H^+ and PO_4^{--}. The H^+ formed by metabolism in the tissues is in large part hydrated to H_2CO_3 and the total H^+ load from this source is over 12 500 mmol/day. Most of the CO_2 is excreted in the lungs, and only small amounts of the H^+ ions from this source are excreted by the kidneys. Common sources of excessive acid loads are strenuous exercise (lactic acid) and diabetic ketosis. Failure of diseased kidneys to excrete a normal acid load is also a cause of acidosis.

Alkalosis is less of a problem than acidosis but the body has a much more limited power of compensation. In surgery the most common cause of alkalosis is loss of acid from the body due to vomiting of gastric juice. This is, of course, equivalent to adding alkali to the body.

The Henderson–Hasselbalch equation

The principal buffers in the extracellular fluid are haemoglobin, protein and carbonic acid H_2CO_3.

As a buffer, the position of H_2CO_3 is unique because it is converted to H_2O and CO_2 and the CO_2 is then excreted in the lungs.

The function of this principal buffer system is expressed in the Henderson–Hasselbalch equation, which defines the pH in terms of the ratio of the salt and acid:

$$pH = pK + \log \frac{[HCO_3^-]}{[H_2CO_3]}$$

The equation shows that the pH of the extracellular fluid is determined primarily by the ratio of base bicarbonate (mainly sodium bicarbonate) to the amount of carbonic acid (related to the CO_2 content of alveolar air) present in the blood. The symbol $[H_2CO_3]$ stands for the concentration of carbonic acid plus dissolved CO_2. In normal subjects the ratio $\frac{[HCO_3^-]}{[H_2CO_3]}$ is 20 : 1 and the pK 6.1. Thus:

$$pH = 6.1 + \log [20_{10}] = 7.4$$

The amount of carbonic acid and dissolved CO_2 is proportional to the $P\text{CO}_2$. The plasma HCO_3^- (which cannot be measured directly) is the total measurable CO_2 of plasma minus the dissolved CO_2, the carbonic acid and the carbamino–CO_2. Constants have been derived experimentally such that the Henderson–Hasselbalch equation for the bicarbonate system in plasma can be written in the following form:

$$pH = 6.1 + \log \left[\frac{HCO_3^-}{0.03 P\text{CO}_2} \right]$$

(0.03 is the solubility coefficient of CO_2)

This is the clinically applicable form of the equation, because HCO_3^- cannot be measured directly but pH and $P\text{CO}_2$ can be measured with suitable accuracy using pH and $P\text{CO}_2$ glass electrodes and HCO_3^- can then be calculated.

Four types of acid base disorder

When acid is added to the buffer system just described (metabolic acidosis), the concentration of bicarbonate (the numerator in the Henderson–Hasselbalch equation) will decrease. Ventilation will immediately increase to eliminate larger quantities of CO_2 with a subsequent decrease in the carbonic acid (the denominator in the Henderson–Hasselbalch equation) until the 20 : 1 ratio is reestablished. Slower more complete compensation is effected by the kidneys with increased excretion of acid salts and retention of bicarbonate. The reverse will occur if *an alkali is added to the system (metabolic alkalosis). Respiratory acidosis and alkalosis* are produced by disturbances of ventilation with an increase or decrease in the denominator and the resultant change of the 20 : 1 ratio. Compensation is primarily renal, with a retention of bicarbonate and increased excretion of acid salts in respiratory acidosis and the reverse process in respiratory alkalosis. The four distinct types of acid base disturbances are shown in Table 4.5. Looking at this table it can be seen that the pH and $P\text{CO}_2$ from a freshly drawn arterial blood sample are necessary for diagnosis. *Thus measurement of pH and* $P\text{CO}_2$ *and calculation of bicarbonate concentration are required for a complete understanding of the acid base status of a patient.*

Anion gap

In the body, electrical neutrality is maintained by balancing the total number of cations with the total number of anions. This principle can be utilised clinically in patients with suspected acid base disorders by measuring the serum sodium, chloride and bicarbonate concentrations. Normally the extracellular concentration of the cations (mainly sodium) equals the sum of the extracellular concentrations of the anions (chloride and bicarbonate) plus a constant. This constant equals about 8 mmol/L. If the sum of the concentrations of these two anions plus 8 is less than the serum sodium concentration, an anion gap is said to exist. Determination of the anion gap may prove quite helpful in assessing the cause of metabolic acidosis. Metabolic acidosis (resulting in an anion gap) may occur in patients with renal insufficiency in which phosphate and sulphate as well as organic acid anions are retained, or in ketoacidosis in which ketoacids accumulate in the blood, or lactic acidosis as arises in hypoxia.

SECTION IV
THE METABOLIC RESPONSE TO INJURY

In Chapters 1 and 2 we outlined the characteristic physiological changes which follow serious sepsis, major trauma or surgical operation and pointed out that most of the metabolic effects observed can be reproduced by infusion of the 'stress hormones', cortisol, epinephrine and glucagon (Bessey et al 1984). The release of these, and other hormones, in major injury is described in terms of a reflex arc (Gann & Lilly 1983). The reflex is initiated by fear, pain, hypovolaemia, hypoxia, tissue injury and/or sepsis (afferent limb) and serves the body by means of metabolic and circulatory adjustments (efferent limb) which lead to correction of the initial disturbance. The sum of all these effects needs to be appreciated in order to manage patients with problems of volume, concentration or composition of body fluids.

NEUROENDOCRINE RESPONSES TO INJURY

Afferent limb

Surgical operation or other forms of trauma cause a series of physiological derangements which

Table 4.5 Four basic types of acid base disorders — before and after partial compensation

	Metabolic				Respiratory			
	Acidosis		*Alkalosis*		*Acidosis*		*Alkalosis*	
	uncompensated	compensated	uncompensated	compensated	uncompensated	compensated	uncompensated	compensated
pH	↓↓	↓	↑↑	↑	↓↓	↓	↑↑	↑
$P\text{CO}_2$	N	↓	N	↑	↑↑	↑↑	↓↓	↓↓
Plasma HCO_3^-	↓↓	↓	↑↑	↑	N	↑	N	↓

N = No change

activate a number of different *afferent pathways*. The neuroendocrine response to trauma can be blocked by section of the nerves to the area being traumatised. Although conscious perception of pain is not necessary for the neuroendocrine response the central nervous connections to the hypothalamus are essential (Hume & Edgahl 1959, Edgahl 1959). Although reception of pain at the site of injury and afferent impulses related to changes in effective circulating blood volume play the overriding roles in the early neuroendocrine response to trauma, as injury progresses, other stimuli such as acidosis, hypoxia, hypercapnia, changes in body temperature as well as the release of local factors from injured tissues may all come into play.

Efferent limb

The efferent arc of the reflex response to injury arises in basically two locations: the pituitary and the brain stem. The output of the *pituitary* is a set of hormones that act either directly on effector organs or via the release of mediating hormones. The efferent fibres of the parasympathetic nervous system and sympathetic nervous system carry the outflow of the *brain stem* to the periphery either directly, or indirectly by affecting the release of peripheral hormones.

Pituitary hormones involved in the metabolic response to injury include ACTH, vasopressin, endorphins, and encephalins, growth hormone and prolactin.

Corticotrophin releasing factor is secreted from the median eminence. This compound is carried by the vessels of the hypothalamo-hypophysial portal system into the anterior pituitary, where it acts upon the chromophobe cells to release ACTH. *ACTH* acts on the cells of the zona fasciculata in the adrenal leading to the biosynthesis of cortisol. *Cortisol* is required for the complete restitution of blood volume after haemorrhage. It appears to be involved in a shift of fluid from the intracellular compartment into the interstitial space. Cortisol also has wide ranging metabolic actions including inhibition of glycogenolysis and increase in gluconeogenesis from muscle amino acids. It inhibits the action of insulin and may affect the immune system.

The prime stimuli that lead to secretion of *vasopressin* are increased osmolality of the plasma and reduction of effective blood volume. In the early response to injury blood volume changes take precedence over tonicity. Vasopressin has several major areas of activity, the most important of which is to control renal free water handling. It increases permeability of the collecting system and this is the prime determinant of renal free water clearance.

There are two main group of *opiate peptides* that are released from the pituitary in injured patients — endorphin and the encephalins. They probably inhibit sympathetic tone and modulate sympathetic activity at the spinal level.

Increased circulating *growth hormone* occurs in response to the stress of surgery and trauma. The effects of this increase are either direct or through the action of *somatomedins*, a family of hormones which possess insulin-like activity. The important actions of growth hormone in the post-traumatic patient are metabolic rather than on fluid and electrolyte metabolism. Growth hormone inhibits the action of insulin in muscle, thereby decreasing net glucose uptake. *Prolactin*, like growth hormone, has mainly metabolic effects in injured patients. *Thyroid hormones* and *thyroid stimulating hormones* are unaffected by injury or surgery. *Luteinising hormone* and *follicle stimulating hormone* are suppressed after surgery.

Hormones under autonomic control. There are also hormones under autonomic control which are released as a response to injury or sepsis. There is an increase in *catecholamines*, *renin*, *aldosterone* and alteration in the *glucagon–insulin* ratio in septic and injured surgical patients. Catecholamines affect tissues through interaction with specific cell surface receptors and affect heart rate and blood pressure.

Catecholamines also act in a wide variety of tissues through stimulation of other hormones; renin is increased and hence renal handling of water and sodium, and insulin and glucagon secretion are also altered by catecholamines. There is an increase in circulating glucagon and a relative decrease in insulin secretion. In haemorrhage, and particularly when there is hypovolaemia, *renin* and hence angiotensin are released. The latter is a potent vasoconstrictor and also has direct chronotropic and inotropic effects on the myocardium. It also acts on the median eminence and pituitary to increase secretion of vasopressin and ACTH. Angiotensin 2, is a major stimulus to secretion of aldosterone by the cells of the adrenal zona glomerulosa. Aldosterone acts on the renal tubule, the colon, terminal ileum, salivary glands and sweat glands to retain sodium.

Autonomic nervous activity. Following trauma the effects of autonomic nervous activity and increased circulating catecholamines on the pancreas result in the release of glucagon and inhibition of insulin secretion. There is a relative hypoinsulinaemia with respect to the circulating glucose concentrations. The ratio of insulin to glucagon which is presented to the liver is the critical determinant of the balance of hepatic anabolism and catabolism.

RESPONSES TO MAJOR INJURY AND SERIOUS SEPSIS

When injury is not great, as in well performed elective surgery, the metabolic response is small and short lived. The central nervous system alone appears to play the major regulatory role. When injury is greater, particularly when combined with sepsis, the response is greater with haemodynamic changes, fever, leukocytosis, hypermetabolism, increased glucose production and muscle proteolysis. If these responses are severe or prolonged they are associated with organ failure. The neuroendocrine response is necessary but not completely responsible for these increased responses (Long & Lowry 1991). It appears that in critical illness cytokines, particularly tumour necrosis factor and interleukin-2, initiate and propagate the metabolic responses. These complex interrelationships which have not yet been fully worked out are under active investigation (Flores et al 1989a, Fong & Lowry 1990a, Michie et al 1988a, Watson et al 1989, Fong et al 1989b, Marano et al 1990, Uehara et al 1987, Beach et al 1989) and in Figure 4.5 a simplified schema describing them is shown.

SECTION V
CLASSIFICATION OF BODY FLUID CHANGES

Shires & Canizaro (1977) have evolved the clinically useful concept that body fluid and electrolyte disorders can be classified into *volume changes, concentration changes* and *compositional changes.*

VOLUME CHANGES

Volume deficit

By far the commonest fluid and electrolyte disorder encountered in surgical practice is a deficit of extracellular fluid. Intestinal obstruction, vomiting, excessive diarrhoea, severe trauma, major surgery associated with an extensive dissection, fluid loss from an enterocutaneous fistula, extensive burns, sepsis and shock, all result in a *net loss of extracellular fluid.* This, in the acute phase, cannot be diagnosed from laboratory information, for plasma sodium (and total body osmolality) have not been altered. Over a longer period of time, laboratory tests will show a rising blood urea and plasma creatinine, due to reduced glomerular filtration. The signs and symptoms of extracellular fluid volume deficit are set out in Table 4.6. Clinically it is quite useful to know that these symptoms and signs roughly equate to the size of the deficit sustained by the patient. Body composition studies in patients with deficits of extracellular fluid suggest that the deficit can be mild (1–2 L of ECF) moderate (2–4 L of ECF) or severe (5 or more L of ECF).

Volume excess

Apart from pulmonary oedema associated with heart failure, extracellular fluid volume excess is caused either by the administration of large quantities of sodium-containing fluids (which is sometimes necessary to preserve renal function in septic patients, see Ch. 19) or is secondary to renal or hepatic failure. The plasma volume, or

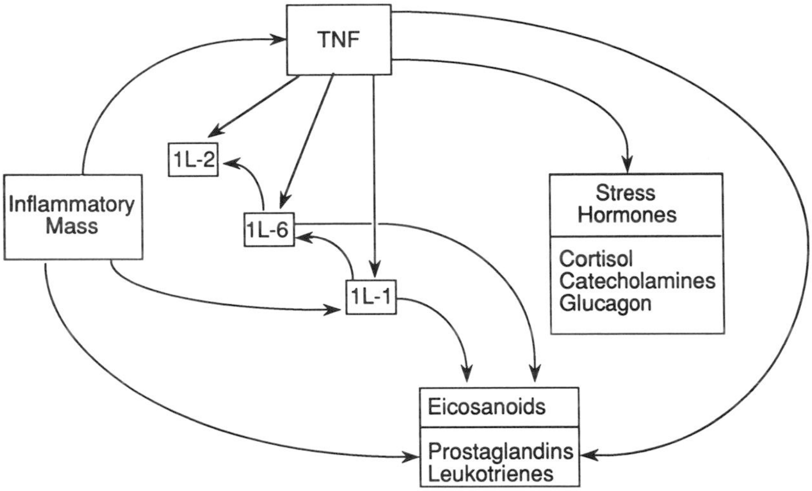

Fig. 4.5 The complex self propagating interrelationship between peptide regulatory factors and the stress hormones (simplified schema). The inflammatory mass releases cytokines which potentiate release of other cytokines and the stress hormones. Key: TNF = tumour necrosis factor; IL = interleukin.

the interstitial volume, or both, are increased. The sign of interstitial volume overload is oedema and the signs of plasma volume overload are hypertension, tachycardia, and increased venous pressure. It is important to stress that very depleted patients, particularly those with hypoalbuminaemia who ordinarily have a large extracellular water volume are not tolerant of excesses of sodium-containing fluids and may readily become overloaded. The surgeon will find such patients who have excessive amounts of extracellular fluid administered prior to surgery, have oedema of the wall of the stomach, colon and small bowel. This makes suturing more difficult, increasing the likelihood of anastomotic disruption.

CONCENTRATION CHANGES

Tonicity of the body fluids is a reflection of the plasma sodium concentration. Hyponatraemia or hypernatraemia in their early stages are not recognisable clinically. Nevertheless abnormal concentrations of plasma sodium should be noted

Table 4.6 Signs and symptoms of extracellular fluid deficit

Deficit	Mild (1–2 L ECF)*	Moderate (2–4 L ECF)*	Severe (5–9 L ECF)*
Symptoms	Gives history of recent loss of ECF	Apathy, anorexia Tachycardia Collapsed veins	Stupor or coma Ileus, Pale, hypotensive, Cold extremities, Absent pulses
Signs	Usually no signs	↓Blood pressure ↓Tissue turgor Dry tongue	↓↓Blood pressure ↓↓Tissue turgor Sunken eyes

* Calculated for 70 kg subject with normal body fat stores

and appropriate corrections made before clinical signs are seen.

Hyponatraemia

Most patients with hyponatraemia are hypotonic due to overhydration plus antidiuresis. Overhydration is due to excessive water administered orally or parenterally (e.g. 5% dextrose in water), and oxidation of fat or protein with production of free water. Vasopressin, as discussed above, is increased in patients suffering from acute surgical illness, immediately after surgical operation or tissue injury, and in chronic wasting disease. In surgical practice hyponatraemia is not uncommonly caused by the replacement of salt-rich losses with salt-poor fluid, i.e. there is a sodium lack with a 'relative' water retention.

Hyponatraemia, defined as serum sodium less than 130 mmol/L, is clinically characterised by signs which reflect excessive intracellular water. When severe, the patient may have signs of central nervous system dysfunction including confusion, areflexia and later convulsions. Many hyponatraemic states are asymptomatic until the serum sodium level falls below 120 mmol/L. Following closed head injury, mild hyponatraemia is more serious because increased intracellular water adds to the problem caused by an increase of intracranial pressure. Most hyponatraemic states are dealt with by withholding water but when severe and associated with symptoms hypertonic salt solutions should be given cautiously, perhaps with frusemide or mannitol to promote water loss.

Hypernatraemia

The patient with hypernatraemia usually presents with dry sticky mucous membranes, a red swollen tongue and flushed skin. The common clinical cause is water deficit. This is true dehydration whereas 'surgical dehydration' is most often extracellular fluid depletion. The treatment of hypernatraemia is to encourage water drinking or to add free water intravenously as dextrose in water. It is important not to correct a hyperosmolar state too rapidly as this may lead to brain oedema.

COMPOSITION CHANGES

Compositional abnormalities, which are clinically important, include changes in *acid base balance* and concentration changes of *potassium, magnesium* and *calcium.*

Acid base changes

In Table 4.5 a broad outline of each of the four main types of acid base disorder before and after partial compensation was shown. The clinical manifestations and the treatment of these compositional disorders will now be discussed.

Respiratory acidosis. This condition is due to alveolar hypoventilation leading to retention of CO_2. There may be depression of the respiratory centre from drugs, injury, and some forms of chronic pulmonary disease. In such patients the $P\text{CO}_2$ is chronically elevated and the bicarbonate concentration rises to compensate for this. Such patients need special management in the operative and postoperative period. Atelectasis, pneumonia and hypoventilation due to pain from the abdominal incision may exacerbate respiratory acidosis. At operation, infiltration of the incision site with local anaesthetic agents and transverse incisions are used by some surgeons to lessen wound pain. Postoperative management includes measures to ensure adequate ventilation, analgesia (via 'pain pump'), bronchodilators, physiotherapy, and incentive spirometry. The management of patients with very large upper abdominal incisions may be helped by the use of epidural anaesthesia, although intensive care with mechanical ventilation may be required.

Respiratory alkalosis. Respiratory alkalosis is due to hyperventilation and is sometimes seen on surgical wards and in intensive care units. Apprehension, pain, hypoxia and acidosis are the usual causes. Deliberate mechanical hyperventilation is used in the management of patients with severe head injury. In other intensive care patients who have respiratory alkalosis, this may be due to the improper use of the mechanical ventilator. There is a depression of the arterial $P\text{CO}_2$ and an elevation of the pH. The bicarbonate falls to compensate if the condition persists. The dangers of severe respiratory alkalosis are those due to impaired oxygen delivery and hypokalaemia such as ventricular arrhythmias. Hypokalaemia occurs because potassium ions enter cells in exchange for hydrogen ions and there is an excessive urinary potassium loss in exchange for sodium. Treatment is primarily directed towards preventing the condition by the proper use of mechanical ventilators and correcting any pre-existing potassium deficits.

Metabolic acidosis. This may result from the retention of acid (diabetic acidosis, lactic acidosis) or the loss of bicarbonate as occurs in diarrhoea, the short gut syndrome, pancreatic fistulas or high output enterocutaneous fistulas. There is a low arterial pH and bicarbonate concentration. The initial compensation is an increase in rate and depth of breathing and reduction of the arterial $P\text{CO}_2$.

A common cause of severe metabolic acidosis in surgical patients is acute circulatory failure causing tissue hypoxia and accumulation of lactic acid. Acute haemorrhagic shock may result in a rapid and profound drop in the arterial pH. Another cause of metabolic acidosis in surgery is the replacement of chloride ion in excess of that which has been lost. The use of a large volume of 'normal saline' (154 mmol of chloride ion/L) to replace extracellular fluid deficits or losses from the small intestine may provide excessive chloride. The treatment of metabolic acidosis should be towards correction of the underlying disorder when possible. In hypovolaemic patients, the use of lactated Ringer's solution (Hartmann's) and blood to restore tissue perfusion results in a rapid reversal of the problem. It is recommended that bicarbonate therapy should be reserved for the treatment of severe metabolic acidosis, particularly when associated with circulatory impairment, e.g. following cardiac arrest when partial correction of the pH may be essential to restore myocardial function. The initial dose of bicarbonate should be 1 mmol/kg/body weight of HCO_3^- as $NaHCO_3$ and the decision for additional bicarbonate should be based on measurements of pH and $P\text{CO}_2$.

Metabolic alkalosis. Metabolic alkalosis results from the loss of acid or the gain of bicarbonate. Both the pH and plasma bicarbonate concentration are elevated. Compensation for metabolic alkalosis is primarily by renal mechanisms, since respiratory compensation is very small. The majority of patients with metabolic alkalosis have some degree of hypokalaemia resulting from an entry of potassium into cells in exchange for H^+ and an excessive urinary potassium loss in exchange for sodium.

The commonest cause of metabolic alkalosis in surgical patients is loss of gastric juice from persistent vomiting or gastric suction. It is also an accompaniment of untreated pyloric stenosis. There is loss of fluid with a high chloride and hydrogen ion concentration. Initial compensation is by the loss of sodium and bicarbonate in the urine but as extracellular fluid is lost there is an attempt to conserve sodium by the kidney and potassium and hydrogen ions are excreted into the urine in increasing quantities, resulting in an uncompensated alkalosis and profound hypokalaemia. The initially alkaline urine therefore becomes acid after a period of time, due to hydrogen ion excretion. Management includes replacement of the extracellular fluid volume deficit with 0.9% sodium chloride solution (N saline), in addition to replacement of potassium. It is important to remember that potassium should never be given to patients until volume repletion has been obtained and a good urine output has been established. The vast majority of patients with metabolic alkalosis and normal renal function can be treated with 0.9% saline and potassium alone. A very small number of patients with severe hypochloraemia and excessive nasogastric drainage may be refractory to even large amounts of 0.9% saline and potassium. In the past ammonium chloride was recommended in such circumstances but more recently 0.1N–0.2N hydrochloric acid has been shown to be safe and effective therapy for correction of very severe metabolic alkalosis. A solution of 150 ml of 1N hydrochloric acid added to 1 L of sterile water gives an isotonic solution containing 150 mmol of hydrogen ion and 150 chloride ion. The solution is administered over a 12-hour period with frequent measurements of pH and $P\text{CO}_2$. Usually 1 or 2 L is sufficient to correct the immediate problem and this gives the surgeon time to correct the underlying cause.

Clinical steps for evaluating a patient with a suspected acid base disorder. A properly taken *history* should give a fairly clear idea of the type of acid base disorder that might be encountered. Evaluation of the *clinical signs* may also be useful, for example, tetany may be a manifestation of alkalosis; cyanosis may reflect respiratory failure. The *routine laboratory data*, i.e. venous blood electrolytes and bicarbonate, should be evaluated before an arterial puncture is decided upon. First the serum *bicarbonate* concentration should be looked at. An elevation represents either a metabolic alkalosis or a metabolic compensation for a respiratory acidosis, and a depression signifies either a metabolic acidosis, or a metabolic compensation for respiratory alkalosis. Next the concentration of serum potassium is noted. If plasma chloride has been measured a high level suggests hyperchloraemic metabolic acidosis and a low level suggests metabolic alkalosis.

The *anion gap* may then be calculated. If the sum of the concentration of serum chloride and serum bicarbonate plus 8 is less than the serum sodium concentration then an anion gap is present. This suggests a metabolic acidosis (Clark & Walker 1983).

Frequently, adequate assessment of a patient's acid base status can be made in this way from history, physical examination and an analysis of the data from a venous blood sample. The decision to determine *arterial* blood pH and $P\text{CO}_2$ depends on the need to confirm the clinical impression; in very sick patients, the determination is essential. Measurements of pH and $P\text{CO}_2$ are also necessary to document a mixed disturbance of acid base balance and determine the extent of acidosis or alkalosis upon which the need for treatment should be based.

Composition changes due to abnormal concentrations of potassium, magnesium, and calcium

Hyperkalaemia. Significant quantities of intracellular potassium are released into the extracellular space in response to severe injury, surgical stress or acidosis. In these situations dangerous hyperkalaemia (greater than 6 mmol/L) is rarely encountered if renal function is normal. The patient may suffer from nausea and vomiting, small bowel colic and diarrhoea. The electrocardiogram may show high peaked T waves, widened QRS complex and depressed ST segments. Heart block and asystolic cardiac arrest may develop with increasing concentrations of serum potassium.

Treatment of hyperkalaemia consists of immediate measures to reduce the serum potassium level, withholding of all administered potassium and correction of the underlying cause if possible. If the plasma level is very high, e.g. >7 mmol/L and there is ECG or clinical evidence of cardiac malfunction, treatment should include the administration of glucose and insulin (100 ml 50% dextrose + 10 units of insulin), calcium (10 ml of 10% calcium gluconate by slow intravenous infusion) and if there is acidosis 1 ml/kg of $NaHCO_3$. Such patients may require urgent haemodialysis. Lesser degrees of hyperkalaemia can usually be managed by K^+ restriction, glucose and insulin, and cation-exchange resins administered either orally or by rectum in doses of 15–30 g every 12 hours.

Hypokalaemia. Patients presenting for surgery may have been taking diuretics for long periods and have low levels of plasma potassium as a consequence. More commonly hypokalaemia occurs in surgical patients with alkalosis, after massive isotonic sodium replacement and when there have been large losses of gastrointestinal fluids. Increased renal loss of potassium occurs with both respiratory and metabolic alkalosis. Potassium is in competition with hydrogen ion for renal tubular excretion in exchange for sodium ion. Renal tubular excretion of potassium is increased when large amounts of sodium are infused and when there is renal tubular dysfunction. The development of hypokalaemia in patients with high losses of intestinal fluid is caused by renal loss of potassium occurring secondary to sodium retention which occurs in response to the loss of sodium from the gut.

The signs of potassium deficit are related to failure of normal contractility of skeletal muscle, smooth muscle and cardiac muscle. They include weakness that may progress to flaccid paralysis, diminished or absent tendon reflexes and paralytic ileus. Sensitivity to digitalis with atrial tachyarrhythmias and ventricular premature beats may occur. In addition the ECG may show flattening of T waves, the development of U waves and depression of ST segments. The treatment of hypokalaemia involves intravenous administration of K^+ at a rate of administration which should not exceed 20 mmol per hour. Figure 4.6 shows that when acid base disturbances are not present, serum potassium concentration is related to the degree of depletion of the total body potassium. It can be seen that a loss of 10% of total body potassium drops the serum potassium from 4 to 3 mmol at normal pH. This can be a useful guide to deciding on the initial rate of replenishment of a patient with hypokalaemia, although the situation should be reassessed every 6 hours.

Magnesium deficiency. Alcoholic patients, or those with high output ileostomies, enterocutaneous fistulas or severe diarrhoea may suffer from magnesium deficiency. The signs and symptoms of magnesium deficiency are clinically the same as calcium deficiency including hyperactive tendon reflexes, muscle tremors and tetany. Hypocalcaemia is usually noted particularly in those patients who have symptoms of tetany. The diagnosis may be missed if the clinician is not aware that neuromuscular symptoms occurring in patients with high intestinal losses are more likely to be due to magnesium deficiency than calcium deficiency. Plasma magnesium levels are usually low, but they are not wholly reliable. Treatment of magnesium deficiency is by the parenteral administration of magnesium sulphate or magnesium chloride solutions (20–40 mmol of $MgSO_4$ per litre of intravenous fluid). When large doses are given, the heart rate, blood pressure, respiration and electrocardiogram should be monitored closely.

Magnesium excess. Symptomatic hypermagnesaemia is rare, but is occasionally seen in patients with renal failure.

Hypocalcaemia. Hypocalcaemia occurs in hypoparathyroidism, severe pancreatitis, renal failure, severe trauma, and overwhelming sepsis. Except in patients with hypoparathyroidism, it is not treated for the condition is most often self limiting. Intravenous calcium, as calcium gluconate or calcium chloride, may be needed for acute symptoms as after parathyroidectomy. More chronic problems are dealt with by giving oral vitamin D supplements and calcium.

Hypercalcaemia. In surgical patients hypercalcaemia is most frequently caused by cancer with bony metastases, hyperparathyroidism, ectopic production of parathormone, hyperthyroidism, prolonged immobilisation and Paget's disease of bone. Hypercalcaemia may impair renal concentrating mechanisms resulting in polyuria. Severe hypercalcaemia can cause coma and death. The treatment of severe hypercalcaemia is to expand the extracellular fluid with isotonic saline and enhance calcium excretion by diuretics. Mithramycin is used when hypercalcaemia is associated with metastatic cancer.

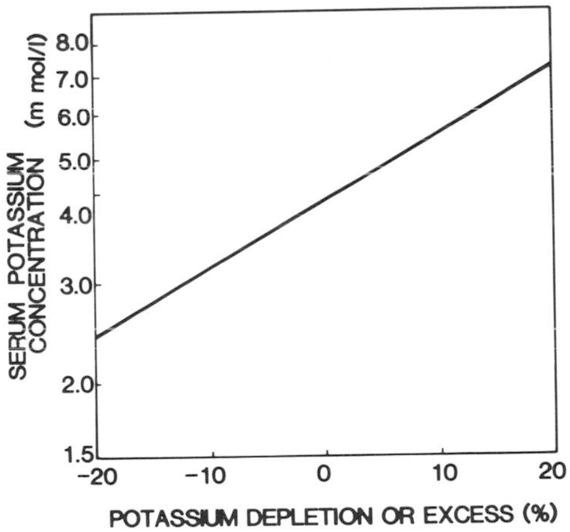

Fig. 4.6 The relationship of the serum potassium concentration to the total body content of potassium when the pH is within normal limits. With excessive external losses of potassium the serum K^+ falls: a loss of 10% of total body K^+ (i.e. about 350 mmol in a young man of normal build) drops the serum K^+ concentration from 4 to 3 mmol/L at normal pH.

SECTION VI
FLUID AND ELECTROLYTE THERAPY

PARENTERAL SOLUTIONS

The composition of various intravenous fluids

Table 4.7 Composition of commonly used parenteral fluids (electrolyte content mmol/L)

	Cations				Anions			Energy
	Na^+	K^+	Ca^{++}	Mg^{++}	Cl^-	HCO_3^-	HPO_4^{--}	kcals
ECF	142	4	2.5	1.5	103	27	3	—
Ringer's lactate (Hartmann's solution)	130	4	3		109	28	—	—
0.9% Sodium chloride	154	—	—	—	154	—	—	—
5% Dextrose	—	—	—	—	—	—	—	200/L
Hypotonic ($\frac{1}{5}$ N saline) (0.18% saline + 4.2% dextrose)	30	—	—	—	30	—	—	168/L
Potassium chloride (20% KCl)	25 mmol K^+ in 10 ml of 20% solution				25 mmol Cl^- in 10 ml of 20% solution			

which are commonly used, is shown in Table 4.7. A good isotonic salt solution for replacing gastrointestinal losses and repairing pre-existing volume deficits in the absence of gross abnormalities of concentration and composition is *Ringer's lactate* or Hartmann's solution. This solution contains 130 mmol of sodium, balanced by 109 mmol of chloride and 28 mmol of lactate and has minimal effect on normal body fluid composition and pH even when infused in large quantities. The chief disadvantage of Ringer's lactate solution is that its sodium concentration is lower than that of plasma. This rarely presents a clinical problem, provided it is remembered in extreme situations that the solution furnishes approximately 100 ml of free water for each litre administered. The remainder of the solutions shown in Table 4.7 are used to correct specific deficits. Choice of a particular fluid depends on the volume state of the patient and the type of concentration or compositional abnormality present.

Isotonic sodium chloride (0.9% of saline or N saline) which contains 154 mmol of sodium and 154 mmol of chloride per L, may under some circumstances provide excessive chloride ion and metabolic acidosis may develop. This solution is ideal, however, for the initial correction of an extracellular fluid volume deficit in the presence of hyponatraemia, hypochloraemia, and metabolic alkalosis. Water and sugar can be supplied as *5% dextrose in water* or hypotonic sodium solution with sugar which is usually given as so called *'fifth normal saline'* (0.18% saline, 4.2% dextrose).

MAINTENANCE, REPLACEMENT AND REPAIR

All good fluid therapy requires attention to three areas:

- maintenance of daily requirements of fluid and electrolyte
- replacement of ongoing losses
- repair of deficits of volume, concentration or composition.

Maintenance of daily requirements of fluid and electrolyte

In Tables 4.2 and 4.3, the normal daily exchanges of water and sodium are shown. In temperate climates the daily maintenance requirement of an adult patient for water is 2500 ml. Different populations vary in their salt intake, but a good rule of thumb is that normal patients require 1 mmol of sodium per kg of body weight per day. Looking at the available solutions, these daily requirements can be usefully provided in one of two ways:

- 500 ml of N saline (0.9% saline) plus 2 L of 5% dextrose or
- 2500 ml of fifth N saline (0.18% saline + 4.2% dextrose).

To each of these regimens K^+ is added at the rate of 1 mmol/kg of body weight/24 h.

Two notes of caution must be observed when supplying maintenance needs after a surgical operation:

1. Potassium is usually unnecessary and may prove dangerous if given during the first 24 hours following surgery. The obligatory breakdown of cells releases potassium after surgery, flooding the extracellular fluid and providing sufficient quantity during the early postoperative period.

2. The stress of operation stimulates the release of aldosterone and vasopressin with the accompanying retention of sodium and water, which may prove harmful to the patient with compromised renal or cardiac reserve, if restriction of fluid administration is not made. Roberts et al (1985) suggested that adequate intraoperative maintenance of extracellular fluid volume will overcome this postoperative need for fluid restriction, but nevertheless the surgeon should be ready to restrict intravenous fluids for the first 24 hours or so (Lancet 1990b). This is especially important in patients who are nutritionally depleted.

Replacement of ongoing losses

In surgical patients the commonest losses are from the gastrointestinal tract. Vomiting, biliary or pancreatic fistulas, enterocutaneous fistulas or severe diarrhoea all necessitate replacement of fluid over and above maintenance requirements. From Table 4.4 it can be seen that the majority of gastrointestinal secretions can be replaced by an isotonic saline solution. If the losses are from vomiting then replacement is best litre for litre with 0.9% saline to which 15 mmols of potassium chloride have been added. Losses from other sites lower in the gastrointestinal tract can be usefully replaced by Ringer's lactate solution, litre for litre.

If losses from the gastrointestinal tract are greater than a litre each day for several days, these should be pooled and sent to the laboratory for more specific electrolyte analysis of sodium, chloride and potassium so that appropriate adjustments can be made to ensure more precise replacement.

Abnormal losses can also occur in two other situations:

1. *Evaporation*
The patient with a high fever, or a respiratory rate of 35 respirations or more may lose from evaporation from the skin or respiratory tract an additional 500 ml or more of water each day. Thus in writing fluid orders an extra 500 ml of 5% dextrose in water will be necessary for patients of this type.

2. *Sequestration*
A number of surgical conditions lead to sequestration of extracellular fluid such that it is unavailable for normal exchange. When the *intestine is obstructed* the bidirectional movement of sodium and water across the intestinal mucosa is altered such that there is a net secretion of fluid (which resembles extracellular fluid) into the lumen of the intestine. In prolonged obstruction this may amount to a quantity of extracellular fluid equivalent to 5–10% of the body weight. This is best replaced by Ringer's lactate solution.

Sequestration of extracellular fluid also occurs at the site of operative trauma. It thus depends on the degree and magnitude of the surgery. Only several hundred ml of fluid are lost in an inguinal hernia repair and this is of no importance physiologically. On the other hand, extracellular fluid sequestered after a complex operation involving lysis of extensive adhesions, or a total gastrectomy or proctocolectomy may be substantial. It has been shown that when lactated Ringer's solution is given at a rate of about 500 ml per hour during major abdominal surgery of this type, the problem of postoperative renal failure is almost entirely eliminated. Thus, in major abdominal surgery it is recommended that Ringer's lactate solution should be continuously administered at this rate throughout the operative procedure and an additional 500 ml of Ringer's lactate solution should be provided each day to the maintenance needs in the early postoperative period (Thoren & Wiklund 1983). The response to this treatment is judged according to the urine output which should be around 50 ml/h.

In patients with hypoalbuminaemic malnutrition, extracellular fluid is already expanded and such a regimen must be administered with considerable caution. We have already seen that such patients may be intolerant of extra sodium.

Repair of volume deficits

The most common volume change, indeed the most common fluid and electrolyte problem encountered in surgical patients is extracellular fluid deficit. Depletion of the extracellular fluid compartment without changes in concentration or composition is a problem found in many acutely ill surgical patients. For instance, in patients with complete small bowel obstruction, there may be a massive shift of extracellular fluid volume into the lumen of the intestine. The patient with massive ascites, burns or crush injuries, or peritonitis has a translocation of extracellular fluid into a so called 'third space'. This fluid is non-functional because it is no longer able to participate in the normal functions of the extracellular fluid and it may just as well have been lost externally. It is helpful to be able to roughly estimate extracellular fluid deficits to give confidence in replenishment and in this context the signs and symptoms in relation to these deficits as shown in Figure 4.6 are a good starting point.

It must be stressed that plasma volume should be restored rapidly to improve oxygen delivery but interstitial fluid replacement should be repleted at a slower rate. Patients with strangulating bowel obstruction, peritonitis from a perforated diverticulum, or a perforated duodenal ulcer may need more urgent replenishment of interstitial fluid volume. In these circumstances rapid replacement of fluid deficit with good urine flow may be accomplished in 1–3 hours, following which laparotomy is performed.

The rate of repletion in other patients depends to some extent on the rate of the development of the deficit. Also an elderly patient adapts more slowly. Reassessment of the clinical situation is mandatory before giving more fluid. An especially helpful guide to fluid balance is the hourly measurement of urine volume. In the absence of diuretics or glycosuria, an adult patient who excretes 50 ml of urine per hour is in satisfactory equilibrium.

The type of fluid replaced will depend in most cases on how it has been lost and the serum electrolyte profile. If electrolytes are relatively normal in the face of obvious volume depletion, losses can be assumed to have been isosmotic with plasma and should be replaced with Ringer's lactate solution. In contrast, if chloride losses exceed sodium losses, as occurs with vomiting, isotonic saline is generally preferred as replacement fluid. Potassium should not be added to any of these fluids until adequate urine output of 50 ml/h is obtained.

Repair of concentration and compositional deficits

The treatment of hyponatraemia, hypernatraemia and alterations in acid base balance has been discussed above.

ESTABLISHING FLUID BALANCE

So-called fluid balance is potentially one of the most abused techniques in surgical practice. Extensive analytical facilities and a complete metabolic balance study are usually quite unnecessary in ordinary clinical practice. What is necessary, is a concept of the broad principles of water and electrolyte balance and the ability to correlate this with the patient's symptoms and signs. Using established data for the electrolyte content of different gastrointestinal fluids, it is possible to carry the management along on a daily basis with the patient in reasonable water and sodium balance and acid base regulation. A simple record is kept of intake and output by all routes, using approximations where daily analysis would not be justified. An accurate record of the volume and nature of the 24 h oral and i.v. intake is made and the 24 h outputs from nasogastric tubes or other losses from drains or fistulas and volume of urine excreted are measured. In order to put such management into effect, some sort of record or chart of the gains and losses should be kept. The exact form of this chart is immaterial. As part of the clinical balance procedure the patient's weight should be followed closely.

In patients suffering from acute disease or injury any rapid gain in weight may be assumed to be due to the addition of water and salt to the body. Only under the circumstances of treating serious sepsis or major trauma, established dehydration, desalting water loss, or interstitial sequestration oedema does one expect weight gain to occur.

By the same token, excessive or sudden losses of weight indicate loss of salt and water from the body; sudden loss of weight in the region of 500–1000 g or more in a 24 h period means quite serious underadministration of fluid. On the other hand the brisk diuresis and natriuresis that occur during recovery from serious surgical illness result in a rapid weight loss that heralds a return to normal function.

Acknowledgement

We are indebted to Butterworth-Heinemann for permission to reproduce much of the material which was contained in our chapter in *Essential Surgical Practice*, 3rd edition 1992.

PART 2

Nutritional Care

Part 2 Contents

5. Understanding protein energy malnutrition

INTRODUCTION

Protein energy malnutrition (PEM) is common. The World Health Organization has suggested that at least 500 million children in the world suffer from it. It is also found in surgical wards (Bistrian et al 1974). One survey of the entire surgical population of a large teaching hospital found that nearly 1 in 5 patients suffered from PEM (Pettigrew et al 1984). In general surgical patients presenting with major gastrointestinal disease, 1 in every 2 or 3 patients shows evidence of PEM although this may be mild and of no clinical significance (Windsor & Hill 1988d). Where hospital stay has been prolonged due to postoperative complications PEM has been documented in more than 50% of patients (Hill, Blackett et al 1977).

SECTION 1
DEFINITIONS

Protein energy malnutrition is a relatively new term and is used to describe a broad spectrum of clinical conditions ranging from mild to very severe. Severe PEM presents an unmistakable picture. The patient is skin and bones; he or she is a walking skeleton. The severe wasting and loss of subcutaneous tissue makes the shoulder girdle and ribs prominent and the skin, particularly over the buttocks, hangs in wrinkles. The skull and cheek bones are prominent and the eyes are sunken. This is cachexia or severe wasting to the surgeon but because it is so like the condition called nutritional marasmus that is seen in starving children, it is called *adult marasmus* (Fig. 5.1). Severely malnourished children also present with oedema and when this is present the condition is called kwashiorkor. Although *adult kwashiorkor* has been described in hospital patients, it is almost unknown for the full clinical picture (oedema, hepatomegaly, hair and skin changes) to be present. There is, however, a resemblance between childhood kwashiorkor and

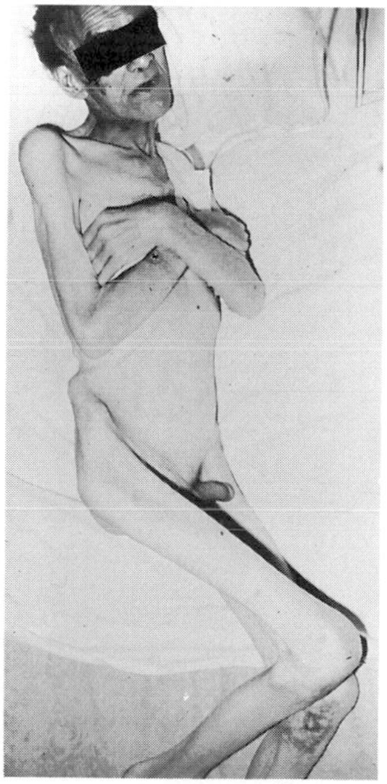

Fig. 5.1 Adult marasmus. The effects of wasting on both fat and muscle are most apparent where these tissues give the figure its rounded appearance.

protein malnutrition of the type that is seen in surgical patients. The resemblance is in three areas: in both there is hypoalbuminaemia, in both there is depressed cellular immunity and in both there is expansion of extracellular water. This expansion of extracellular water presents as oedema in children although clinical oedema is present less often in surgical patients with protein malnutrition. Bistrian (1990) does not use the term kwashiorkor for this adult variant, preferring the name *hypoalbuminaemic malnutrition*. In this book we persist with the term *adult kwashiorkor* rather than use the term *hypoalbuminaemic malnutrition* which we feel does not highlight the important clinical fact that the main compositional disorder in these patients is a marked expansion of extracellular water. Intermediate forms of PEM are common in surgery, i.e. *marasmic kwashiorkor* (wasting with hypoalbuminaemia with or without oedema; Fig. 5.2) which is much more common than kwashiorkor.

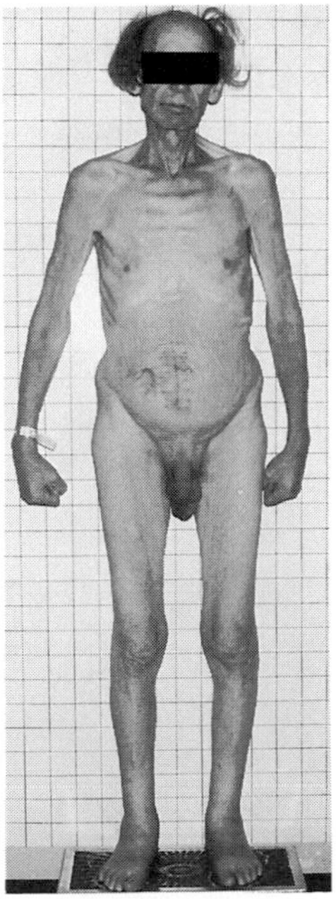

Fig. 5.2 Marasmic kwashiorkor. This patient has lost 25% of his body weight and his plasma albumin is 25 g/L. There is mild ankle oedema. Subcutaneous tissues appear to be relatively preserved.

SECTION II
WHY IS PROTEIN ENERGY MALNUTRITION IMPORTANT TO THE SURGEON?

CLINICALLY SIGNIFICANT PEM

PEM is important surgically when it is severe enough to impact on physiological function sufficiently to increase operative risk and/or prolong postoperative recovery and convalescence. *In this book this intensity of malnutrition is termed moderate–severe PEM. If PEM does not impact on physiological function it is termed mild PEM.*

THE CONCEPT OF CRITICAL PROTEIN LOSS

The physiological impairments found in moderate–severe PEM are associated with a loss of total body protein. There is a close relationship between the body's store of protein and physiological function (Windsor & Hill 1988a). When more than 20% of body protein has been lost most physiological functions are significantly impaired (Fig. 5.3). Such patients have more postoperative complications and a longer hospital stay as a consequence (Windsor & Hill 1988b).

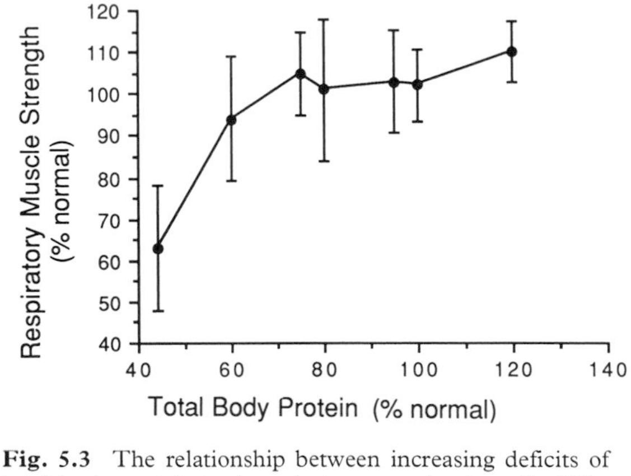

Fig. 5.3 The relationship between increasing deficits of total body protein and respiratory muscle strength. 101 patients presenting for major surgery were ranked according to total body protein and divided into equal groups. It can be seen that when more than 20% of body protein is lost, respiratory muscle strength falls precipitously ($p < 0.05$). Other physiological dysfunctions appear also when total body protein falls below 80% of the predicted normal value (data from Windsor 1989).

THE CONCEPT OF CRITICAL WEIGHT LOSS

It is not possible to demonstrate that weight loss less than 10% affects physiological function to a degree that is clinically important. On the other hand, when more than 20% of body weight has been lost, moderate to severe PEM with accompanying physiological impairments is invariably present. Many, but not all, patients with losses between these two limits have clinically significant PEM. We studied a consecutive group of patients awaiting a major gastrointestinal resection: 43% had less than 10% weight loss and no physiological impairments could be detected on objective measurement, 17% had sustained more than 10% weight loss and also had no demonstrable functional impairments, the remaining 40% who had lost more than 10% of body weight had marked impairments in liver function, skeletal muscle function, respiratory function and some aspects of psychological function. It was this latter group who suffered from more postoperative complications and who had a longer postoperative stay (Windsor & Hill 1988d).

THE RELATIONSHIP BETWEEN WEIGHT LOSS AND PROTEIN LOSS

In a study of hundreds of patients who had both measurements of weight loss and total body protein loss we found that there was a significant correlation between weight loss and protein loss ($r = 0.6$, $p < 0.0001$). Table 5.1 shows this relationship in clinical terms. It can be seen that if 100 patients have lost 10% of their body weight the 95% confidence limits for their total body protein loss is 15.2–20.8%. If 100 patients have lost 20% of their body weight the 95% confidence limits for their total body protein loss is 23–29%. *These data confirm again the high likelihood that patients with more than 15% weight loss are likely to have clinically significant (i.e. 20%) loss of body protein.*

Table 5.1 The relationship between body weight loss and loss of total body protein in 624 patients

Weight loss (%)	Confidence limits (95%) for protein loss (%) in 100 patients
5	11.2–16.8
10	15.2–20.8
15	19.2–24.8
20	23.0–29.0
25	26.8–33.2

SECTION III
SPECTRUM OF PEM IN SURGICAL PATIENTS

PATHOGENESIS

We have already seen in Chapter 1 how prolonged starvation is accompanied by an adaptive response which results in a reduction of loss from body protein stores. However, when major injury or serious sepsis supervenes, this adaptive process is lost and massive losses of body protein may occur. The scheme shown in Figure 5.4 illustrates how two variables, semistarvation and stress (sepsis or injury) determine the degree and type of PEM. A patient with normal fat and

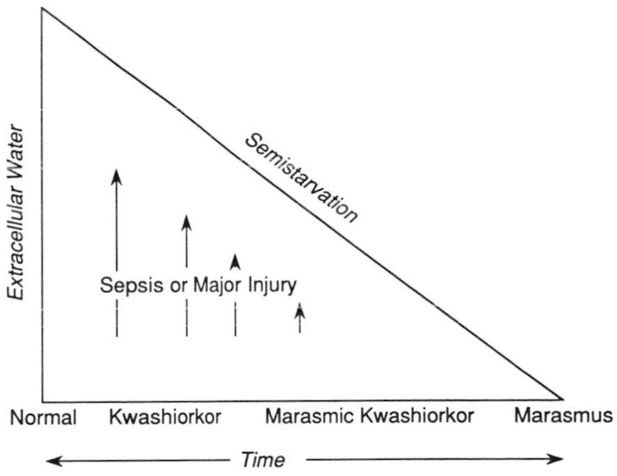

Fig. 5.4 This scheme, developed from the concept of Viteri et al 1964, shows how semistarvation eventually leads to severe PEM (Marasmus). Severe stress, from serious sepsis or major injury leads to rapid consumption of host tissues and an expanded extracellular water (Kwashiorkor). Intermediate stages (Marasmic Kwashiorkor) are common.

protein stores and normal physiological function who undergoes semistarvation will eventually develop severe PEM with impaired physiological function (marasmus). Severe stress (that is from serious sepsis or major trauma) results in expansion of extracellular water, hypoalbuminaemia and rapid consumption of protein stores. A severely stressed patient who is well nourished does not present at first with the physical findings of PEM for the loss of fat and protein is masked by an expanded extracellular water (kwashiorkor). Stress of lesser severity (such as major elective surgery, pneumonia, pancreatitis) may produce extracellular water expansion and hypoalbuminaemia in a patient with moderate–severe marasmus — this is marasmic kwashiorkor. Intermediate states are, of course, common.

THREE BASIC TYPES OF PEM IN SURGICAL PATIENTS

Marasmus

Definition. Marasmus is malnutrition in a patient who has sustained more than 10% weight loss and has clinical signs of reduced stores of fat and protein with accompanying physiological impairments. There is no evidence of recent injury or sepsis. Metabolic expenditure is normal or low.

Other names:

- Moderate to severe PEM without stress
- Moderate to severe protein depletion without raised metabolic expenditure
- Resting semistarvation
- Resting total starvation.

Clinical examples. Oesophageal stricture, carcinoma of proximal stomach, carcinoma of gastric antrum, pharyngeal pouch, short gut syndrome, chronic intestinal obstruction.

Marasmic kwashiorkor

Definition. Marasmic kwashiorkor is malnutrition in a patient who has sustained more than 10% weight loss, has clinical evidence of reduced stores of fat and protein and has accompanying physiological impairments. There has been a major injury or the patient is septic or has been so in the recent past. Metabolic expenditure is usually raised. Plasma levels of albumin are low or are falling.

Other names:

- Moderate to severe PEM with stress
- Moderate–severe protein depletion with raised metabolic expenditure
- Septic starvation.

Clinical examples. Depleted patient with carcinoma of oesophagus or stomach who develops septic complications after oesophagectomy or gastrectomy, late stage of pancreatitis with complications, chronic colitis with a prolonged acute exacerbation, depleted patient with acute attack of Crohn's disease.

Kwashiorkor

Definition. Kwashiorkor can be said to be present in a hypermetabolic patient early after major injury or serious sepsis when there is bodily oedema and hypoalbuminaemia. Clinical evidence of depleted protein and fat stores or abnormal physiological function may not be apparent in the early stage. Metabolic expenditure is raised.

Other names:

- Hypoalbuminaemic malnutrition
- Protein depletion with raised metabolic expenditure
- Early post-traumatic catabolic weight loss
- Early septic starvation
- Protein malnutrition — kwashiorkor-like.

Clinical examples. Acute attacks of severe inflammatory bowel disease in some non-depleted patients, acute severe pancreatitis, major trauma, serious sepsis.

SECTION IV
SPECTRUM OF MICRONUTRIENT DEFICIENCIES IN SURGICAL PATIENTS

Biochemical evidence of deficiencies of important vitamins such as vitamin A, vitamins of the B group, folic acid, vitamin C, vitamin K or of minerals such as iron, magnesium or zinc are frequently present in surgical patients with moderate–severe PEM (Table 5.2). All of these deficiencies are accompaniments of the disease causing PEM or of a grossly inadequate diet (Zak et al 1991). They are not usually the cause of PEM. The specific deficiencies and their clinical manifestations are discussed in Chapter 8. In Table 5.2 are shown measurements of the levels of some common vitamins that were measured during a nutritional survey of the general surgical population of a large teaching hospital. It can be seen that postoperative patients in particular had low levels of white blood cell vitamin C and red blood cell vitamin B_2. Overall, 1 in 5 patients in this study were found to have vitamin deficiencies with 46% of the patients who had suffered a postoperative complication having low levels of vitamin C.

SECTION V
THE DISORDER OF METABOLISM THAT OCCURS IN PEM

MEASURING THE WHOLE BODY CARBOHYDRATE, FAT AND PROTEIN METABOLISM

Using infusions of isotopically labelled glucose, glycerol, free fatty acids, urea, alanine and lysine and taking blood samples 2–3 hours later for isotopic enrichment measurements an integrated analysis of glucose, fat and protein metabolism can be obtained (Wolfe 1984). The total loss of protein from the body, calculated from the urea appearance data, is termed *net protein catabolism.* The algebraic difference between *whole body protein catabolism,* calculated from the lysine

Table 5.2 Indices of nutritional state and vitamin deficiencies measured in the entire general surgical population of a large hospital (reproduced from Hill et al 1977 Lancet 1: 689, with permission)

Category	Statistical data	Weight loss (%)	Arm-muscle circumference (cm)	Plasma albumin (g/dl)	Haemoglobin (g/dl)	Plasma transferrin (mg/dl)	White blood cell vitamin C μg/10^8	Folate (ng/ml)	Vitamin B_2* (saturation ratio)	Vitamin B_6* (saturation ratio)
Controls	Mean	0	25.9	42.3	14.4	281	20.1	252	1.01	1.78
	s.d.	0	±2.4	±2.7	±1.6	±25	±8.1	±125	±0.12	±0.34
	n	21	18	21	21	18	21	21	21	18
All patients	Mean	9.9	23.4	39.7	12.5	223	17.0	199	1.15	1.78
	s.d.	±9.0	±3.8	±5.1	±1.8	±60	±11.6	±135	±0.15	±0.31
	n	91	97	103	104	54	47	46	45	47
	$p^†$		<0.01		<0.001	<0.001			<0.001	
Minor surgery	Mean	5.9	23.9	41.2	13.0	243	17.4	175	1.15	1.78
	s.d.	±6.6	±3.6	±4.0	±1.8	±44	±11.5	±99	±0.16	±0.20
	n	35	36	39	39	19	17	16	16	17
	$p^†$				<0.01				<0.01	
Before major surgery	Mean	11.7	23.3	39.2	13.2	239	22.5	268	1.09	1.65
	s.d.	±10.0	±4.5	±5.0	±1.9	±73	±19.0	±221	±0.12	±0.31
	n	18	20	20	21	11	8	8	8	8
	$p^†$									
<1 week after major surgery	Mean	10.3	24.3	41.6	12.2	222	17.5	231	1.20	1.73
	s.d.	±8.7	±3.5	±5.6	±1.2	±57	±8.1	±133	±0.17	±0.32
	n	16	16	17	17	13	11	11	10	11
	$p^†$				<0.001	<0.005			<0.005	
>1 week after major surgery	Mean	13.9	22.2	36.9	11.5	174	12.5	158	1.17	1.94
	s.d.	±9.3	±3.7	±4.9	±1.5	±54	±6.8	±87	±0.13	±0.42
	n	22	25	27	27	11	11	11	11	11
	$p^†$		<0.005	<0.001	<0.001	<0.001	<0.025		<0.005	

† Calculated by comparison with control group–only values <0.025 given
* Levels in red blood cells

appearance data, and the rate of net protein catabolism is the *whole body protein synthesis*.

DEFECTS IN FAT AND PROTEIN METABOLISM IN PEM

Semistarvation results in a decrease in energy expenditure accounting for increasing tiredness and the need for more rest. When this decrease in active energy expenditure cannot compensate for the inadequate energy intake lipolysis occurs (as reflected by glycerol flux) resulting in a visible loss of subcutaneous tissue. Protein loss occurs at a slower rate and is mainly from net catabolism of muscle protein with increased flux of amino acids that contribute to energy sources. Visceral protein is preserved longer, especially in marasmus. In surgical patients with major trauma or serious sepsis, marked metabolic changes occur with an enhanced reliance on fat as an energy substrate; lipolysis is increased two or three times as reflected by increased glycerol flux (Shaw & Wolfe 1987b). There is increased glucose production from amino acids, glycerol and lactate. The rate of glucose recycling is increased threefold (Shaw & Wolfe 1989). Most of the loss of total body protein is due to a marked increase in whole body protein catabolism which in part is offset by an increased rate of whole body protein synthesis (Birkhahn 1980).

SECTION VI
THE DISORDER OF BODY COMPOSITION THAT OCCURS IN PEM

MEASURING THE COMPARTMENTS OF THE BODY

In recent years there has been renewed interest in measuring the compartments of the body. It is now possible to break down the total body, even in critically ill patients, in terms of fat, protein (and its compartments), water (and its compartments), glycogen and minerals (Beddoe et al 1984, Knight et al 1986). Figure 5.5 shows our in vivo neutron activation analysis (IVNAA) facility which measures body composition within

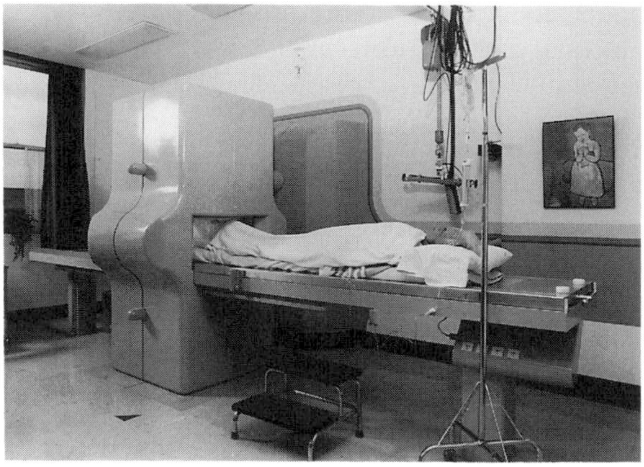

Fig. 5.5 A prompt 'gamma' neutron activation facility designed for clinical use. The patient enters the scanner 'feet first' with all lines (TPN, catheters, drains, ECG leads etc.) following, with monitors placed at the head of the counter. The scan takes a total of 35 minutes.

a clinical setting. The patient is passed between stationary neutron beams, irradiating him in his entirety. The patient is first injected with tritiated water which is diluted within the body to give a measure of total body water. In a similar way extracellular water is measured by bromide dilution. He is then weighed on a hoist weighing system consisting of an electrically operated block-and-tackle system attached via a load cell to a frame which supports a canvas sheet on which the patient lies; the system transfers the patient from his bed to the scanning couch, weighing him during transfer. The patient enters the scanners 'feet first' with all lines (TPN, catheter, drains, ECG lead etc.) following, with monitors placed at the head of the couch and with the respiratory trolley following alongside.

The gamma-radiation emitted by radionuclides induced by the neutrons is specific for various elements in the body, the complex spectrum from the patient is measured and analysed to give counting rates due to nitrogen ($g\ N \times 6.25 = g$ protein), hydrogen and chlorine. Calculations can then be made to give the total content in the body of fat, protein, minerals and water. A recent innovation has been to combine the neutron scan with dual energy X-ray absorptiometry (DEXA), which gives more precise measurements of fat and minerals and eliminates the need to use tritiated water. This system and other similar ones have now reached a high level of sophistication and comparisons with chemical carcass analysis have shown a considerable degree of accuracy (Knight et al 1986). The scientific background of the combined scanning facility is to be found in Appendix I at the end of the book.

Using these techniques the detailed body composition of patients with PEM has been characterized.

THE BODY IN TERMS OF FAT, WATER, PROTEIN, GLYCOGEN AND MINERALS

Total body fat and the fat free body

Total body fat is defined as all the non-aqueous neutral fat of the body. Fat stores in man are in the form of triglyceride and are stored mainly in specialized cells, the adipocytes. The fat free body is obtained by adding together the measured total body protein, minerals, glycogen and water and when this is subtracted from the measured body weight total body fat is obtained. Almost all surgical illness results in the oxidation (consumption) of body fat.

Body water and the fat free body

With measurements of total body water and extracellular water the hydration of the fat free body in terms of total and extracellular water can be obtained. These are some of the most remarkably constant values found in biology. The hydration of the fat free body throughout the animal kingdom in health is around 73% and similarly the extracellular water content of the fat free body in health is very close to 35%. Another remarkable feature about these relationships is that nearly all sickness is associated with an increased hydration of the fat free body — in kwashiorkor it may go as high as 80% and this is mainly due to the extracellular water content of the fat free body rising as high as 43–46% (Moore & Boyden 1963, Beddoe et al 1985, Streat et al 1985a).

Total body protein

More than half (~55%) of the total body content of protein is inside cells. The rest is in the supporting structures of the body (tendon, fascia, connective tissue, dermis) and here it is probably not involved in rapid metabolic interchanges. Cellular protein is the most important component of body composition. Here all the energy interchange of the body occurs. Oxygen is consumed, carbon dioxide is produced and the work of the body is generated. This is the engine room of the body and if eroded there is always a loss of some physiological function.

Total body glycogen

Glycogen is stored in muscle and liver cells as a gel of glycogen and water. The long branching-chain molecules of glucose that make up glycogen are stored inside cells with water and electrolyte between the chains. As the cell accumulates glycogen 2–4 g of potassium-rich (150 mmol K^+ per litre) water are stored per gram of glycogen.

Total body minerals

This is the total mineral content of the body which comprises mainly bone calcium and phosphorus although there is a small amount of potassium, sodium, chlorine and traces of other elements.

COMPOSITIONAL DEFECTS

The whole body

In Table 5.3 the changes in body composition that have occurred in association with each of the three basic types of PEM are presented. The patient with marasmus has marked deficits of total body fat (28%) and protein (36%) with a very modest relative increase in extracellular water (6%). Plasma albumin is in the normal range although the levels of the short half life plasma proteins, transferrin, and prealbumin have fallen by 25%. Metabolic expenditure is not raised. The severe protein depletion observed is associated with physiological dysfunction (~30%).

The patient with marasmic kwashiorkor has similar deficits of total body fat (31%) and protein (35%) but there is a marked relative increase in extracellular water (23%). Plasma

Table 5.3 Nutritional assessment profile of 3 patients with moderate-severe PEM; one with marasmus, one with marasmic kwashiorkor and one with kwashiorkor. Stress index = measured resting metabolic expenditure:predicted metabolic expenditure

	Marasmus			**Marasmic Kwashiorkor**			**Kwashiorkor**		
	Est. value when well	Measured value	% change	Est. value when well	Measured value	% change	Est. value when well	Measured value	% change
Body composition									
Body weight (kg)	63.0	52.0	−18	70.1	56.6	−19	82.3	90.1	+9
Total body fat (kg)	14.8	10.7	−28	16.0	11.1	−31	19.0	16.5	−13
Total body protein (kg)	9.8	6.3	−36	10.0	6.5	−35	13.8	12.8	−7
Total body water (L)	34.5	30.6	−11	40.1	34.4	−14	45.6	55.9	+23
Extracellular water (L)	17.0	15.3	−10	19.0	19.6	+3	21.9	31.9	+46
TBW:FFM	0.72	0.74	+3	0.74	0.76	+3	0.72	0.76	+6
ECW:FFM	0.35	0.37	+6	0.35	0.43	+23	0.35	0.43	+23
Plasma proteins									
Albumin (g/L)	38	36	−5	39	29	−26	39	31	−21
Transferrin (mg/dl)	230	176	−23	240	110	−54	240	160	−33
Prealbumin (mg/dl)	22	16	−29	26	8	−61	27	12	−56
Physiological function									
Grip strength (kg)	36	28	−22	40	26	−35	—	—	—
Resp muscle strength (cm H_2O)	93	69	−26	104	65	−38	—	—	—
Forced expiratory volume$_{1\ sec}$ (L)	3.6	3.2	−11	4.0	3.0	−25	—	—	—
Vital capacity (L)	4.3	3.6	−17	4.8	3.6	−25	—	—	—
Peak expiratory flow rate (L/min)	513	385	−25	576	428	−26	—	—	—
Metabolic expenditure									
Resting metabolic expenditure (kcal/day)	1209	1140	−6	1289	1277	−1	1414	1800	+27
Activity energy expenditure (kcal/day)	1059	524	−34	1515	500	−67	1898	125	−93
Total energy expenditure (kcal/day)	2268	1164	−21	2804	1777	−37	3312	1925	−42
Stress index	1.0	1.02	+2	1.0	1.09	+9	1.0	1.3	+30

albumin is low as are the plasma levels of transferrin and prealbumin. Physiological dysfunction is marked (~30%).

The patient with kwashiorkor is hypermetabolic (RME raised 30%) but deficits of fat and protein are not yet marked (13 % and 7% respectively). Total body water, extracellular water and the proportion of extracellular water in the fat free body are all raised, The patient is hypoalbuminaemic. Unfortunately physiological measurements were not performed on this very sick patient.

It is important to understand that these fundamental compositional changes also occur in the vascular compartment. Associated with the expanded extracellular water volume is an expanded plasma volume. Red cell mass is smaller, sharing its shrinkage with the shrinkage of body protein generally.

Hypoalbuminaemia and expanded extracellular water

The physiological role and the distribution of plasma and interstitial fluid albumin is not fully understood (Doweiko & Nompleggi 1991). From a clinical point of view, however, hypoalbuminaemia is usually associated with an expanded extracellular water. In Figure 5.6, 34 patients, all with moderate–severe PEM (i.e. weight loss greater than 20%) have been arrayed according

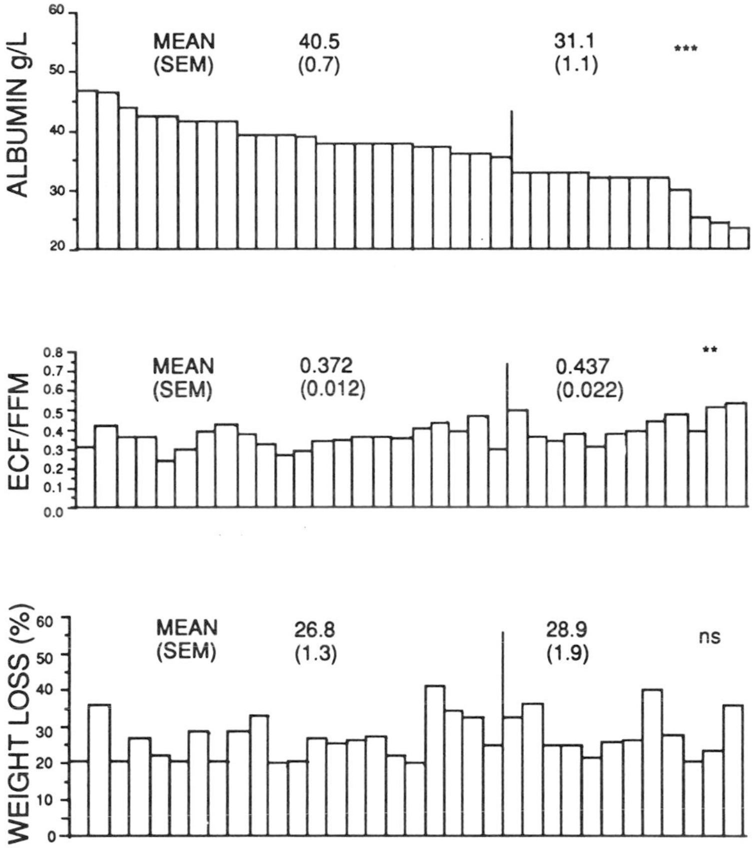

Fig. 5.6 Malnourished surgical patients (all with more than 20% weight loss) ranked by plasma albumin. The corresponding values for extracellular fluid/fat free mass and percentage weight loss are shown. Mean values for each subgroup significantly lower than for patients with albumin greater than 35 g/L are indented — $^{**}p < 0.01$, $^{***}p < 0.001$.

to their level of plasma albumin. It can be seen that those with the lowest levels of plasma albumin had the largest increases in extracellular water — this was independent of the degree of weight loss. Children with kwashiorkor have greatly expanded water volumes and present with clinical oedema; *surgical patients with moderate–severe PEM with hypoalbuminaemia seldom have clinical oedema but the fundamental defect of an overhydrated fat free body is there nevertheless.* In patients with protein malnutrition of the kwashiorkor type overhydration with clinically obvious tissue oedema is more common. In 8 such patients with serious sepsis and multiorgan failure we found an average overexpansion of 9.7 L of total body water (Streat et al 1987).

The organs

The degree of wasting of various organs of the body that accompanies body weight loss has been calculated by comparing weights of different organs in patients with severe PEM subjected to necropsy with normal standards. Unfortunately many of the standards are unsatisfactory and proper longitudinal studies are lacking. Nevertheless available data are instructive. Results of the autopsy studies of Krieger (1921) are given in Table 5.4 and show that most organs have a percentage mass loss roughly similar to that of the total body, the exception being the brain. Generally speaking, skin, muscle and particularly liver waste more than the heart, although it must

Table 5.4 Percentage losses of weight of the body and various organs in autopsies of malnourished subjects (data from Krieger 1921)

	Marasmus (% loss)	Septic starvation (% loss)
Body weight	39	44
Heart	35	31
Liver	42	28
Kidney	36	16
Spleen	47	—
Brain	5	3
Pancreas	—	31

be said that there is great variability among individuals.

The tissues

Water content has been measured in biopsy samples of muscle, skin and liver in both children and adults with PEM. Total water and extracellular water were higher than normal in all forms of PEM with the highest values in the oedematous (Frenk et al 1957, King et al 1978). Intracellular potassium is usually low and membrane pump activity is impaired with accumulation of sodium in the cell. There are also defects in muscle fibre types, with associated reductions in key enzymes of glucose oxidation and intracellular substrates. Table 5.5 shows the muscle fibre size and distribution in the vastus lateralis muscle of 14 patients with moderate to severe PEM (average weight loss 26%, plasma albumin 33 g/L). It can be seen that both type I (high oxidative and low glycolytic capacity) and type II fibres (low oxidative and high glycolytic capacity) were smaller in patients than in controls and there was a smaller proportional number of type II fibres in patients.

This loss of type II fibre numbers and preferential type II atrophy results in a depression in key enzymes of glucose oxidation. Fructose bisphosphatase, phosphofructokinase and hexokinase activities were reduced by 40% in malnourished patients. This loss of type II fibres may be responsible for the syndrome of impaired glucose tolerance, muscle weakness and fatigue that is seen in malnourished patients (Church et al 1984).

SECTION VII
THE DISORDER OF PHYSIOLOGICAL FUNCTION

HYPOTONICITY AND SODIUM INTOLERANCE

Sodium, chloride and water excretion in malnourished patients is dependent on dietary intake. During a complete fast, sodium, chloride and water excretion is excessive. When 150 g of glucose are given the excretion of sodium and water is much less — probably through a tubular effect of insulin. This may lead to hyponatraemia in some surgical patients (Katz et al 1968). The erosion of the body's cellular protein stores and the oxidation of fat and protein also produce free water which when added to the extracellular water results in further bodily hypotonicity and a tendency to overhydration with oedema. This problem of hypotonicity and overexpanded extracellular water means that the patient with PEM is intolerant of salt and water loads and may be quite easily oversalted and overwatered. The surgeon, while operating on an overwatered and oversalted patient, may find the gastrointestinal wall oedematous to a degree that can make suturing a hazard or it may be found that the injudicious use of saline postoperatively may cause the patient with PEM to develop pulmonary oedema more readily than usual.

SKELETAL MUSCLE DYSFUNCTION

In nutrition and metabolic studies measurements of muscle function have assumed new importance and have added much to our understanding of the effects of protein depletion in malnourished patients. The important tests that have been developed for clinical use are:

Maximum voluntary grip strength

Maximum voluntary grip strength can be measured with small error by isokinetic dynamometry or a simple bulb vigorimeter. The results obtained are closely related to the proportion of protein loss in surgical patients (Windsor & Hill

Table 5.5 Muscle fibre size and distribution in the vastus lateralis muscle of depleted patients and normal controls — values are mean ± s.e.m. (from Church J M, Choong S Y, Hill G L, 1984 Br J Surg 71: 563, by permission of the publishers)

	Cross-sectional area ($\mu m^2 \times 10^{-2}$)		**Proportional number (percentage total fibres counted)**		**Proportional area (percentage total area)**		**Number of fibres per mm² of muscle**	
	I	II	I	II	I	II	I	II
Controls (n = 13)	73.3 ± 0.6	72.5 ± 0.5	35.4 ± 2.7	64.6 ± 3.1	38	62	37 ± 5	67 ± 7
Patients (n = 13)	41.4 ± 0.4	27.7 ± 0.4	52.2 ± 2.7	47.8 ± 3.1	65	35	92 ± 9	81 ± 10
p	<0.001	<0.001	<0.001	<0.001	—	—	<0.001	N.S.

1988a) and have been shown to be important indicators of postoperative risk (Klidjian et al 1982).

Electrical stimulation of the ulnar nerve

A controlled and objective method of stimulating muscle that does not depend on voluntary effort has been developed for use in clinical nutrition by Jeejeebhoy (1988). The ulnar nerve is electrically stimulated at the wrist and the contraction–relaxation characteristics of the adductor pollicis muscle are measured. The measurements obtained from the adductor pollicis give the same results as measurements obtained from muscles as diverse as quadriceps, sternomastoid, and the diaphragm — i.e. the function of adductor pollicis is considered to be representative of muscle function in general. In patients with PEM a slower maximal relaxation rate and increased muscle fatiguability has been demonstrated (Lopes et al 1982). These physiological findings have been related to the fibre abnormalities mentioned above and also to alterations in intracellular enzymes (Church et al 1984), intracellular substrate (Jeejeebhoy 1986) and energy (Kobayashi et al 1991), and cellular chemistry (Russel et al 1984).

DISORDERS OF RESPIRATORY FUNCTION

Respiratory muscle function

Respiratory muscle strength (RMS) can be assessed by measuring mouth pressure with a bi-differential pressure transducer during maximal static expiration at functional residual lung capacity and during maximal static expiration at total lung capacity. The value of RMS is the average value of maximal inspiratory pressure and maximal expiratory pressure expressed in centimetres of water. Forced expiratory volume in one second (FEV_1), vital capacity (VC), and peak expiratory flow rate (PEFR) are measured by standard spirometric techniques. Table 5.6 shows that all these aspects of respiratory function are adversely affected in surgical patients with PEM.

Table 5.6 Respiratory function data (mean ± s.e.m.) for protein depleted (>20% below predicted total body protein) and non protein depleted surgical patients, (data from Windsor J A and Hill G L 1988 Ann Surg 207: 290, by permission of the publishers, J B Lippincott & Co)

	Non protein depleted patients (n = 41)	Protein depleted patients (n = 39)	*p*
Measured total body protein (kg)	9.67 ± 0.49	6.28 ± 0.31	<0.005
Predicted total body protein (kg)	9.82 ± 0.37	9.73 ± 0.33	NS
Respiratory muscle strength index (% predicted)	95.3 ± 6.9	78.9 ± 6.7	<0.025
FEV_1 (% predicted)	98.5 ± 3.8	89.2 ± 4.8	NS
VC (% predicted)	91.2 ± 2.5	83.8 ± 3.5	<0.05
PEFR (% predicted)	89.3 ± 2.7	77.2 ± 3.6	<0.005

Ventilation

Ventilation is not just a matter of respiratory muscle strength. It is the result of an integrated system involving ventilatory drive (brain) and mechanical work (through muscles) and gas exchange (the lung). Patients with severe PEM have been shown to have a reduced capacity to sustain adequate levels of ventilation from effects on both the central nervous system and respiratory muscles. As well as the demonstrated inspiratory and expiratory muscular weakness neural ventilatory drive is also impaired (Arora & Rochester 1982).

IMPAIRED WOUND HEALING

Subcutaneously implanted Goretex tubing can be used to monitor and detect variations in wound healing potential in patients (Haydock & Hill 1986). To monitor wound healing response 5 cm lengths of 1 mm diameter Goretex tubing are implanted in the subcutaneous tissues over the deltoid muscle. A 13 gauge spinal needle is pushed through a fold of subcutaneous tissue and this acts as the wound. Implanted in the needle track is the Goretex tubing which lies in the subcutaneous tissue for 7 days. At the end of that time the tube is removed and its hydroxyproline content, a measure of collagen deposition, is measured. Segments of the tubes can also be prepared for histological examination to determine the extent of the cellular response and degree of collagen fibroplasia (Haydock et al 1988).

Although there is ample evidence that protein deficiency is associated with impaired wound healing in animals, it has been much more difficult to obtain objective data which suggests the same holds true for adult surgical patients. The wound healing response in malnourished surgical patients as assessed by this microimplant technique demonstrates that the response appears to be impaired in malnourished patients although the effect is seen at a much earlier stage than had previously been supposed (Haydock & Hill 1986). It is probably more related to deficiencies in dietary intake than to absolute amounts of body protein that have been lost (Table 5.7).

Table 5.7 The wound healing response in 83 patients undergoing major gastrointestinal surgery. The patients were divided into 2 groups: those who had been eating normally up to the time of surgery (n = 59) and those who had a reduction of at least half their normal food intake over the week before surgery, (n = 24). There was no difference between these two groups in terms of nutritional status but the group with impaired food intake had a reduced wound healing response. (Adapted from Windsor J A, Knight G S, Hill G L 1988 Br J Surg 75: 135, by permission of the publishers.)

	Patients with adequate food intake* n = 59	Patients with inadequate food intake* n = 24	*p*
Wound healing response			
Hydroxyproline (nmol/mg Goretex)	1.81 ± 0.16	1.04 ± 0.22	<0.005
Nutritional status			
Weight loss (%)	9.01 ± 1.14	11.05 ± 1.67	NS
Protein index†	0.82 ± 0.03	0.74 ± 0.03	NS
Fat index ‡	1.05 ± 0.08	0.98 ± 0.10	NS
Plasma Proteins			
Albumin (g/L)	39.5 ± 0.63	38.2 ± 1.07	NS
Transferrin (mg/dl)	246.2 ± 8.5	214.7 ± 14.5	<0.05
Prealbumin (mg/dl)	19.6 ± 1.1	17.5 ± 1.6	NS

* Values are mean ± s.e.m.
† Protein index — measured total body protein divided by predicted total body protein
‡ Fat index — measured total body fat divided by predicted total body fat

IMMUNE DYSFUNCTION

Delayed hypersensitivity responses, such as allergic reactions of the skin, involve T-D cells. Skin reactions are relatively easy to test; therefore, delayed hypersensitivity is a convenient clinical measurement of the functional capacity of cell mediated immunity. Another common measurement of the functioning capacity of cellular immunity is the stimulation of T cells to blast transform and function as activated T cells. Concanavalin A and phytohemagglutinin are plant mitogens that cause the blastogenesis of T cells.

The consensus of many studies shows that PEM is commonly associated with an acquired immune deficiency (Law et al 1973). Of the two recognised, extreme variants of PEM, kwashiorkor as characterised by a depression of serum albumin levels has relatively severe immune deficiencies (Bistrian et al 1975). Where both protein and energy deficits occur as in marasmus, the serum albumin levels are better maintained, and immune function appears to be less severely affected (Bistrian et al 1975).

PSYCHOLOGICAL DYSFUNCTION

Psychological fatigue can be measured using a questionnaire called the profile of mood score which was derived at the Education and Industrial Testing Service in San Diego. Moderate to severe PEM has been shown to be associated with impairment of psychological function in surgical patients (Windsor & Hill 1988d).

6. Metabolic, physiological and pharmacological effects of nutritional therapy

INTRODUCTION

There is wide variation of opinion about the efficacy of nutritional support in clinical surgery. While there is no doubting that in some clinical settings nutritional support can be life saving, and in others hospital stay is reduced and convalescence is shortened by its use, it has been overused in the past. In this chapter we will look at objective evidence for the efficacy of current methods of nutritional therapy.

SECTION I
THE EARLY FUNCTIONAL RESPONSE TO NUTRITIONAL REPLETION

In Chapter 5 we saw the widespread defects in cellular chemistry and physiologic function that occur in patients with protein energy malnutrition; it is these defects that lead to the organ dysfunction observed. After 3 or 4 days of nutritional repletion (it occurs both with enteral and parenteral feeding), long before there is any demonstrable gain in tissue protein, there is an improvement (10–20%) in many physiological functions (Christie & Hill 1990, Stokes & Hill 1992).

Table 6.1 shows the early effects of total parenteral nutrition (TPN) on respiratory and skeletal muscle function that occurred in 7 patients who had moderate to severe PEM second ary to attacks of inflammatory bowel disease. It can be seen that the maximal functional improvement occurred by the fourth day of feeding and there were no statistically significant improvements from then on up to the last measurement on day 14. These favorable effects of TPN on physiological function occurred long before there was any detectable change or improvement in body protein stores.

Figure 6.1 shows sequential measurements of skeletal muscle function and respiratory function in 19 patients with marasmic kwashiorkor secondary to acute attacks of inflammatory bowel disease. Each received 2 weeks of TPN. Compared to a group of matched controls they had lost approximately 35% of their body protein stores with accompanying physiological impair-

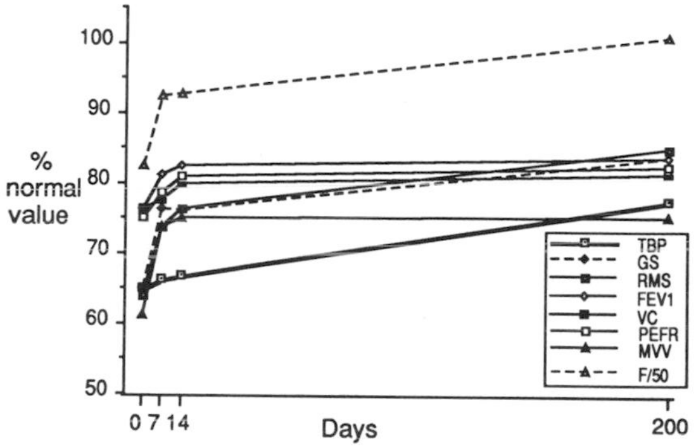

Fig. 6.1 The average changes in physiological function and total body protein that occurred in 19 patients who received TPN for a 2-week period whilst in hospital and who were then measured again when they had fully recovered 200 days later. Key: TBP = total body protein; GS = maximal voluntary grip strength; RMS = respiratory muscle strength; FEV_1 = forced expiratory volume in 1 second; VC = vital capacity; PEFR = peak expiratory flow rate; MVV = maximal voluntary ventilation; F50 = force at 50 Hz or maximal involuntary force. (Redrawn from Christie P M & Hill G L 1990 Gastroenterology 99:730, by permission of the publishers, W B Saunders & Co.)

Table 6.1 Effect of TPN on respiratory and skeletal muscle function — timing of early improvement in 7 surgical patients with protein energy malnutrition (mean ± s.e.m.). Key: RMS = respiratory muscle strength: FEV_1 = forced expiratory volume; PEFR = peak expiratory flow rate; GS = maximal voluntary grip strength: F10/20 = force at 10 HZ : force at 20 HZ; F10/50 = force at 10 HZ : force at 50 HZ; F5O = force at 50 HZ or maximal involuntary force (Reproduced from Christie P M & Hill G L 1990 Gastroenterology 99: 730, by permission of the publishers, W B Saunders & Co.)

	Day 0		Day 2		Day 4		Day 7		Day 14
RMS (cm H_2O)	50 ± 7		50 ± 8		61 ± 8		60 ± 8		62 ± 9
		NS		xxx		NS		NS	
FEV_1 (L)	3.3 ± 0.3		3.3 ± 0.3		3.4 ± 0.2		3.4 ± 0.3		3.5 ± 0.3
		NS		NS		NS		NS	
PEFR (L/min)	419 ± 42		411 ± 39		447 ± 32		444 ± 31		442 ± 30
		NS		x		NS		NS	
GS (kg)	26 ± 4		26 ± 4		31 ± 5		32 ± 5		33 ± 4
		NS		xxx		NS		NS	
F10/20 (%)	57 ± 3		52 ± 4		44 ± 3		44 ± 3		46 ± 3
		NS		xxx		NS		NS	
F10/50 (%)	40 ± 4		36 ± 4		34 ± 2		34 ± 3		31 ± 3
		NS		NS		NS		NS	
F50 (kg)	5.6 ± 0.8		5.6 ± 0.8		5.3 ± 0.4		6.0 ± 0.5		6.0 ± 0.5
		NS		NS		NS		NS	

paired t test x = $p<0.05$, xxx $p < 0.005$

ments of 20–40%. After a few days of TPN there were improvements in all the physiological measurements (approximately 12%) but no significant changes in total body protein. These patients were measured again as outpatients after recovery, approximately 200 days later. It can be seen from the figure that during convalescence there were further improvements in physiological function which were accompanied by an increase in body stores of protein.

Thus there is an early and rapid improvement in physiological function that occurs in malnourished patients being treated with TPN even though this is not accompanied by demonstrable protein gain. From Figure 6.2 it can be seen that a similar improvement occurs in patients receiving enteral nutrition.

After these early improvements in physiological function further improvements and restoration to normality depend on accretion of total body protein. This early improvement of approximately 12% is probably sufficient to be of clinical benefit. The cellular mechanisms responsible for this early improvement have not been fully worked out. It has been shown, however, that the considerable decreases in muscle ATP and ADP that occur in malnourished surgical patients are returned to normal with nutritional repletion (Kinney & Furst 1988).

SECTION II

THE METABOLIC RESPONSE TO NUTRITIONAL REPLETION

METABOLIC EXPENDITURE

There is a rise in resting energy expenditure of 10–20% in patients receiving nutritional support. This is due to diet-induced thermogenesis and is more prominent when glucose is the dominant energy source (Fig. 6.3).

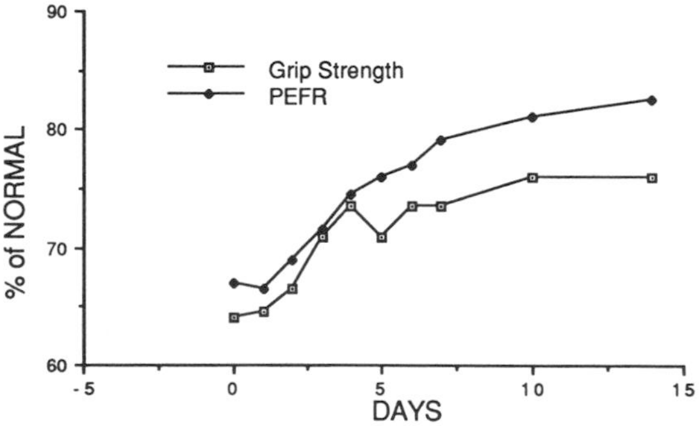

Fig. 6.2 Average changes in grip strength and peak expiratory flow rate (PEFR) that occurred in 11 malnourished surgical patients receiving a 2-week course of enteral nutrition. (Redrawn from Strokes 1991.)

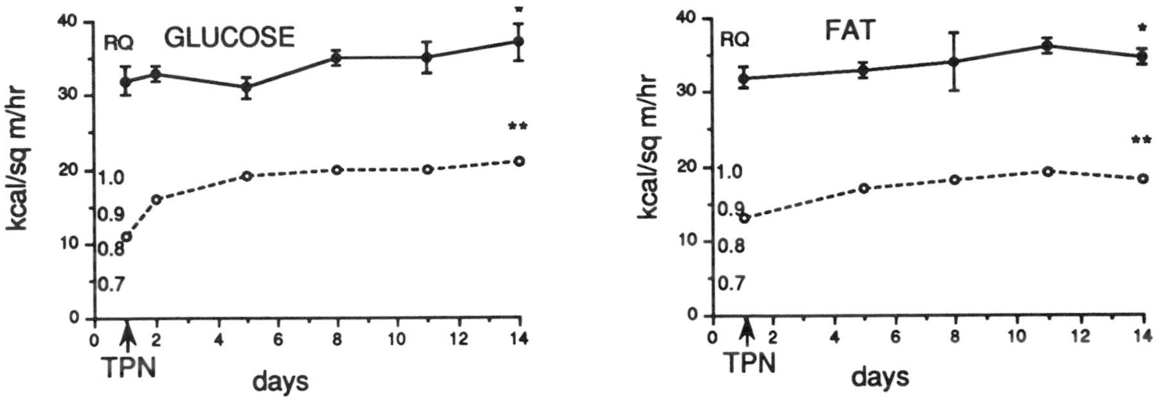

Fig. 6.3 Serial measurements of resting energy expenditure (—●—) and respiratory quotient (RQ) (---○---) with TPN using either glucose alone or glucose in combination with fat as the energy source (*significantly different from value on day 1). (Redrawn from MacFie J, Holmfield J, King R, Hill G L 1983 J Parenter Enter Nutr 7: 1, by permission of the publishers.)

It can be seen that the use of glucose as the only energy source during TPN is associated with a greater rise in energy expenditure than is observed when a glucose fat regimen is used. In this study, where hypercalorific energy intakes were given, glucose was also associated with persistent elevation of the RQ above 1, indicating lipogenesis.

PROTEIN METABOLISM

There is an improvement in whole body protein synthesis with nutritional support

The net change in total body protein during nutritional support depends on the algebraic difference between two opposing processes: an obligatory whole body breakdown of protein and a simultaneous whole body synthesis of protein. In normal circumstances, whole body breakdown of protein is exactly balanced by an equal amount of protein being synthesised and the total amount of body protein remains unchanged. Patients undergoing semistarvation have rates of whole body protein breakdown and synthesis which are reduced and net protein catabolism occurs but it is small. Provision of food to such patients results in an increased whole body synthesis of protein with an overall net gain in total body protein. Even in patients with serious sepsis, very major trauma or metastatic cancer where whole body rates of protein breakdown are high and uninfluenced by any nutritional therapy the provision of nutrients results in increased synthesis usually of sufficient degree to halve the total amount of body protein that is broken down. *Thus, although in many surgical diseases protein losses are large and nutritional therapy is unable to achieve net protein anabolism, losses are reduced in many situations to less than half of those that would occur without the added nutritional support* (Fig. 6.4).

Response is determined by protein status and metabolic expenditure

Net changes in total body protein that occur with TPN are determined by the relative effects of two competing processes: protein depletion and raised metabolic expenditure. In a recent study of a large number of surgical patients receiving a 2-week course of TPN those patients with moderate–severe protein depletion (approximately 30% depletion in body protein stores) had a marked tendency to gain protein with TPN. When similar patients had a raised metabolic expenditure this tendency to gain protein was still present but it was less (Fig. 6.5). Patients with mild protein depletion (approximately 10% depletion) who had increases in metabolic expenditure had continuing losses of protein in spite of

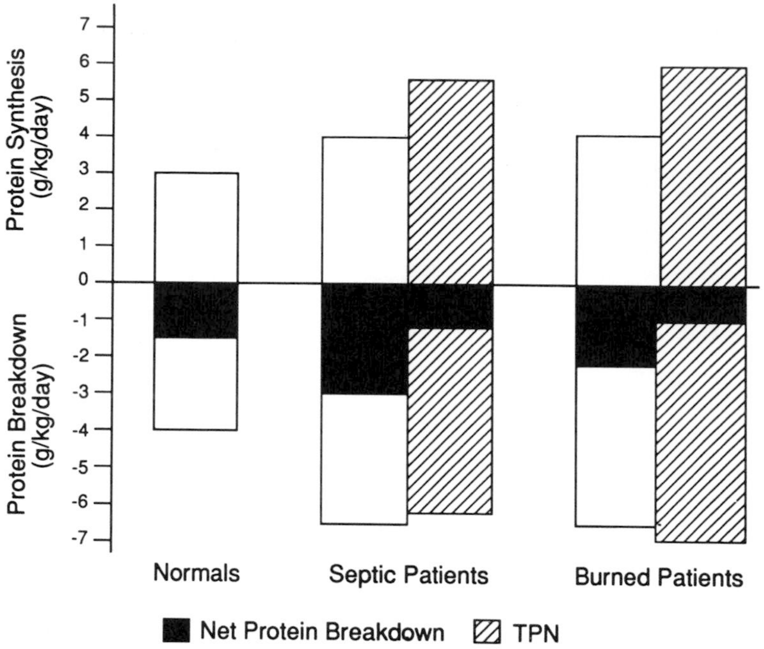

Fig. 6.4 Rates of total body protein synthesis, total body protein breakdown and net protein breakdown in normal volunteers, septic patients and burned patients. In septic and burned patients the rate of net protein breakdown is significantly greater, ($p < 0.05$) than in normals. Providing TPN reduces net protein breakdown by significantly increasing total body protein synthesis, the rate of total body protein breakdown remains unchanged. (Redrawn from Douglas R G, Shaw J H F 1989 Br J Surg 76: 115, by permission of the publishers.)

aggressive nutritional support. It has long been recognised that the efficiency of protein retention at a given level of protein and energy is increased in protein depleted subjects. The mechanism for this is not completely understood. The labile protein pool possibly remains depleted as long as the body's protein stores are depleted, providing a potential mechanism for this increased protein avidity (Hoffer 1988).

Other factors influencing response

The ability of patients to retain administered protein depends on other factors including the biological value of the protein being administered, and also the elemental balance achieved during feeding. Negative mineral balances during refeeding result in an inability to gain total body protein (Rudman et al 1975). In gastrointestinal surgery this situation is classically seen in patients convalescing after the establishment of an ileostomy. With a high volume output salt depleting ileostomy the patient continues to lose weight, and is unable to increase muscle mass while sodium and water balance are negative. Correction of the body sodium deficit results not only in normal hydration being restored but also in a rapid accretion in total body protein appropriate to the patient's dietary intake. Rudman et al (1975) using elegant elemental balance studies showed that not only a sodium deficit caused an inability to accrete protein but negative balances of potassium and phosphorus had the same effect.

CARBOHYDRATE METABOLISM

In a normal subject who is starving the administration of total parenteral nutrition completely eliminates endogenous glucose production. In marasmic patients the same suppression of

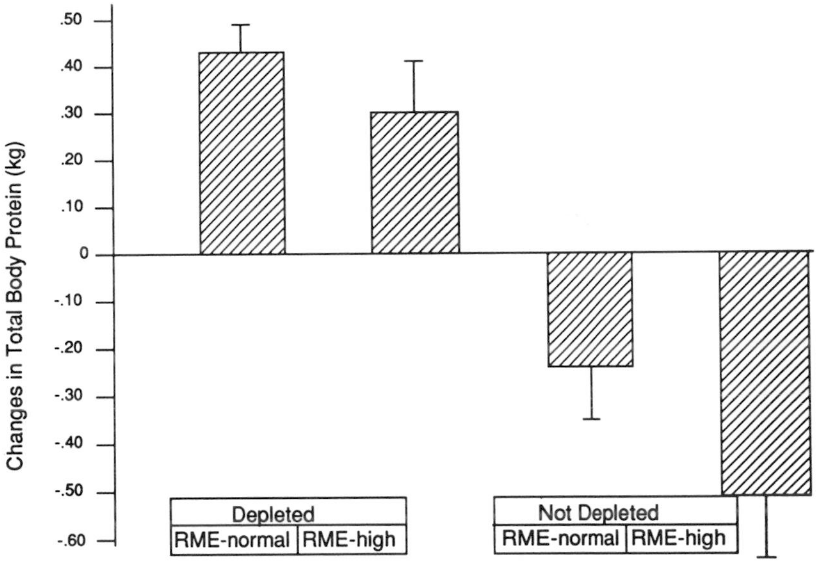

Changes in Total Body Protein with 2 weeks TPN
Fig. 6.5 Surgical patients who are depleted of body stores of protein have a marked tendency to gain protein with TPN. When metabolic expenditure is raised in similar patients this tendency to gain protein is still present but it is less (data from Hill et al 1991).

endogenous glucose production occurs, but patients with major injury or serious sepsis have suppression of glucose production to a limited extent only (Shaw & Wolfe 1986). When glucose is infused as the only calorie source as part of a TPN regimen muscle glycogen accumulates slowly and increasingly with time (King et al 1981). The total amount of glycogen laid down generally speaking is small and in one study the total amount of glycogen that accumulated in the body was calculated to be little over 100 g. In seriously septic and critically ill patients fed with hypercalorific glucose regimens, however, there is some evidence to suggest that hepatic glucose accumulation is much greater than this (Nordenstrom et al 1981). Hypercalorific glucose intakes induce different effects in patients with marasmus and those with kwashiorkor. In marasmic patients a large glucose load has no significant effect on oxygen consumption but induces a marked elevation in CO_2 production. The RQ value increases above 1, indicating that sufficient energy is being provided and that the excess glucose energy is being converted into fat. In hypermetabolic patients a large glucose load includes a significant increase in oxygen consumption accompanied by a marked increase in CO_2 production. The RQ, however, remains below 1 indicating persistent net oxidation of fatty acids. This suggests that there is a significant proportion of non-oxidised glucose which cannot be converted into fat which is stored as glycogen. This inability of hypermetabolic patients to utilise large glucose loads is accompanied by a further increase in the already elevated levels of catecholamines. Thus, excess glucose loads in critically ill patients may act as a metabolic stress.

In both depleted and hypermetabolic patients the higher CO_2 production in response to an excessive glucose load induces a marked increase in minute ventilation; this response can precipitate pulmonary decompensation in patients with impaired or limited ventilatory function (see p. 91).

FAT METABOLISM

The effect of TPN on fat metabolism has not been fully worked out (Kinney 1990). In starving normal subjects TPN which is glucose based suppresses glucose production as well as fat oxidation. In patients with serious sepsis or major injury TPN is much less effective. Excessive amounts of TPN whatever the energy source result in the accumulation of body fat. The metabolism of administered fat emulsion is of considerable interest and it is clear that new forms of intravenous fat are required to overcome some of the potential problems that have been uncovered (Jensen et al 1990). Lipid emulsions can affect lipid transport in the plasma (Carpentier 1990), can alter cell membrane composition to begin to resemble the composition of the administered lipid emulsion (Bernardier 1988) and can influence prostaglandin metabolism (Oates et al 1988) and surfactant production (Rhoades 1975). Having said that, parenteral lipid emulsions have been demonstrated to be important metabolic fuels which make management of hypermetabolic patients more straightforward. We will see later that the inclusion of a substantial amount of lipid in the nutrient regimen in patients with borderline respiratory function maintains carbon dioxide production at a manageable level.

SODIUM, WATER AND ELECTROLYTES

In very depleted patients refeeding is associated with major shifts of minerals to intracellular spaces, and serum levels may plummet. Body fluid compartments redistribute as intracellular fluid increases. If these changes occur rapidly life-threatening complications may arise; this may occur if the provision of nutrients is too rapid or the composition is inappropriate (Solomon & Kirby 1990). Common problems include: excessive glucose loads with the rapid development of hypokalaemia (due to glycogen being laid down), hypophosphataemia, which may occur in very depleted patients receiving glucose based nutrient solutions without sufficient phosphate, hypomagnesaemia (in patients with gastrointestinal losses) and so-called 'refeeding oedema'. Although refeeding very malnourished patients with sodium-rich glucose based TPN regimens may result in extracellular fluid retention (Bloom 1967) it can be avoided by leaving sodium out of the nutrient solution for the first few days of refeeding. Avoidance of hypokalaemia is also important in preventing sodium retention (Friedberg et al 1991).

SECTION III
EFFECTS OF NUTRITIONAL REPLETION ON SKELETAL MUSCLE FUNCTION

The early functional effects of nutritional therapy we saw earlier are particularly obvious in skeletal muscle. The explanation for these changes may be related to immediate restoration of cellular phosphate levels. True and sustained improvements in physiological function, however, are related to both restoration of muscle fibres and the enzymes within them associated with an increase in total muscle bulk. In Figure 6.1 we saw how restoration of body protein stores were necessary to obtain physiological improvements after the early functional improvement had been attained. In Table 6.2 the results of our study of muscle histochemistry during nutritional repletion are shown. After two weeks of TPN there is a partial restoration of type II muscle fibres associated with an increase in the activity of a key enzyme of glucose utilisation — phosphofructokinase. The data suggest that as protein is being laid down there is a slow restoration of muscle fibre types and distribution although quite long periods of refeeding are necessary to achieve normality. The increase in phosphofructokinase activity with TPN may account for the apparent increase in insulin sensitivity shown in patients after TPN (Greenberg et al 1981).

SECTION IV
EFFECTS OF NUTRITIONAL REPLETION ON RESPIRATORY FUNCTION

From Figure 6.1 we can see the early improvement in respiratory function that occurred within a few days of commencing TPN and the continuing slow improvement that continued for months as total body protein stores were replenished. These effects are due to improvements in skeletal muscle which are demonstrated in Table 6.2. We have seen, however, that ventilation is not just a matter of respiratory muscle strength, it involves ventilatory drive and gas exchange as well. TPN with hypercalorific amounts of glucose causes increased ventilatory demand and respiratory distress in very ill surgical patients (Askanazi et al 1980). Since CO_2 is produced in greater quantities with glucose, glucose based TPN systems increase demand for minute ventilation. Energy intake may be increased without a major increase in CO_2 production by adding lipids to a glucose, amino acid TPN system.

The arterial CO_2 tension 'set point' is regulated by the respiratory control centre; if the set point is lowered, ventilatory demand increases. Amino acid infusions tend to lower the set point and enhance the ventilatory response to high CO_2 tensions in malnourished patients. Clearly increased ventilatory demands induced by TPN due either to increased CO_2 production or lowered CO_2 set point may be important in the management in patients with borderline respiratory function and those with problems in weaning from mechanical ventilation. The practical lessons are that nutrient intake should match energy expenditure in such patients and 50% of the energy source should be provided as lipids (Skeie et al 1988).

SECTION V
EFFECTS OF NUTRITIONAL REPLETION ON WOUND HEALING

Using the Goretex micro implant technique we were able to demonstrate an improvement in the wound healing response with TPN (Haydock and Hill 1987).

- We found that in 47 malnourished patients presenting for TPN the wound healing response was less (0.34 ± 0.23 μg of hydroxyproline/cm of Goretex tubing) than that of 36 normally nourished subjects (0.49 ± 0.30 μg/cm; $p < 0.01$). After TPN it rose to 0.88 ± 0.62 μg/cm, $p < 0.005$.
- In 29 surgical patients, two sequential studies of wound healing were conducted over a 14-day period of TPN. The mean accumulation of hydroxyproline during the first week of TPN was 0.36 ± 0.24 μg/cm and this was increased significantly over the second week of TPN to 0.78 ± 0.67 μg/cm, $p < 0.005$.
- The wound healing response that occurred in wounds made after a period of preoperative nutrition was better than that which occurred when only postoperative nutrition was given ($p < 0.02$).

Table 6.2 Maximal activities of the rate determining enzymes of glycolysis and the Krebs cycle in the vastus lateralis muscle of malnourished surgical patients together with the size and proportional numbers of muscle fibre types I and II from the same biopsy specimen. Shown are values before and after 2 weeks of TPN in 11 patients. (Adapted from Church J M, Choong S Y, Hill G L 1984 Br J Surg 71: 563, by permission of the publishers.)

	Hexokinase	**Phosphofructokinase**	**Fructose bisphosphatase**	**Oxoglutarate dehydrogenase**
Before TPN*	0.81 ± 0.08	19.62 ± 1.85	0.41 ± 0.04	0.26 ± 0.06
After TPN*	0.97 ± 0.08	30.74 ± 2.99	0.47 ± 0.03	0.30 ± 0.05
p	NS	< 0.01	NS	NS

	Proportional number of fibre types (%)†		**Cross-sectional area of fibre types ($\mu m^2 \times 10^2$)**†		**Proportional area of biopsy occupied by fibre types (%)**	
	I	II	I	II	I	II
Before TPN	58 ± 6	42 ± 6	49 ± 19	40 ± 18	63	37
After TPN	45 ± 5	56 ± 5	50 ± 5	47 ± 20	46	54
p	<0.05	<0.05	NS	<0.05		

* Values are mean ± s.e.m.
† Values are mean ± s.d.

From these data we have concluded that an improvement in the wound healing response occurs after only 1 week of TPN and before there is a measurable improvement in nutritional status. The improved wound healing response is more marked when TPN is given before, rather than after the surgical procedure (Haydock & Hill 1987).

There are, however, two major clinical studies which have shown improved wound healing in *postoperative patients* receiving additional nutrition. A 2-week course of TPN administered postoperatively seemed to be associated with improved perineal wound healing after rectal excision (see Ch. 10, Fig. 10.3), and another study of postoperative enteral feeding was found to be associated with an improved wound healing response as assessed by the Goretex implant method (Schroeder et al 1991). Thus, evidence suggests that wound healing is improved by TPN in malnourished patients, it is seen after only 1 week of nutrition and is independent of any measurable change in nutritional status.

The tide is coming in rapidly for the use of recombinant growth factors in wound healing. New advances in the future will see not only nutrients but growth preparations being used and applied to wounds to accelerate healing (Kingsnorth & Slavin 1991).

SECTION VI
EFFECTS OF NUTRITIONAL REPLETION ON IMMUNE FUNCTION

The relationship between PEM and impaired cell mediated immunity has been established in both children with kwashiorkor and in adult hospitalised patients with PEM of the kwashiorkor type. In pure marasmus seen classically in patients with anorexia nervosa anergy to skin test antigens may be seen but normal cell mediated immunity with normal T lymphocyte function is the rule (Bistrian et al 1975). On the other hand, absolute numbers of T lymphocytes are decreased and anergy is common in kwashiorkor and marasmic kwashiorkor. In one study, nutritional repletion was associated with recovered skin reactivity in half the patients after 4 weeks while skin tests were restored to normal in all patients after 6 weeks (Twomey 1982).

SECTION VII
EFFECTS OF NUTRITIONAL REPLETION ON PSYCHOLOGICAL FUNCTION

In protein energy malnutrition the intellect remains clear but there is a personality change with inability to concentrate, irritability and apathy. In a study of preoperative patients awaiting major gastrointestinal surgery the fatigue/inertia score was found to be raised (Windsor & Hill 1988d). Furthermore, patients being fed intravenously seemed to have improvement in mood and become more cheerful and energetic. In Table 6.3 which shows the results of our study of 32 surgical patients with protein energy malnutrition it can be seen that, after a 2-week course of TPN the clinical impression of mood improvement and increased cheerfulness with nutritional support has been validated objectively.

Table 6.3 Psychological scores before and after 2 weeks of nutritional support in 32 surgical patients. The values given are the mean ± s.d. score. Significance was determined using the Wilcoxon signed-rank test for paired non-parametric variables. (Data from Stokes 1991.)

	Before	After	Significance
Poms*			
Tension–anxiety	8.6 ± 6.4	4.1 ± 5.1	$p < 0.001$
Depression–dejection	12.9 ±10.1	8.0 ± 7.4	$p < 0.001$
Anger–hostility	6.8 ± 8.9	4.5 ± 6.4	$p < 0.05$
Vigour	9.3 ± 7.5	13.2 ± 6.2	$p < 0.005$
Fatigue	16.1 ± 7.8	10.2 ± 6.6	$p < 0.001$
Friendliness	16.3 ± 5.6	19.4 ± 4.6	$p < 0.001$
SCL†			
Somatisation	1.15 ± 0.61	0.74 ± 0.48	$p < 0.001$
Depression	1.47 ± 0.69	0.92 ± 0.65	$p < 0.001$
Anxiety	0.76 ± 0.64	0.45 ± 0.39	$p < 0.005$
Hostility	0.61 ± 0.62	0.26 ± 0.27	$p < 0.001$
Global severity	0.28 ± 0.10	0.20 ± 0.10	$p < 0.001$
Fatigue score‡	6.9 ± 2.0	5.1 ± 1.8	$p < 0.01$

* Profile of mood states (McNair et al 1971)
† Symptom check list (Derogatis 1978)
‡ Fatigue scale (Christensen et al 1982)

We have found that this positive effect occurs whether the route of feeding is parenteral or enteral.

SECTION VIII
NUTRITIONAL PHARMACOLOGY

It is now realised that nutrients may serve a pharmacological role. For instance, it has been shown that the following nutrients act as pharmacological agents:

Arginine supplementation has metabolic and immune modulatory effects. It appears to improve nitrogen balance (Daly et al 1982), enhance wound healing (Barbul et al 1990), and increase lymphocyte mitogenesis in response to phytohaemagglutinin and concanavalin A (Barbul 1990).

Glutamine supplementation is associated with improved growth and repair of the gut mucosa, attenuation of the loss of intestinal immune function associated with standard nutrient formulations, improved survival of severe abdominal sepsis, increased gut villus height and mucosal thickness, and maintenance of intestinal integrity. It has been shown to be essential for lymphocyte proliferation and macrophage secretory activity (Fox et al 1988, Burke et al 1989, Souba 1988, Newsholme et al 1988, Newsholme & Parry-Billings 1990, Wan et al 1989, Klimberg et al 1990, Wilmore 1991).

Branched-chain amino acids may improve protein synthesis in catabolic patients (Bower et al 1986a).

Dietary RNA is beneficial in stimulating immune function — it improves delayed hypersensitivity responses and maintains cell mediated immune responses (Pizzini et al 1990).

n-3 (omega-3) polyunsaturated fatty acids. There are a number of beneficial health effects from dietary intake of n-3 polyunsaturated fatty acids — of particular relevance here is the recent study which showed that the synthesis of IL-1 and TNF was suppressed by dietary supplementation with marine lipid concentrate (rich in eicosapentaenoic and docosahexaenoic acids) (Endres et al 1989). The mechanism for this suppressive effect remains unknown, although alterations in the type of arachidonic acid metabolites produced during stimulation of mononuclear cells may explain in part the decreased production of these two cytokines.

It is clear that the future will see nutrient solutions enriched with, or composed of, some or all of these agents. In this way a new era of nutritional support may open up (Bower 1990b). An enteral diet with supplemental arginine, RNA and omega-3 fatty acids is now available. In a preliminary trial (Daly et al 1992) 85 patients with upper gastrointestinal cancer were randomised to receive for 7 days post-operatively the new diet or Osmolite-HN. Immunological, metabolic and clinical outcome parameters were measured. In the patients who received the new diet, infectious and wound complications occurred significantly less than in those who received Osmolite-HN (11% versus 37%). The results of a multicentre trial are awaited with considerable interest (Bower 1990a).

7. Assessment of nutritional status

INTRODUCTION — THE OBJECTIVE OF THE NUTRITIONAL ASSESSMENT

We have found the 'concept of circles' developed by Heymsfield and Williams (1988) to describe body composition and physiological function to be a most helpful way of understanding the objective of nutritional assessment. Figure 7.1 describes this concept. Circle A is thought of as encompassing the body composition and physiological function of a normal healthy subject. Disease causes negative energy and protein balance with accompanying changes in body composition and physiological function. Circle B is where all reserves of fat and protein have been utilised and physiological function is barely compatible with life. An alternative outcome is for major injury or serious sepsis to intervene causing not only consumption of host tissue but also an expansion of extracellular water and profound deficits in physiological function (circle C). The objective of the nutritional assessment is to determine the location, direction and rate of change of the patient between circles A, B and C. For the proper assessment of nutritional status, therefore, four components are necessary, *energy and protein balance*, *body composition*, *physiological function* and *degree of metabolic stress (injury or sepsis)*.

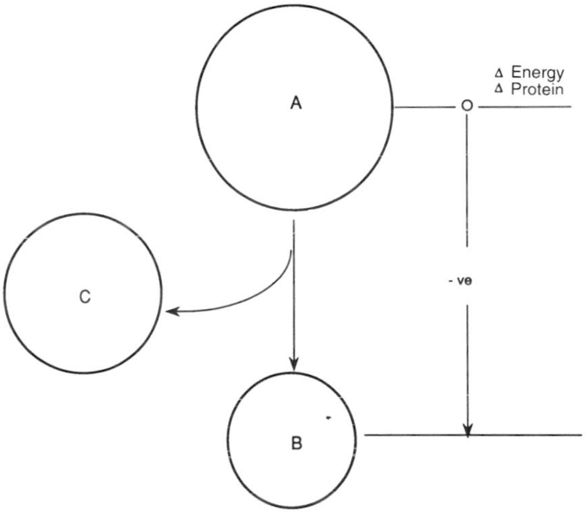

Fig. 7.1 The 'concept of circles' (Heymsfield) is used to describe changes in energy and protein balance, and body composition and function in protein energy malnutrition. Circle A is the range of body composition and physiological function of a normal subject. Weight is stable and energy and protein balance is zero. Surgical disease causes negative energy and protein balance with accompanying changes in body composition and physiological function. Circle B is the minimal range of body composition and function that is compatible with life. The deterioration in the state of a patient passing between A and B may be interrupted by major injury or serious sepsis and the result is depicted by circle C. Assessment of nutritional state aims to determine the location, direction and rate of change of the patient between circles A, B and C.

SECTION I
ASSESSMENT OF ENERGY AND PROTEIN BALANCE

CLINICAL

In practice the clinician can obtain an overview of energy and protein balance by assessing the frequency and size of the patient's meals and comparing the results obtained with an estimate of rate of loss of body weight. Table 7.1 shows the relationship between meal size and loss of body weight over time (data come from the

Table 7.1 Relationship between meal size and loss of body weight over time

Meal size (% of normal)	Weight loss* (%) over time 3 months	6 months	12 months
20	30	45	—
30	25	35	40
50	15	25	30
70	10	15	20
80	8	12	15

* Weight loss expressed as a percentage of original body weight.

Minnesota starvation experiment Keys et al 1950). It can be seen that if meal size has been only 50% of normal over a period of 3 months the patient will have a weight loss of 15%. If energy intake is 20% of normal over a period of 6 months then the patient will suffer from near lethal loss of body weight (45%).

Over shorter time periods changes in body weight reflect either overhydration or the combined effects of starvation and major metabolic stress (Fig. 7.2). With major injury or serious sepsis, negative energy and protein balance are the rule, but simple bedside assessment of the magnitude of this imbalance is almost impossible.

OBJECTIVE

A more comprehensive assessment of *energy and protein intake* is performed by a dietitian (Morgan et al 1978). A 24 h recall with a food frequency cross check is the technique used most frequently although an analysis of a food record diary or a calorie count are also used. Once the diet information is collected the data are processed by a computer using food composition tables, and the amount and adequacy of the total energy intake and protein intake are assessed by comparison with recommended daily allowances.

For clinical purposes, *energy and protein output* in surgical patients is calculated at the bedside; 40 kcal/kg/body weight and 1.5 g of protein/kg/

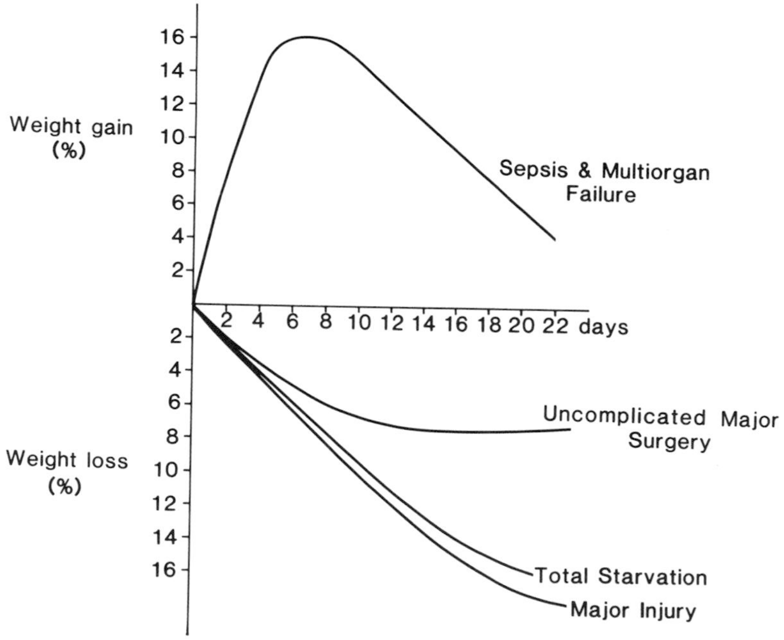

Fig. 7.2 Changes in body weight that occur in serious sepsis (after resuscitation), uncomplicated surgery and major injury compared to the rate of loss of body weight that occurs with total starvation. (Reproduced from Hill G L, Beddoe A H 1988 Dimensions of the human body and its compartments. In: Kinney J M et al (eds) Nutrition and metabolism in patient care, W B Saunders, Philadelphia, ch 4, by permission of the publishers.)

day are reasonable approximations of energy and protein requirements (see Ch. 8). When the output calculated in this way is related to dietary assessment of intake then an approximation of the caloric and protein deficit is obtained. From Chapter 8 it can also be seen that basal energy expenditure, diet induced thermogenesis, activity energy expenditure and the expenditure due to metabolic stress may, if required, be estimated in the clinical setting.

RESEARCH TECHNIQUES

For the accurate calculation of energy and protein balance, such as that required for research purposes, a metabolic ward is used. All nutrient intake is precisely and accurately measured and all losses from the body are collected and analysed. Whole body calorimetry (Pullicino et al 1991), energy balance techniques using body composition methodology (Stokes & Hill 1990b) and isotopic methods using double labelled water (Schoeller & van Santen 1982) all allow direct and fairly accurate measurements of energy balance to be made.

SECTION II
ASSESSMENT OF BODY COMPOSITION

CLINICAL

Body weight

In the assessment and subsequent evaluation of patients with nutritional and metabolic disorders measurements of body weight should always be made (Table 7.2). Body weight can be measured on chair-type ward scales to the nearest 0.1 kg. In some cases chair scales can not be used for acutely ill patients and bed-type scales on to which the patient can be moved can be used. Other scales are available which make it possible to weigh the patient without moving the bed but here it is important to ensure that the same 'patient extras', such as sheets and pillows are included in exactly the same way at each weighing.

Table 7.2 Protocol for measuring body weight

- The measurement is made at approximately the same time each day (best first thing in the morning)
- The patient should be weighed in the same clothing each day and the bladder should be emptied immediately before weighing
- Weighing should always be made on the same properly calibrated scales
- If there are any gross or unexpected inconsistencies the measurement should be checked by a second observer

Weight loss can be determined easily if a patient's weight before and after the occurrence of the loss has been measured. Usually, however, patients have already lost weight when they are first seen and the size of the weight loss then needs to be evaluated by comparing the measured weight with some other estimate of well weight. The accuracy of the result depends on the accuracy with which well weight can be measured. There is a lot of research on the measurement of well weight (ideal weight) and it is now clear that it is more reliable to estimate weight loss by using the patient's recalled well weight than by using published tables of ideal weight (Morgan et al 1980). Even then, estimating weight loss can be quite misleading in individual subjects and it is important therefore to relate the estimate of weight loss obtained to the physical examination of the patient.

General appearance

The appearance of the marasmic patient has already been described. There are marked decreases in muscle tissue and subcutaneous fat with the patient losing the rounded contours of the body. The face is thin and the cheekbones are prominent, the patient looks haggard and emaciated. The wasting of soft tissues is particularly marked in the region of the buttocks which are thin and flat. The shoulder girdle is square and prominent. Patients after major injury and serious sepsis may be profoundly protein depleted with severe erosions of muscle mass, yet without this classical appearance due to a relative preservation of body fat mass and an overlying layer of extracellular water.

Body fat stores

Gross loss of body fat can be observed not only from the patient's appearance but also by palpating a number of skinfolds between the finger and thumb. When the dermis can be felt between the finger and thumb on pinching the triceps and biceps skinfolds then one can be sure that considerable losses of body fat have occurred. *We call this a positive finger–thumb test.* Body composition studies have shown that the body mass when this physical sign is present is composed of less than 10% fat (Stokes 1991).

Body protein stores

In a similar manner protein stores may be assessed by inspection and palpation of a number of muscle groups. The temporalis muscles, deltoids, suprascapular and infrascapular muscles, the bellies of biceps and triceps and the interossei of the hands should all be looked at and palpated. The long muscles in particular are considered to be profoundly protein depleted when the tendons are prominent to palpation. Body composition studies have shown that when the tendons are prominent to palpation and the bony prominences of the scapula are obvious then patients have lost more than 30% of their total body protein stores (Stokes 1991). *We call this a positive tendon–bone test.*

Hypoalbuminaemia and excess body water

Plasma albumin levels are of fundamental help in determining the type of protein energy malnutrition. Although albumin is affected by a host of factors unrelated to nutrition, when a patient with protein energy malnutrition has low levels of plasma albumin it usually indicates an expanded extracellular fluid space which may be large enough to be clinically detectable as pitting oedema (Ch. 5).

OBJECTIVE

Anthropometry

Many nutritionists use anthropometry routinely to measure body fat and the fat free mass. Two types of measurement are usually made: skinfold thicknesses and limb circumferences. Triceps skinfold in particular is used in the clinical setting and the result obtained is compared to reference tables and an estimate of fat depletion made. A single skinfold thickness is, however, a relatively poor predictor of the absolute amount and rate of change in total body fat in an individual (Collins et al 1979, Streat et al 1985a). Combining a limb skinfold thickness with a corresponding circumference allows the calculation of limb fat areas. It is also possible to measure a number of skin folds (usually triceps and biceps and subscapular) and to derive from them an estimate of total body fat (Durnin & Womersley 1974). This estimate of total body fat is subtracted from body weight giving an estimate of the fat free body mass.

There are limitations in using anthropometry routinely in nutritional assessment because of the large errors both in accuracy and precision which are involved in individual patients (see Streat et al 1985a). Nevertheless such measurements can be very valuable in patients undergoing long term nutritional follow-up over months or years, or in identifying patients who are profoundly depleted. They can also be used in assessing the incidence of malnutrition in a patient population (Bistrian et al 1974).

Chemical methods

Apart from plasma albumin assay which is an indispensable chemical method for identifying the type of malnutrition present, other chemical methods used for nutritional assessment include 24-hour urea/creatinine, and creatinine/height index (Bistrian 1977). The levels of plasma transferrin, plasma prealbumin and retinol binding protein are affected by recent changes in energy intake and are also highly correlated with all other commonly used methods of assessing nutritional state (Young & Hill 1978). They are also valuable in following the nutritional status of a patient longitudinally (see p. 103).

RESEARCH TECHNIQUES

Physical techniques

There are a number of research techniques for measuring body composition and some of the more simple ones may soon be applicable to the daily care of the sick. These include bioelectrical impedance analysis (BIA), dual energy X-ray absorptiometry (DEXA) and total body potassium measurements (TBK). BIA measures the resistance and reactance of a current passed through the body between the wrist and the contralateral leg. From the data obtained total body water may be estimated and by using assumptions as to the relationship between body water and the fat free body mass the latter can be estimated. Some suggest that extracellular water can also be estimated by these techniques (Lukaski & Bolunchuk 1988). The simplicity and low cost of BIA have made some nutritionists advocate its widespread use (Shizgal 1991). We ourselves have reservations, however, and advocate its use for estimating the fat free body mass, while at the same time advising caution in using the technique for following the patient on treatment (Schroeder et al 1990).

Dual energy X-ray absorptiometry is a technique which was developed to measure skeletal mineralisation but more recently further development has enabled measurements of body fat and total body soft tissue as well as of skeletal mass to be obtained. DEXA gives very precise estimates of total body fat (Mazess et al 1990, Heymsfield et al 1989).

In Appendix I the technique of combining DEXA with in vivo neutron activation analysis, to give a comprehensive assessment of body composition is described. Although this is the ideal for a research based nutritional assessment the cost and sophistication of the combined technique restricts its use clinically. There are also potential developments in in vivo neutron activation analysis (associated particle technique) which may add a new dimension to the precision and accuracy of the measurements of protein and extracellular water. Isotopic dilution methods using tritium and radioactive sulphate are used to measure body water and its compartments. All these are research techniques and due to their expense and sophistication have not yet found a place in routine patient care.

Growth hormone — somatomedin axis

Undernutrition reduces the hepatic release of somatomedins even though growth hormone levels may be raised. Phillips (1986) argues that this is a metabolic adaptation allowing reduced growth processes from decreased somatomedin activity while direct actions of growth hormone spare muscle protein and mobilise fat. This sensitivity to alterations in nutritional state has led to the use of somatomedin-C (insulin like growth factor-I or IGF-I) as a marker of malnutrition (Unterman et al 1985).

In patients who developed PEM following biliopancreatic bypass for morbid obesity IGF-I levels were low, increased with nutritional repletion and predicted body composition changes better than transferrin levels (Minuto et al 1989). A further study by Phillips' group (Donahue & Phillips, 1989) showed that 85% of malnourished hospital patients had reduced levels of IGF-I and when short term repletion was obtained IGF-I proved to be a better indicator of changes in nutritional status than transferrin. Clearly more work needs to be done but IGF-I might prove to be an important practical tool for nutritional assessment of hospitalised patients.

SECTION III
ASSESSMENT OF PHYSIOLOGICAL FUNCTION

CLINICAL

Functional impairment secondary to loss of body protein is the most important part of the assessment of nutritional status. The loss of function to be noted is that which is clinically quite obvious and which has occurred over the same time period as the loss of body weight. The patient should be questioned about unhealed scratches or sores, easy tiredness or substantial changes in exercise tolerance. Weight loss without evidence of physiological abnormality is probably of no consequence (Windsor & Hill 1988d). Function is observed whilst performing the physical examination and by watching the patient's activity around the ward. Grip strength can be assessed by asking the patient to squeeze strongly the surgeon's index and middle fingers for at least 10 seconds. Impairment is judged in the light of the patient's age, sex and body habitus. Respiratory muscle function is assessed by asking the patient to blow hard holding a strip of paper 10 cm from the lips; this should normally be blown away with some force. Severe impairment is present when the paper does not move. Shortness of breath is noted at rest. Severe impairment is indicated when normal conversation is not possible. Respiratory excursion is noted by asking the patient to take as deep a breath as possible. When there is virtually no chest expansion, severe impairment exists.

OBJECTIVE

We have seen in Chapter 5 that it is possible to measure the wound healing response directly by the Goretex microimplant technique and in the same chapter we saw how skeletal muscle function and respiratory function can also be assessed objectively. In clinical practice objective measurement of grip strength by the use of a hand held vigorimeter has, in some nutritional assessment programmes, become a regular and valuable part of nutritional assessment (Klidjian et al 1982).

RESEARCH

Comprehensive assessments of physiological function such as that shown in Appendix I of this book are valuable in research directed at relating body compositional deficits to functional impairment. They are, however, expensive to develop and time consuming to perform.

SECTION IV ASSESSMENT OF METABOLIC STRESS

CLINICAL

A history and physical examination will reveal evidence of metabolic stress. It is present if the patient has had major trauma or major surgery in the previous week or there is evidence of serious sepsis according to the criteria shown in Table 7.3.

Table 7.3 Markers of metabolic stress

- Highest temperature in the last 24 hours >38°C
- Pulse rate >100 per min in the last 24 hours
- Respiratory rate >30 per min in the last 24 hours
- White cell count >12 000 or <3000 in the last 24 hours
- Positive blood culture
- Active inflammatory bowel disease
- Defined focus of infection

OBJECTIVE

Indirect calorimetry

Direct measurement of resting metabolic expenditure by indirect calorimetry is the best way of quantifying the intensity of metabolic stress. This is then related to estimated values when well. These are best related to an anthropometric measurement of metabolic body size. Although measurements of total body potassium and through them estimates of the body cell mass are the gold standard for metabolic body size (Kinney et al 1963), fat free body mass is more practical in the clinical setting. Fat free mass may be measured either by skinfold measurements, or simply by electrical impedance. In normal subjects resting metabolic expenditure is related closely to the size of the fat free body regardless of age and regardless of sex (Roza & Shizgal 1984).

From a normal population in our own laboratory the following regression equation was obtained:

RME (kcal/24 h) = 13.6 FFM + 550
(males and females)
(RME = resting metabolic expenditure, FFM = fat free body mass in kg)

The mean (S.D.) ratio of the measured RME to predicted RME for normal subjects was:

1.00 ± 0.09

and so patients with a ratio greater than 1.18 are considered in our laboratory as having a raised RME and to suffer from metabolic stress.

Catabolic index

This index separates urinary urea excretion into urea excretion due to dietary protein intake and urea excretion due to increased protein catabolism (Bistrian 1979). Measurements required are 24-hour nitrogen intake and 24-hour urinary urea over the same time period.

The catabolic index (CI) is then calculated as follows:

$$CI = \text{urinary urea N (g)} - \left(\frac{\text{dietary N (g)}}{2} + 3\right)$$

If	CI < 0	no stress
	CI 0–5	moderate stress
	CI > 5	severe stress

Scoring systems

There are physiological scoring systems such as the APACHE II score which give a general measurement of disease severity (Kraus et al 1985).

RESEARCH

Levels of counter-regulatory hormones, acute phase reactants and quantification of circulating cytokines are used by some to estimate the degree of metabolic stress, or presence of invasive sepsis (Michie et al 1988).

SECTION V **PUTTING THE COMPONENTS OF THE ASSESSMENT TOGETHER**

From the measurements of the separate components of the assessment, that is, energy and protein balance, body composition, physiological function and metabolic stress, the surgeon will be able to:

- identify the type of malnutrition present
- quantify the intensity of the malnutrition
- decide whether metabolic stress is present or not.

THE TYPE OF MALNUTRITION PRESENT

Marasmus. Patients with marasmus will be found to have an overall deficit in their intake and/or utilisation of food. They will also have weight loss of greater than 10% or more, marked by clinical evidence of subcutaneous fat loss and wasting of muscle bellies. Plasma albumin remains normal but plasma prealbumin and plasma transferrin may be low. The patient, if the condition is severe, looks like a walking skeleton. Indirect calorimetry will demonstrate that resting metabolic expenditure is low-normal or low and urinary nitrogen loss will be found to be small.

Marasmic kwaskiorkor. Patients with this type of PEM will be found to have an overall deficit in their intake and/or utilisation of food. They will also have weight loss of 10% or more, marked by clinical evidence of subcutaneous fat loss and wasting of muscle bellies. Indirect calorimetry may give normal values if the metabolic stress causing the malnutrition has been dealt with. If there is continuing stress indirect calorimetry will show an increase in the measured RME compared with the predicted RME. Plasma albumin levels are low as also are levels of plasma transferrin and prealbumin. There may be evidence of pitting oedema.

Kwashiorkor. These patients are easily picked out because they are suffering from major trauma or serious sepsis or have been so in the recent past. They are not eating. Massive weight loss may not yet be a feature and clinical examination will find near normal stores of muscle and fat but there will be clear signs of sepsis or major metabolic stress. Plasma levels of albumin will be low as well as those for transferrin and prealbumin. Oedema is frequently present. If this situation persists, muscle wasting follows and extracellular fluid accumulates further, although fat stores are (clinically) relatively preserved.

INTENSITY OF MALNUTRITION

We have defined moderate–severe protein energy malnutrition as that which is of sufficient intensity to impact on physiological function. The definition requires this impact to be clinically obvious. *It is important for the examiner to have very strict criteria for the clinical assessment of physiological dysfunction.* In a recent study we found that of those patients said to have impaired physiological function only 48% actually did so on objective measurement (Stokes 1991).

ASSESSMENT OF METABOLIC STRESS

The importance of identifying metabolic stress is that:

- it gives a clue as to the type of malnutrition that is present or soon will be present
- it indicates that extracellular water is expanded or will be expanding
- the response to nutritional support will be impaired in those in whom metabolic stress is present.

METABOLIC STRESS

We have seen in Chapter 6 how patients with metabolic stress have a blunted ability to retain administered protein because of continuing catabolism. Protein synthesis can be increased in stressed patients with adequate nutritional support but whole body protein catabolism goes on unabated and is not affected by known nutritional or pharmacological regimens. Assessment of metabolic stress directly enables the patient's energy requirements to be calculated accurately.

SECTION VI
IMPLICATIONS FOR PATIENT MANAGEMENT

THE TYPE OF PROTEIN ENERGY MALNUTRITION

The surgeon needs to identify the type of malnutrition in order to set appropriate nutritional/metabolic goals for treatment. The marasmic patient has less distortion of body compartments but the malnutrition may have developed over a long period of time and hence considerable caution must be taken over the rate of repletion to avoid complications (Weinsier et al 1981, Heymsfield et al 1978). The patient with marasmic kwashiorkor has an overexpanded extracellular water as well as erosion of body stores and needs careful restriction of sodium and free water to normalise body hydration and avoid the possibility of oversalting and overwatering. The patient with kwashiorkor has a catastrophic illness with massive proteolysis and expansion of extracellular water. The surgeon's eye must be to dealing with the metabolic stress causing this, as well as dealing with the developing compositional defect.

THE SEVERITY

There is ample evidence now to suggest that patients without physiological impairment or in whom physiological impairment is not expected to occur do not need nutritional repletion.

SECTION VII
FOLLOWING THE PATIENT ON TREATMENT

CLINICAL RESPONSE

For nutritional therapy to be effective it is necessary to ensure that the nutrients being provided are adequate and are being utilised effectively. There are a number of studies which show that wound healing (Haydock & Hill 1987, Hadley & Fitzsimmons 1990), muscle function (Christie & Hill 1990) and psychological function (Ch. 6) may be measurably improved with total parenteral nutrition, resulting in the clinical observation that the patient looks and feels better and on examination he or she is physically stronger.

NITROGEN BALANCE

On the laboratory side nitrogen balance is sometimes used as a marker of dynamic nutritional assessment but in clinical practice the performance of a nitrogen balance is full of difficulties (Konstantinides et al 1991) unless very strict attention is paid to measuring *all* losses. In many surgical patients this is quite impractical. If, however, the surgeon can be sure that there has been a complete 24-hour collection of urine a fair approximation of all nitrogen losses from the body can be made. Generally speaking though, all 'clinical nitrogen balances' tend to have cumulative errors which err on the side of being optimistic and the patient needs to be in a positive nitrogen balance of +5 g N/day to be certain that nitrogen accretion is occurring (Streat et al 1986). The technique of performing a 'clinical nitrogen' balance is as follows:

- The amount of urea passed in the urine in a 24-hour period is calculated by multiplying the 24-hour urine output by the urine urea concentration
- Urea with a molecular weight of 60 is, by weight, about 50% nitrogen
- Urea accounts for ~80% of N in urine and therefore the urea N must be increased by 20%
- In addition, 2 g/day of N are added to account for stool N and integumentary losses
- N balance (g/day) = N intake – N output
- If nitrogen balance is > 5 g per day the patient is in +ve N balance.

PLASMA PROTEINS

As practical alternatives to nitrogen balance, four serum transport proteins have been suggested as markers of nutritional progress and are now being used in some nutritional assessment programmes (Bernstein et al 1989, Ota et al 1985, Winkler et al 1989). These are *albumin, transferrin, prealbumin* and *retinol binding protein*. Table 7.4 shows the predictive value of three plasma proteins, plasma albumin, transferrin and prealbumin in determining the likelihood of adequate protein retention. It can be seen that in patients requiring TPN for two weeks a positive nitrogen balance was reflected by a rise of prealbumin in 88% of cases, whereas a negative nitrogen balance was associated with a falling prealbumin in 70%. Predictive values in the group indicate that 93% of patients with a rising plasma prealbumin level had a positive nitrogen balance.

Table 7.4 Sensitivity, specificity and predictive value of weekly rise in plasma protein levels in detecting positive nitrogen balance: patients receiving 2 weeks of TPN (adapted from Church J M, Hill G L 1987 J Parenter Enter Nutr 11: 135, by permission of the publishers)

	Albumin	Prealbumin	Transferrin
Sensitivity (%)	61	88	67
Specificity (%)	45	70	55
Positive predictive value (%)	86	93	87
Negative predictive value (%)	17	56	27
Prevalence of rising nitrogen balance	61/72	90/108	90/108

8. Assessment of nutritional requirements

INTRODUCTION–THE IMPORTANCE OF SETTING NUTRITIONAL/METABOLIC GOALS

From Chapters 5 and 6 we learnt that by the end of a thorough clinical assessment of the nutritional state of a patient the surgeon needs to be able to answer the following questions:

- What type of protein energy malnutrition is this (marasmus, marasmic kwashiorkor, or kwashiorkor)?
- Is the intensity of the protein energy malnutrition sufficient to adversely impact on the patient's clinical course?
- Is the patient metabolically stressed (i.e. is the resting metabolic expenditure raised above normal)?

By answering these three questions realistic nutrition/metabolic goals can be set according to the following guidelines.

Nutritional support is indicated when PEM is already or soon will be of sufficient intensity to impact adversely on the course of the patient's illness. If after proper dietetic assessment it is clear that oral food intake is insufficient or unable to restore the patient's nutritional status to normal then enteral or parenteral nutrition will be required.

The type of malnutrition present and whether the patient is metabolically stressed have important implications for management. For the surgical patient with nutritional marasmus, the goal is restoration of fat and protein stores and the normalisation of body hydration. For the patient with major trauma or serious sepsis (kwashiorkor) the goal is more limited. No matter what nutritional therapy is given, protein repletion cannot be obtained and the best that can be hoped for is the limitation of protein losses, partial normalisation of body hydration and moderate improvement in physiological function. For those patients with intermediate degrees of marasmic kwashiorkor who are not septic the goal is protein accretion, with normalisation of body hydration and physiological function. On the other hand, when such patients are septic the goal must first be to control the sepsis, if possible, before nutritional therapy is started. Thus for each patient nutritional therapy is grounded on a clear diagnosis of the type of malnutrition present and a realistic idea as to what nutritional therapy is likely to achieve. Later (in Ch. 11) we will present some clinical examples of the nutritional management of each of the main types of clinically significant malnutrition.

SECTION I
ENERGY REQUIREMENTS

TOTAL ENERGY REQUIREMENTS

For some time it was thought that energy requirements for sick surgical patients were very high and that large energy intakes (described as hyperalimentation) were necessary in order to gain protein and fat. It is now realised that, apart from being wasteful of resources and money, excessive energy intakes can, by raising the level of catecholamines, be the source of added metabolic stress (Nordenstrom et al 1981). Hypercaloric feeding may also increase ventilatory demand which may be important in patients with borderline respiratory function and imminent respiratory failure and in those with problems in weaning from mechanical ventilation (Askanazi et al 1980, Covelli et al 1981). There is therefore a strong argument for tailoring energy intake to the patient's requirements.

The total energy requirements of a patient in metabolic balance are the same as his or her total energy expenditure. This includes basal requirements (i.e. the energy necessary for the work of the heart and lungs, work for the synthesis of new chemical bondings and work to maintain electrochemical gradients in cells), the increased energy requirements brought about by the patient's disease, the energy expended during the process of assimilation of nutrients and the energy expended on physical work. The only direct way to measure all these components together is by means of a direct calorimeter which measures all the heat produced by the patient in a 24-hour period (Webb 1984, Pullicino et al 1991). A direct calorimeter is in reality a huge airtight insulated box which completely isolates the patient, and it is therefore quite impractical for day to day patient management. Total energy requirements may also be measured by the double labelled water technique (Schoeller & van Santen 1982, Mathews & Heymsfield 1991), but this is prohibitively expensive. In order to understand how total energy requirements are calculated in clinical practice some definitions are required.

DEFINITIONS

Terms currently used by clinical nutritionists for the calculation of total energy expenditure include:

Basal metabolic rate (BMR)

This is the lowest or basal metabolic requirement which occurs for a period of time when the patient is deeply asleep during the early hours of the morning. These conditions are not often available clinically.

Resting metabolic expenditure (RME)

This is a measurement in a fasted patient who has been quietly resting for at least 1/2 an hour in a thermoneutral environment. It is 5–10% higher than BMR and is the measurement used in clinical practice.

Diet induced thermogenesis (DIT)

This is the energy expended in the assimilation of nutrients whether given enterally or parenterally. In a surgical context it is not to be thought of as the energy expended after a bolus of food. It is the energy expended during the assimilation of a diet which is being administered continuously. It varies with the type of diet being infused and the metabolic state of the patient. In surgery when nutritional support is usually given continuously in the form of a balanced mixed diet, DIT is calculated by multiplying the RME by 0.1.

Resting energy expenditure (REE)

This is the same as RME, only the patient is being measured during continuous enteral or parenteral infusion. Thus it includes the additional 10% of RME caused by diet induced thermogenesis.

Activity energy expenditure (AEE)

This depends on the amount of physical work performed and varies in active people from 500 kcals per day in sedentary individuals to 3000 kcals per day in manual labourers. In surgical patients up and about around the ward it is calculated by multiplying the RME by 0.3.

Stress factor

Surgical disease usually raises metabolic rate by a factor of 5–10% for uncomplicated surgery to more than 100% for extensive burns. In practice the stress factors are calculated as follows:

Patient status	Multiply RME by
Skeletal trauma	0.3
Post elective surgery	0.1
Intraabdominal sepsis	0.3–0.5
Head injury	0.6
Serious sepsis or injury in ICU	0.4–0.6
Major burn	up to 1.0

CLINICAL MEASUREMENT OF TOTAL ENERGY REQUIREMENTS

In surgical practice there are three ways in which total energy requirements are calculated:

The surgeon can assume that all surgical patients need 40 kcal/kg/day

Using the energy balance technique, we studied the energy requirements in 106 surgical patients who required TPN (Table 8.1) and found that for a variety of surgical illnesses TEE was about 40 kcal/kg/day. This is explained by the fact that those patients whose REE is raised are usually the most ill and because they are unable to move around the ward their AEE is low. On the other hand those who are up and about around the ward with a higher AEE are less ill and their REE is not raised. The net effect is that all patients have about the same TEE. Close examination of Table 8.1 shows, however, wide confidence limits for the 40 kcal/kg/day estimation suggesting that for individual patients this general rule is subject to wide variation.

Table 8.1 Total energy expenditure in 106 surgical patients receiving 2 weeks of TPN as assessed by the energy balance technique (energy intake – energy stored as fat and protein). The patients were divided into clinical subgroups according to whether metabolic stress was present or not. (Metabolic stress is defined in Ch. 7.)

	n	**Body weight** kg	**Total energy expenditure** kcal/day	kcal/kg/day
Preoperative				
No stress	24	58.6 ± 2.6	2596 ± 280	44.3 ± 4.8
Stress	22	50.2 ± 2.8	2127 ± 244	42.4 ± 4.9
Postoperative				
No stress	28	56.8 ± 2.1	2435 ± 196	42.9 ± 3.5
Stress	14	59.2 ± 3.5	2741 ± 469	46.3 ± 7.9
Intensive care				
Major trauma	10	58.2 ± 4.4	2348 ± 371	40.3 ± 6.4
Serious sepsis	8	75.6 ± 5.5	2646 ± 397	35.0 ± 5.3

The other problem about assuming that all surgical patients require 40/kcal/kg/day is the problem of overprescription due to the varying proportions of body fat between patients. One study showed that of 50 patients given a prescription of 40 kcal/kg/day one third received more than 1000 kcal per day more than they would have received if their energy requirements had been measured directly (Parry 1989).

The surgeon can use standard tables and add factors for DIT, AEE and stress

According to the Harris–Benedict equations the basal metabolic rate can be computed using the following equations:

RME (kcal/day) for males	=	65.5 + 13.8 × W + 5 × H 65.5 – 6.8 × A
RME (kcal/day) for females	=	65.5 + 9.6 × W + 1.9 × H – 4.7 × A

(W = weight in kg, H = height in cm and A = age in years)

Having obtained the RME, requirements for DIT, AEE and stress are added. Thus:

TEE = RME + Stress Factor + DIT + AEE

Most studies show that energy requirements, for groups of patients in particular, can be fairly accurately calculated in this way. The problem arises because body weight is used in the calculation of RME and in individual patients, particularly those who are very thin or very fat or who have abnormal degrees of hydration, the results can be quite misleading. Furthermore, the stress factor is not always easy to calculate leading to a further source of error.

REE and stress factor are measured directly using a metabolic cart and AEE factor is added

There are now a number of indirect calorimeters commercially available which have been specially designed for clinical use (e.g. M.M.C. Horizon Metabolic Cart Sensor-Medics, Anaheim, California). These instruments measure oxygen consumption rate ($V\text{O}_2$), carbon dioxide production rate ($V\text{CO}_2$), and respiratory quotient ($V\text{CO}_2/V\text{O}_2$). From the $V\text{O}_2$ (assuming the RQ is 0.82) REE is calculated, for the caloric value of 1 litre of O_2 consumed at this RQ is 4.825 kcal. This value for REE in surgical patients includes both diet induced thermogenesis and the stress factor for the disease, and TEE is obtained by adding AEE. In practice REE × 1.3 is very close to the true TEE (Long et al 1979, Taggart et al 1991).

The respiratory quotient (RQ) gives an idea of what substrate is being utilised. An RQ of 1.0 is achieved during the oxidation of carbohydrate and an RQ of 0.7 indicates fat oxidation. When energy is given in excess of need an RQ above 1.0 indicates fat synthesis.*

There are a number of studies now showing the cost effectiveness of indirect calorimetry in clinical practice. A recent study of the energy requirements of a large number of patients showed that total energy requirements estimated from the Harris–Benedict equations tended to overestimate energy needs in 90% of patients leading to overfeeding of more than 500 kcal per patient per day. It was shown that considerable cost savings could be made by using indirect calorimetry in patients requiring total parenteral nutrition (Keck Jones et al 1991).

PRESCRIBING ENERGY REQUIREMENTS

Having measured the total energy requirements of a patient the amount of energy prescribed depends on the nutritional/metabolic goal for the individual patient. To preserve total body protein and total body fat at present levels the measured TEE is used. For energy store repletion, that is gain in body protein and body fat, the TEE is multiplied by 1.2.

For those who have a metabolic cart the process is even simpler. For tissue preservation multiply REE by 1.3; for tissue repletion multiply REE by 1.5.

* In patients the oxidation of carbohydrate and fat to CO_2 and water is complete although the oxidation of protein is incomplete. Each litre of O_2 involved in oxidising carbohydrate yields 5.01 kcal. Each litre of O_2 involved in oxidising fat yields 4.65 kcal. The metabolism of protein sufficient to produce 1 g of urinary N results in the production of 26.51 kcal. From the non-protein RQ and reference to standard tables the amount of calories per litre of O_2 used for the oxidation of carbohydrate and fat can be calculated. To calculate REE the amount of energy produced by protein oxidation is added.

ADMINISTERED ENERGY IS INTERCHANGEABLE

A kcal is a kcal whether given via the intestine or intravenously or as fat or as glucose.

SUMMARY

Tables 8.2 and 8.3 summarize the clinical measurement and clinical prescription of energy requirements for surgical patients.

Table 8.2 Clinical measurement of energy requirements

	Comment
Method 1 All patients receive the same TEE = 40 kcal/kg/day	30% of patients have gross overprescription
Method 2 Calculate from tables TEE = RME + Stress Factor + DIT + AEE	Often leads to overprescription in individual patients
Method 3 Indirect calorimetry TEE = measured REE + AEE	Shown to be cost effective and is recommended wherever possible

Table 8.3 Prescribing energy requirements

	Tissue maintenance is required	Tissue synthesis is required
Method 1	Prescribe TEE	Prescribe REE × 1.2
Method 2	Prescribe REE × 1.3	Prescribe REE × 1.5

SECTION II
PROTEIN REQUIREMENTS

TOTAL PROTEIN REQUIREMENTS

Calculating a patient's requirement for protein is a much less precise procedure than that used for the calculation of energy requirements. All current methods are based on body weight and are therefore prone to considerable error.

The recommended daily requirement for protein for healthy adult males is about 50 g per day although the average western diet may contain more than twice this amount. Patients with moderate to severe protein depletion behave as growing children and may gain body protein at intakes far below that which are required in surgical patients who are not as depleted (Elwyn 1980). Patients with major injury or serious sepsis have increased requirements although in such patients continuing whole body protein breakdown means that there is a limit above which increased protein intakes are not utilised.

The biological value of the administered protein (or intravenous amino acid solution) is important. All diets do not have the same biological value. This depends on the detailed amino acid composition of the diet in relation to the amino acid composition of the body. The lack of an essential amino acid can considerably decrease the biological value of an otherwise adequate intake of protein. Egg protein is very effectively utilised by man and supplementation of its amino acid content does not improve its biological value. For this reason egg protein is frequently used as a reference protein and comparisons made between its content of amino acids and those in synthetic amino acid mixtures can give a useful guide when selecting a solution for clinical use.

A number of studies have shown that amino acids or protein hydrolysates administered enterally have an effect similar to that observed when these same amino acids or protein hydrolysates are given intravenously. The precise amount of protein intake that an *individual patient* should receive cannot be measured but there are three principles which apply.

- There is an increasing linear retention of nitrogen with an increasing protein intake over a range of 0.25–2 g/kg/day.
- 1.5 g protein/kg/day is suggested by some to be the upper limit that surgical patients, even those that are severely septic, are able to utilise (Shaw et al 1987).
- Some patients have protein needs over and above those involved in metabolic processes. For instance, patients with inflammatory bowel disease may lose 0.5–1.0 g/kg/day in the stool. (Smiddy et al 1960).

With these principles in mind we recommend:

For maintenance	– prescribe 1.0–1.5 g/kg/day
For repletion	– prescribe 1.5–2 g/kg/day
For those with excessive losses	– prescribe 2–2.5 g/kg/day

These recommendations are used as a first approximation but it is important that the surgeon monitors the response according to the patient's plasma proteins (Ch. 7), or according to nitrogen balance (Ch. 7) or by direct measurements of total body protein (Appendix I).

INTERRELATIONSHIPS OF PROTEIN AND ENERGY

Within certain limits of protein and energy intake there is a region where increases in either will result in protein retention. Normally nourished patients lay down protein only when energy requirements are met but depleted patients retain protein at lesser intakes. In this respect depleted patients behave as growing children. Nevertheless authorities agree that high rates of restoration of fat free mass require high protein intake and that by proper manipulation of energy and protein intake it is possible to increase fat free mass or body fat in proportions appropriate to the individual. We have seen already that depleted patients even with moderate stress continue to retain protein but those with invasive sepsis or major trauma whether depleted or not are unable to be repleted of protein and the best to be expected is that protein losses are halved even with maximal intakes of 2 g/kg/day.

SECTION III
REQUIREMENTS FOR WATER AND ELECTROLYTES

Baseline water and mineral requirements for adult patients are set out in Table 8.4.

These recommendations for water and electrolytes are only approximate for in clinical practice the *water* and *sodium* requirements, in particular, depend on the type of malnutrition present. When there is hypoalbuminaemia there

Table 8.4 Baseline water and mineral requirements for adult patients

Patient groups	Young (16–25 y)	Adults (25–55 y)	Older patients (56–65 y)	Elderly (over 65 y)
Water requirements	40 ml/kg	35 ml/kg	30 ml/kg	25 ml/kg
Sodium	60–100 mmols	60–100 mmols	60+ mmols	50+ mmols
Potassium	60+ mmols	60+ mmols	60+ mmols	50+ mmols
Calcium	15 mEq	15 mEq	15 mEq	10 mEq
Phosphate	20–50 mmols	20–50 mmols	20–50 mmols	20–50 mmols
Magnesium	8–20 mEq	8–20 mEq	8–20 mEq	8–20 mEq

is almost always an expanded extracellular fluid space and initially little or no sodium is required unless there is hyponatraemia. If there is dilutional hyponatraemia free water is reduced and monitored according to plasma osmolality. *Potassium* requirements vary greatly depending on the type of malnutrition present. In severe marasmus the first few days of nutritional replenishment may see profound hypokalaemia develop soon after the nutrient solution has been commenced. This is due to entrance of potassium into cells as potassium-rich water is bound with glycogen as it is being replenished. *Hypophosphataemia* may also occur if phosphorus is not given in sufficient amounts particularly in glucose based nutrient regimens. Tetany may suggest that large intakes of calcium are required but in surgical patients hypocalcaemia is more likely to be secondary to hypomagnesaemia and the patient will respond to the administration of magnesium rather than calcium. Because of these variations in electrolyte requirements it is helpful in critically ill patients to use commercially available nutrient solutions which allow individualisation of water and mineral intakes depending on the clinical state of the patient.

Table 8.5 Recommended allowances for vitamins

	Action	Effect of deficiency	Dietary*	Intravenous†
Water-soluble				
Thiamine (B_1)	Glucose metabolism	Beri beri	1.4 mg	3 mg/day
Riboflavine (B_2)	Energy transfer	Glossitis dermatitis	1.6 mg	3.6 mg/day
Nicotinic acid (niacin) (B_3)	Energy transfer	Pellagra	18 mg	40 mg/day
Pyridoxine (B_6)	Decarboxylation and transamination	Muscle weakness, seizures	2.2 mg	4 mg/day
Pantothenic acid	Component of CoA	Fatigue, muscle cramps	7 mg	15 mg/day
Folate	Coenzyme with B_{12}	Anaemia	400 µg	400 µg/day
B_{12}	Coenzyme with nucleic acid synthesis	Pernicious anaemia	3 µg	5 mg/day
C	Collagen synthesis	Scurvy	60 mg	100 mg/day
Fat-soluble				
A	Glycoprotein synthesis	Night blindness	1000 µg RE‡	2500 iu/day
D	Calcium and phosphate utilization	Rickets	5 µg	5 µg/day
E	Energy transfer	Neurological disorder	10 mg[d]	50 mg§/day
K	Prothrombin synthesis	Bleeding disorder	NR¶	10 mg/week

* Committee on Dietary Allowances (1980) (males 23–50 years old)
† Nutrition Advisory Group (1979)
‡ Retinol equivalents. 1 µg retinol equivalent corresponds to 1 µg retinol or 3.33 iu
§ Alpha-tocopherol equivalents. 1 mg alpha-tocopherol equivalent has the same activity as 0.67 mg d-alpha-tocopherol
¶ No recommendation

SECTION IV
REQUIREMENTS FOR VITAMINS AND TRACE ELEMENTS

VITAMINS

These are organic substances required to maintain normal cellular activity. In clinical surgery deficiency states do not usually single out a particular vitamin and the clinical syndromes observed are often combined with deficiencies of protein and energy and other vitamins. Table 8.5 shows the major vitamins, their normal action, the effects of deficiency and the recommended daily allowances. Recommended intravenous allowances are based on dietary allowances in healthy individuals. The effect of serious illness, sepsis and trauma on these requirements when the vitamins are given by intravenous and commercial enteral feedings is not fully known.

Table 8.6 Recommended daily allowances of trace elements

Element	Effect of deficiency	Dietary*	Intravenous
Iron	Anaemia	2 mg	2 mg
Zinc‡	Impaired wound healing and growth, dermatitis, alopecia	15 mg	4–10 mg††
Copper	Anaemia, neutropenia, bone demineralization	2–3 mg	0.5 mg†
Chromium	Impaired glucose handling	0.05–0.2 mg	10–15 µg†
Iodine	Goitre, hypothyroidism	150 µg	150 µg
Fluorine	Dental susceptibility to caries	1.5–4 mg	0.4 mg
Manganese	Vit K deficiency	2–3 mg	0.15–0.8 mg†
Molybdenum	Neurological abnormalities	100 µg	100–200 µg
Selenium	Muscle weakness and pain	20–50 µg	40–120 µg

* Committee on Dietary Allowances (1980)
† Nutrition Advisory Group (1979)
‡ Excessive losses of zinc are not uncommon in surgical patients and clinical zinc deficiency syndromes were first described in such patients. Patients with diarrhoea or ileostomies lose about 17 mg of zinc per litre of faeces, but for patients with a high small bowel fistula the losses are proportionately less, about 12 mg per litre of fistula discharge.
†† If given as zinc sulphate, this needs to be multiplied by 2.5. As only 20% of orally administered zinc is absorbed a further multiplication by 5 is required if given orally. Zinc levels in the blood reflect zinc ingestion rather than balance. While 4 mg of elemental zinc is sufficient for parenteral regimens to maintain most patients in zinc balance many surgical patients require more than this and 10 mg as a base requirement is suggested.

TRACE ELEMENTS

These are found in micromolar amounts in the tissues and are essential for normal cellular function. The place of iron in haem, cobalt in vitamin B_{12} and iodine in thyroid metabolism has been known for some time. Deficiencies of zinc, copper, selenium, and chromium have also been described and these are listed along with other elements considered essential in Table 8.6.

SECTION V
SOURCES OF NUTRIENTS IN COMMERCIALLY AVAILABLE SOLUTIONS

ENTERAL DIETS

The number of commercially available enteral diets is now more than 100 and the surgeon will be bewildered by the formidable data sheets that accompany each (see Appendix II). In practice the differences lie in their amounts and forms of energy and protein.

Sources of energy

Energy from carbohydrate sources is provided from sucrose, liquid glucose (corn syrup), lactose, maltodextrins and starch. When energy is supplied as fat in an enteral diet it may be in the form of whole milk fat, vegetable oil, coconut oil or hydrogenated soya oil. Medium-chain triglycerides are indicated for some malabsorption states when long-chain fatty acids are contraindicated. Generally speaking most balanced enteral diets provide around 1 kcal per ml. Modular feeds are different being specially formulated to provide either high energy (4–8 kcal/ml) or high protein. Most balanced diets contain around 40 g of protein per litre, but high protein diets have 60 g or more of protein per litre.

Sources of protein

Protein in enteral diets is supplied in the form of sodium caseinates, soy protein isolate, whey protein or lactalbumin. The form of protein can influence absorption in surgical patients. Peptide based diets may be better absorbed than protein diets which in turn may be better absorbed than amino acid diets (Birke et al 1990, Feller et al 1989, Jones et al 1983). Table 8.7 shows the composition of some commonly used balanced enteral formulas. More complete lists are given in Appendix II.

Table 8.7 Composition of three commonly used balanced enteral diets (all lactose free)

Nutrient	Isocal	Ensure	Osmolite
kcal (ml)	1	1	1
mOsmol/kg	300	450	300
kcal : N	167 : 1	153 : 1	153 : 1
Protein (g/L)	33	35	37
Fat (g/L)	41	35	36
Carbohydrate (g/L)	125	137	137
Na (mEq)	23	37	28
K (mEq)	34	40	26
C1 (mEq)	30	30	23
P (mmol/L)	16	16	16
Mg (mEq)	4	4	4
Ca (mEq)	6	6	6
Fe (mg/L)	15	9	9
Zn (mg/L)	13	15	15
Cu (mg/L)	2	1	1
Mn (mg/L)	2	2	2
I (μg/L)	130	75	75

PARENTERAL DIETS

Sources of energy

As for enteral feeding, energy sources come from carbohydrate or fat. For intravenous use, glucose is the safest and most widely used energy source in therapeutic nutrition. Others have advocated alternative carbohydrate energy sources such as fructose, maltose, and the polyols, sorbitol, xylitol and glycerol, but they currently have a very small place in surgical nutrition. Most agree that no more than 30 kcal/kg/day of glucose energy should be used in TPN regimens (Wolfe et al 1979). Glucose is supplied in a variety of concentrations and osmolalities (Table 8.8).

Table 8.8 Concentrations of dextrose solutions

Concentration	Osmolality (mOsmol/L)
5%	250
10%	500
20%	1000
50%	2500
70%	3500

On the other hand, fat also has an important place and must be given to prevent fatty acid deficiency. There is a group of fats with unsaturated bonds in their carbon chains which are precursors of prostaglandins and are considered essential fatty acids. Normal ratios of fatty acids in the blood are maintained if 1–2% of energy is supplied as linoleic acid. Fat is used increasingly as a complementary energy source with glucose. For clinical use intravenous fat is supplied as soy bean or safflower oil emulsions which have the same properties as chylomicrons. If fat is used to supply from 30–50% of the patient's non-protein energy it not only provides essential fatty acid requirements but also is associated with a lesser incidence of metabolic problems than if glucose alone is used. Fat solutions provide energy in concentrated form. For example, 1 L of 20% fat emulsion (isotonic) supplies 2000 kcal, whereas 2000 kcal in 1 L of dextrose solution requires a 59% hypertonic glucose solution (nearly 3000 mOsmol/L). The composition of some commercially available fat emulsions is shown in Table 8.9.

Sources of protein

Intravenous protein requirements can be supplied either as protein hydrolysalates or as synthetic crystalline amino acid solutions. Although protein hydrolysalates may produce positive nitrogen balance they are less effective than crystalline amino acids and have more often been associated with adverse effects. There is at present available a huge number of crystalline amino acid sources for infusions (see Appendix II).

Table 8.10 which is representative of only a few of the solutions available shows that amino acid solutions may be provided with electrolytes or without electrolytes. Also there are specialised amino acid solutions for patients with nitrogen retention disorders such as hepatic and renal failure (Table 8.11). There are also solutions with increased concentrations of branched-chain amino acids. It was thought that these solutions may have a particular role in hypercatabolic states although that view is now losing favour (see Ch. 9).

Table 8.9 Composition of four commonly used lipid emulsions

	10% Intralipid	20% Liposyn	10% Travamulsion	20% Intralipid
Osmolarity (mOsm/L)	280	340	270	330
pH	5.5	8.3	5.5	9.0
Particle size (microns)	0.5	0.4	0.4	0.5
Kilocalories per ml	1.1	2.0	1.1	2.0
Source of fat	Soybean	Safflower	Soybean	Soybean
Linoleic acid (%)	50	77	56	50
Oleic acid (%)	26	13	23	26
Palmitic acid (%)	10	7	11	10
Linolenic acid	9	0.1	6	9
Stearic acid (%)	2.5	2.5	?	2.5
Egg phospholipid (%)	1.2	1.2	1.2	1.2
Glycerol (%)	2.3	2.5	2.3	2.3

Special note

Tables 8.10 and 8.11 which show but a few of the parenteral nutrients on the market may seem to contain information which is beyond the brief of the practising surgeon. It is not necessary for

Table 8.10 Examples of the currently available amino acid solutions. They contain from 50–150 g/L of protein and some include daily requirement of electrolytes

Product (manufacturer)	**Protein g/L**	**Electrolytes (mEq/L)**						
		Na	K	Mg	Cl	Acetate	Phosphate (mH/L)	Osmolality
Crystalline amino acid infusions in which electrolytes have been excluded								
Aminosyn 5%	50	—	5.4	—	—	60	—	500
Travasol 8.5%	85	—	—	—	34	52	—	860
Aminosyn 10%	100	—	5.4	—	—	48	—	1000
Travasol 10%	100	—	—	—	40	87	—	1000
Novamine 15%	150	—	—	—	—	151	—	1388
Crystalline amino acid infusions with electrolytes								
Travasol 5.5% w/Electrolytes	55	70	60	10	70	100	30	850
Fre Amine III 8.5%	85	10	—	—	<2	74	10	810
Travasol 8.5% w/Electrolytes	85	70	60	10	70	135	30	1160

Table 8.11 Specialised amino acid solutions. HepatAmine is formulated for patients with hepatic failure, FreAmine HBC for patients with renal failure and BranchAmin for patients with hypercatabolic states

	Hepat-Amine	Branch-Amin	FreAmine HBC
Protein Concentration (%)	8.0	4.0	6.9
Osmolality (mOsmol/L)	785	316	620
Essential amino acids (g/100 ml)			
Isoleucine	900	1380	760
Leucine	1100	1380	1370
Lycine	610	—	410
Methionine	100	—	250
Phenylalanine	100	—	320
Threonine	450	—	200
Tryptophan	66	—	99
Valine	840	1240	880
Nonessential amino acids (g/10 ml)	3.8	0	2.4
Electrolytes (mEq/L)			
Sodium	10	—	10
Potassium	0	—	0
Magnesium	0	—	0
Chloride	<3	—	<3
Acetate	62	—	57
Phosphate	10	—	0

him or her to know details of the components of these solutions and they have been included only to illustrate the range of nutrients that are now commonly available. A comprehensive list is given in Appendix II at the end of the book. The clinician's task is to set the nutritional goal and calculate the requirements of the patient for energy, protein, water, minerals, vitamins and trace metals. It is then up to the pharmacist, who has special training in this area, to work out the appropriate solution that will enable these requirements to be met properly. The nutrients are mixed together and supplied in a 3 L plastic bag, having been mixed in strict aseptic conditions under a laminar flow hood in the pharmacy and with an eye to possible incompatibilities that may occur. It is almost impossible to manage modern parenteral nutrition without the back up of a highly trained pharmacy staff.

9. Enteral nutrition and tube feeding

INTRODUCTION — WHICH ROUTE — ENTERAL OR PARENTERAL?

When it is clear that the patient needs nutritional therapy and the nutritional/metabolic goal has been set consideration is given to selecting the most appropriate route for the administration of the nutrients. As a general rule, if the gastrointestinal tract is working and access to it can be gained safely, feeding via the enteral route is to be preferred. We have seen that the gastrointestinal tract may atrophy without intraluminal nutrition and the normal barrier to the translocation of endotoxins and bacteria is lost. It is thought that the higher proportion of septic episodes that accompany treatment by the parenteral route is related to gut rest with consequent atrophy and loss of gut barrier function (Alverdy et al 1988, Abad-Lacruz et al 1990). Unfortunately, it is not always possible to use the enteral route in surgical patients and administration of the nutrients via the parenteral route is necessary. Total parenteral nutrition is given when disease or dysfunction of the gastrointestinal tract or impossible access preclude its use, or if the use of the enteral route causes increased morbidity. The algorithm shown in Figure 9.1 helps the selection of the most appropriate method of nutritional support. It is not always as simple as this, however, and choosing the best route for a particular patient may require considerable discussion and consultation before a decision can be made.

SECTION I
ORAL NUTRITION

There is no doubt that the natural route for ingestion and assimilation of nutrients is the cheapest and most efficient. To be effective, an intact gastrointestinal tract, an ability to absorb nutrients, a favourable metabolic environment and a motivated patient are required. There are many surgical disorders where diet modification is an essential part of therapy. The dietitian by taking a diet history determines the nutrient content of the food intake and the appropriateness of that intake for the patient (Mason et al 1977). Modifications to oral intake may be made, for instance, by provision of a high energy, high protein diet. Such a diet needs to be adjusted to the needs and tolerance of the patient. To be sufficient to cause nutritional repletion it needs to supply 1000 kcal or more of supplemental energy and provide a minimum of 1.0 g/kg/day of protein. Additional meat, milk and eggs are included and dietary supplements commercially available as Sustacal (extra calories) or Replete (extra protein) can be added to the meals to provide the extra energy or protein that are required. Despite good dietetic services and ingenious manipulation of the presentation of food, many surgical patients fail to increase energy intake sufficiently to maintain body weight.

It has been shown that supplements similar to Sustacal and Replete given in the post operative phase can decrease the postoperative dietary deficit substantially but whether this is of any measurable clinical benefit has not been proven

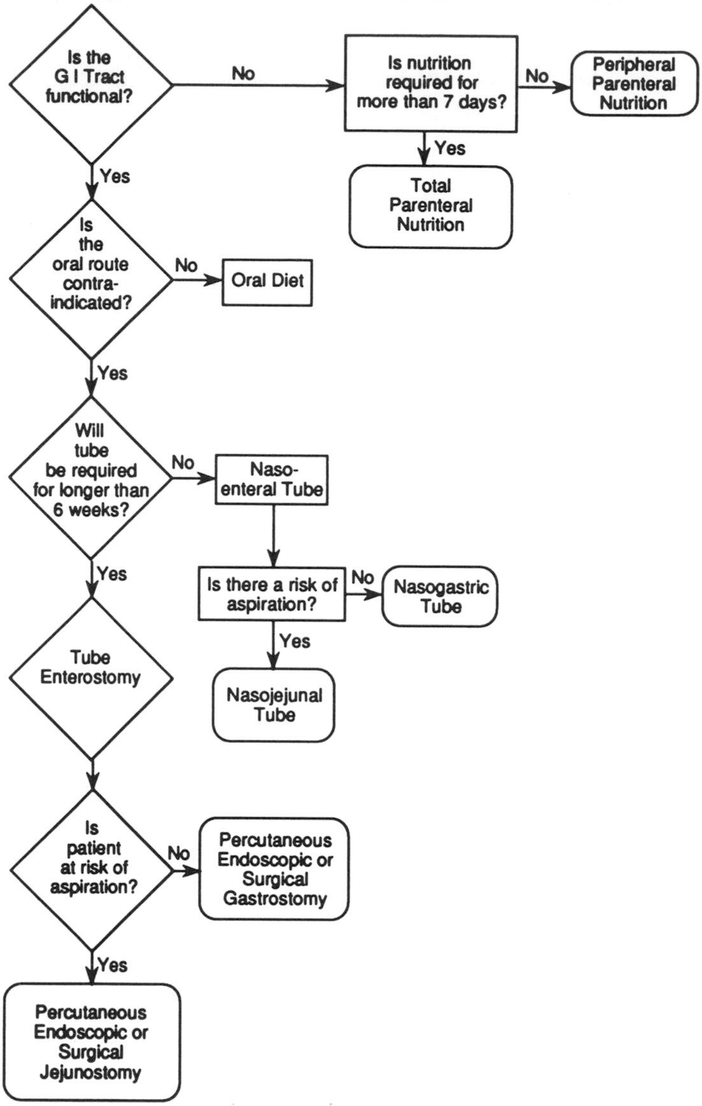

Fig. 9.1 Algorithm for deciding on appropriate feeding route.

(Isaksson et al 1959). Patients with partial obstruction from Crohn's disease (Ch. 13), patients with resection of the terminal ileum (Ch. 17) and patients with the short gut syndrome may all obtain considerable benefit from dietary manipulation and the attentions of a skilled dietitian.

SECTION II
FEEDING INTO THE INTESTINE

Enteral feeding can be used to supplement oral intake or supplement parenteral nutrition, or as a method of using the gastrointestinal tract where disorders of the mouth, oesophagus or stomach prevent natural delivery of food to the small intestine. There is a growing awareness of the importance of enteral nutrition — in its absence there is rapid atrophy of the intestine due mainly to lack of blood flow but also because specific nutrients required by the enterocyte and colonocyte may not be available. As we have seen above (p. 115) absent or inadequate enteral nutrition results in failure of gut barrier function which may lead to translocation of endotoxin and bacteria from the intestine. The gut epithelium prefers certain dietary components. We now know that glutamine and short-chain fatty acids are specific gut fuels. Glutamine is an important fuel for enterocytes and short-chain fatty acids are a preferred fuel source for the colonocyte. There is no doubt that intraluminal nutrients play an integral role in the maintenance of gut structure and the prevention of mucosal atrophy (Saito et al 1987). Moreover, there is an increasing experimental evidence that the earlier the feedings can be started the greater the systemic advantages are to patients with trauma and burns (Mochizuki et al 1984). Studies in the future will focus on the ideal composition of enteral diets with the effects of the nutrients glutamine, fibre, arginine and 3-omega fatty acids being critically analysed as well as evaluating what effects enteral feeding will have on clinical outcome (Bower 1990a). The overall nutritional, metabolic and physiological effects of enteral feeding are the same as those which occur with parenteral nutrition. The same rapid improvement of impaired physiological function is seen and the ability to maintain and accrete body protein is the same (Stokes & Hill 1992, Yeung et al 1979a). Enteral feeding, especially with elemental diets, reduces the volume of chyme and favourably influences the chemical characteristics of fistula drainage (Hill et al 1975c, Hill et al 1976).

INDICATIONS AND CONTRAINDICATIONS FOR ENTERAL NUTRITION

There are three conditions which need to be fulfilled before nutrition via the enteral route should be considered.

- Spontaneous oral intake must be inadequate for nutritional requirements. A careful dietary assessment is needed to determine if energy and protein intake meet estimated requirements.
- The proximal small intestine needs to be functional.
- The gastrointestinal tract needs to be an appropriate route for the administration of nutrients for the patient's condition. This needs careful attention in situations where gut rest is considered part of patient management despite a functional gastrointestinal tract. Acute pancreatitis, or high small bowel fistulas are therefore not appropriately treated by enteral therapy.

Table 9.1 gives a list of the accepted indications and contraindications for enteral nutrition in surgery.

NASOENTERIC FEEDING

Nasoenteric feeding may be used for patients with neoplasms, inflammation or trauma to the oropharynx or oesophagus. In some patients with pancreatitis, inflammatory bowel disease, the short bowel syndrome and low output fistulas it may also be the feeding route of choice. It probably should not be used when it is anticipated that the course of nutritional therapy will be longer than 4–6 weeks.

Table 9.1 Specific indications and contraindications for enteral feeding in surgery

Indications
- Patients with moderate–severe PEM in whom an inadequate oral intake has been received over the previous 3 days
- Patients with mild protein energy malnutrition in whom less than 50% of normal dietary requirements have been taken over the previous 7–10 days
- Dysphagia for all but clear liquids
- Massive enterectomy during recovery period
- Distal enterocutaneous fistulas
- Patients with major trauma in whom it is anticipated that return to full oral intake will be prolonged
- Patients with a prolonged postoperative course
- Some patients with inflammatory bowel disease

Contraindications
- Complete small bowel obstruction
- Ileus
- Severe diarrhoea
- Proximal small bowel fistulas
- Severe pancreatitis
- Shock

Nasogastric tubes may be passed into the stomach or upper jejunum.

The tube lies in the stomach

This is the technique of choice when the risk of aspiration is small or absent. There is no indication for the use of wide bore nasogastric tubes in enteral feeding; they are uncomfortable for the patient and increase the incidence of aspiration and oesophageal ulceration. There are many fine bore tubes on the market with variations of weighted ends, side and end holes, and adaptations to aid placement. Silicone rubber or polyurethane tubes are the most effective because they are soft and well tolerated by most patients. Nevertheless this softness makes them difficult to insert on occasion. Stylets or tube stiffeners are provided with some of these tubes but the whole task is made easier by following a very strict protocol. We use the system advocated by John Rombeau, MD, of Philadelphia (Table 9.2).

Feeding tubes may become blocked when the consistency of the nutrient is too thick for the size of the tube or crushed medicines are passed through it (Fagerman 1988). This problem can usually be prevented by irrigating the tube with 20 ml of normal saline every 6 hours and after each intermittent feeding or use of medications.

Table 9.2 Rombeau's protocol for nasoenteric tube insertion

- Patient in sitting position with neck flexed slightly
- Ensure the stylet can be inserted and removed easily from within the tube
- Measure length of tube required by measuring the length from the tip of the nose to the earlobe and then the earlobe to the xiphisternum — add 50 cm to this length
- Lubricate the end of the tube and pass through patient's nasal passage — ask patient to swallow water to facilitate this
- Once tube is beyond nasopharynx allow patient to rest
- Advance the tube with the patient swallowing, neck is flexed
- If patient begins to cough withdraw the tube back into nasopharynx and start again
- After removal of stylet confirm tube is in stomach by aspiration of gastric contents. If not sure obtain X-ray
- Secure tube to bridge of nose or upper lip with non-allergenic tape
- Tape tube securely to bridge of nose or upper lip

Carbonated beverage is injected down the tube if an obstruction occurs. Very occasionally when this does not work a fine guidewire is passed down the tube under radiological control to break down the blockage (Metheny et al 1988).

Aspiration is the most serious complication of nasogastric feeding. Patients who are confused or have depressed central nervous function are particularly at risk, as are those with known gastro-oesophageal reflux (Cogen & Weinrijb 1989). Nasogastric feeding should not be used in such patients. Aspiration may still occur with fine bore tubes particularly at night and patients should be encouraged to sleep semirecumbent to avoid this potentially serious problem.

The tube lies in the small intestine

Nasojejunal feeding may be used on a short term basis (up to 4–6 weeks) in patients who are at high risk of aspiration. Slightly larger silicone rubber or polyurethane tubes about a metre long with non-absorbable mercury weights at their tips are passed on into the jejunum. It has been shown that the optimal position i.e the one with least risk of aspiration is the proximal jejunum just distal to the ligament of Trietz. A weighted flexible tube of this type lying in the stomach passes into the duodenum within 1–2 days in most patients, particularly so when the patient is encouraged to turn on his or her right side. When this does not occur passage can usually be achieved after one or two doses of 10 mg i.v. metoclopramide. If the tube still will not pass into the duodenum the aid of an endoscopist or interventional radiologist should be sought. After all this, it must be said that there is always the possibility that the tip of a nasoduodenal or nasojejunal tube will reflux or be inadvertently withdrawn back into the stomach where the potential for aspiration is increased.

Tube enterostomy

Small bore gastrostomy, gastroduodenostomy, or jejunostomy tubes have made intubation of the gut possible at any level. This may be done directly via laparotomy in the anaesthetised patient or percutaneously, either with the help of an endoscopist or radiologist in the unanaesthetised patient. Tube enterostomy is used when enteral nutrition is required for longer than 4–6 weeks. When aspiration is a real possibility tube jejunostomy is preferred to tube gastrostomy. Generally speaking tube enterostomy is indicated in patients with upper gastrointestinal obstruction — stricture or neoplasm of the oropharynx, oesophagus, stomach or duodenum — or it is used as an adjunct to major surgery. Such patients may include those who have had laparotomy for very major trauma (see Ch. 20), or oesophagectomy, total gastrectomy, pancreato-duodenectomy or massive enterectomy.

Surgical techniques

Gastrostomy. There are three common types of surgical gastrostomies: Stamm, Witzel and Janeway. The Stamm and Witzel techniques are performed when the gastrostomy is to be temporary whereas the Janeway procedure or a modification of it is used when permanent gastrostomy is required. Figures 9.2, 9.3 and 9.4 show how each of these gastrostomies is formed. The disadvantage of a surgically performed gastrostomy includes the risk of the anaesthetic and the laparotomy and there is the possibility of a wound infection. On the other hand these procedures allow the placement of a bigger tube, more accurate tube placement and if a combined gastrojejunal tube is used more accurate placement of the tube in the upper jejunum.

Jejunostomy. The Witzel technique can also be used for placement of a feeding catheter in the upper jejunum. More popular now is the technique of fine needle catheter jejunostomy (Fig. 9.5). Considerable care in placement and anchoring of these catheters is required for free peritoneal leak, small bowel fistula and pneumatosis intestinalis are complications which have been described. Fine needle catheter jejunostomy has been described mostly as a post-operative feeding technique (Yeung et al 1979b) or as the technique of choice for feeding after laparotomy for trauma (see Ch. 21).

Percutaneous techniques

Percutaneous endoscopic gastrostomy and *percutaneous endoscopic jejunostomy* (PEG and PEJ) are techniques for tube intubation which are still

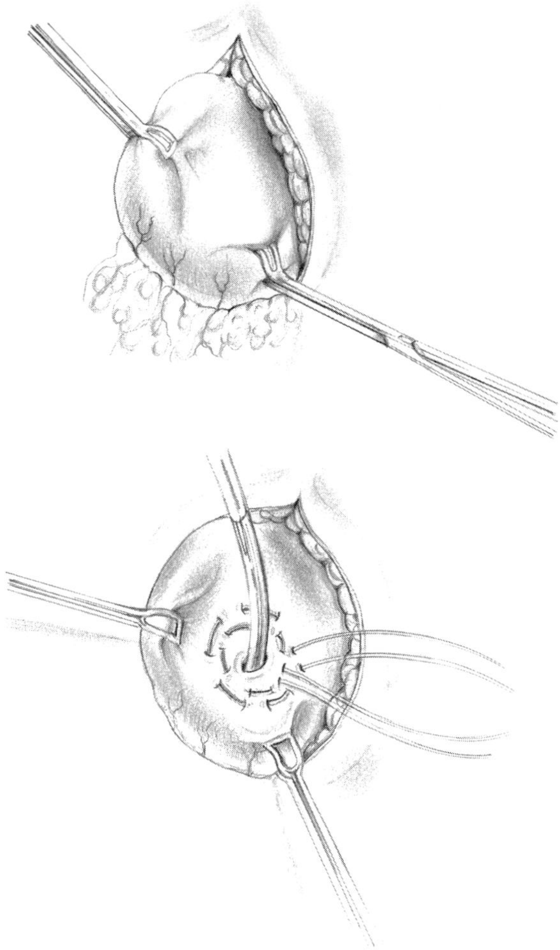

Fig. 9.2 Stamm gastrostomy: provides for temporary placement of a Foley or mushroom catheter into the stomach. This is the technique we use most often for surgical gastrostomy.

being evolved. Their safety and relative ease of insertion have caused a minor revolution in the practice of enteral feeding. For insertion the so-called 'pull method' is the most widely used and reported (Gauderer & Ponsky 1980). The first description of the technique of PEG was by this method in which the gastrostomy tube is pulled retrograde down the oesophagus into the stomach and out through the abdominal wall (Gauderer & Ponsky 1980). Other methods modifying this original technique have been described more recently (Ponsky & Gauderer 1989).

The pull method. The patient is prepared in the usual way as for gastroscopy. Prophylactic

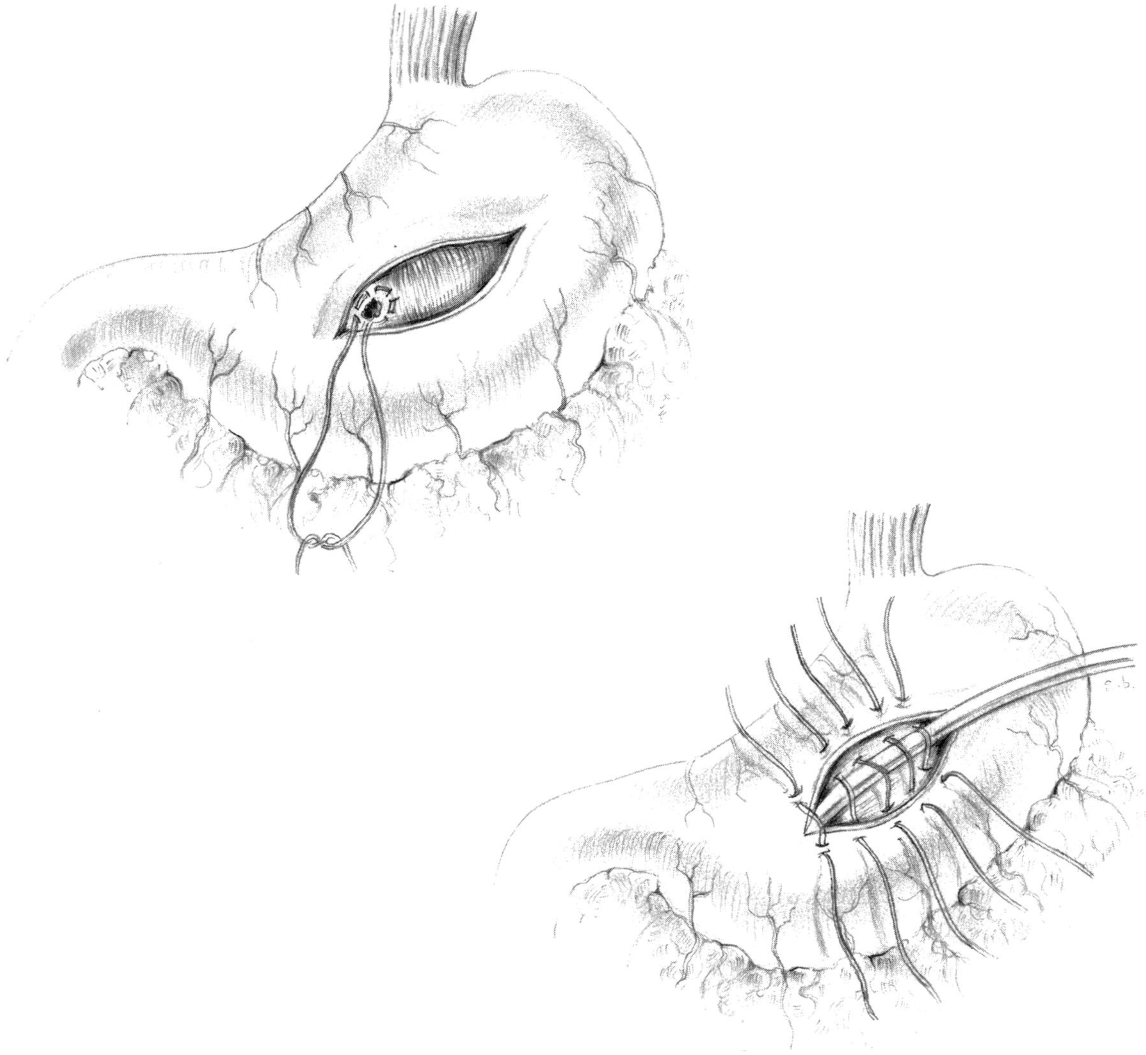

Fig. 9.3 Witzel gastrostomy. An 18F rubber catheter is placed in a submucosal tunnel before passing into the stomach. This is a temporary gastrostomy.

antibiotics are administered half an hour before the procedure. The abdomen is prepared as for a surgical operation and drapes are applied. Various gastrostomy tubes may be used for this procedure but a tube with a compressible–expandable polyurethane balloon is one of the better types (Fig. 9.6).

The endoscope is inserted and passed into the stomach which is fully inflated. The room lights are turned off and as the gastroscope is positioned just proximal to the incisura the assistant observes the transilluminated stomach through the abdominal wall. The point of maximum transillumination is that in which the stomach wall is apposed without the intervention of other organs to the parieties of the abdominal wall. Finger pressure on the abdominal wall at this site allows the endoscopist to see an indentation of the gastric wall. When the correct site, which is usually in the left upper quadrant, is agreed on by both the assistant and the endoscopist the endoscopist opens a polypectomy snare alongside the stomach wall at this site. The assistant infiltrates the area with a local anaesthetic and makes a short incision in the skin and subcutaneous tissue. A 16-gauge intravenous cannula is passed through the

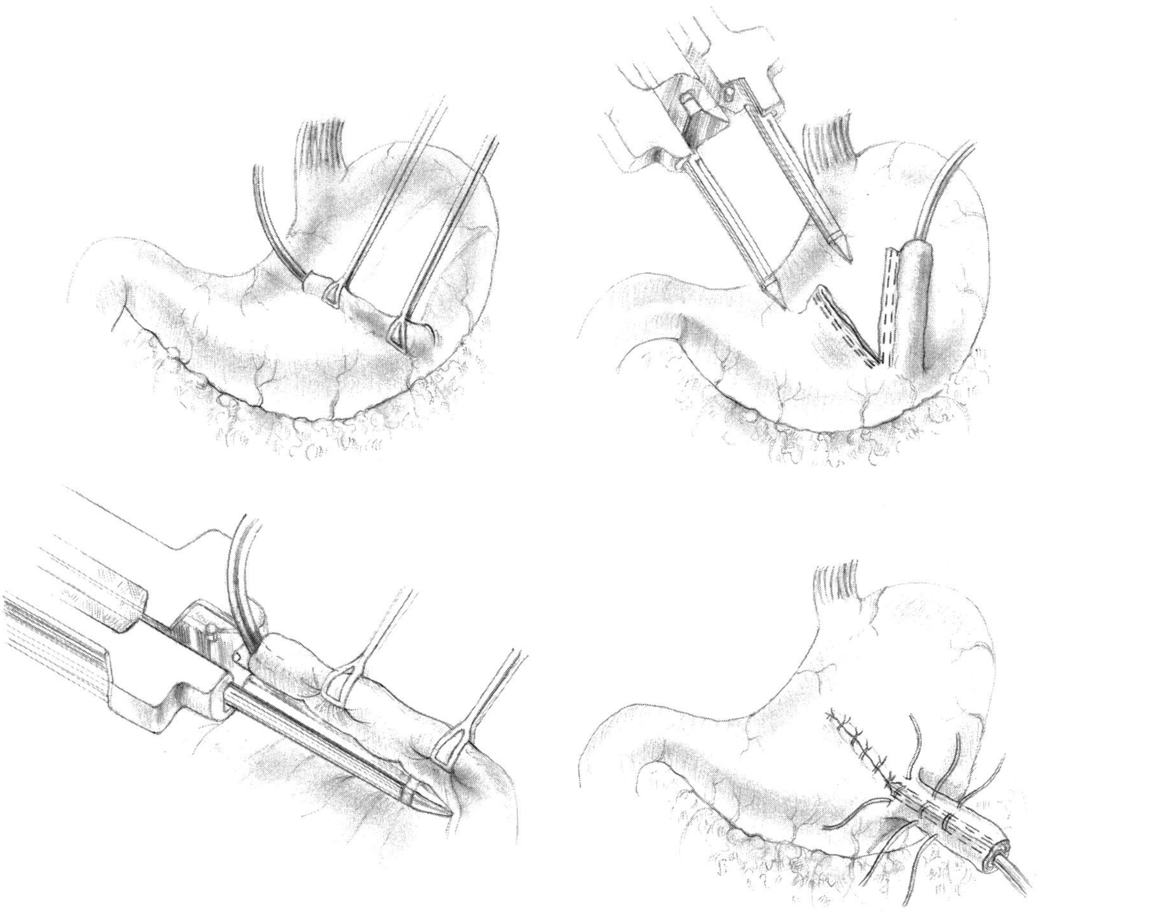

Fig. 9.4 Janeway permanent gastrostomy. A gastric tube is made from the anterior stomach wall using a stapling device. At the skin level a flat stoma is created; the mucocutaneous sutures are silk.

abdominal wall and through the gastric wall into the stomach to lie within the circumference of the snare. The snare is then tightened around the cannula. The needle within the cannula is removed and replaced by a long length of number 2 nylon. The nylon is threaded through the cannula into the stomach where it is grasped by the endoscopy snare. The scope, the snare and its contained suture are pulled up out of the stomach, through the oesophagus and out the patient's mouth. The nylon suture is then attached to the tapered end of the polyurethane gastrostomy tube. Once it is firmly attached and the tube and mouth are sterilised with antiseptic solution the assistant pulls on the nylon suture and the gastrostomy tube proceeds retrogradely down the oesophagus into the stomach and out through its wall and through the abdominal wall. After several inches of the tube have exited through the abdominal wall the gastroscope is once again inserted and the endoscopist looks particularly for the soft balloon of the gastroscopy tube. The assistant tugs externally on the tube and when the endoscopist notes that the balloon lies gently on the gastric mucosa without blanching the pulling ceases and the gastrostomy tube is anchored. Great care is required here to prevent ischaemia and necrosis of the gastric mucosa and gastric wall. Figure 9.6 shows how the gastrostomy tube lies in the stomach and how it is safely applied to the skin of the abdominal wall. It must be remembered that excessive tension will lead to stomach wall necrosis and early extrusion of the tube. During the next few days

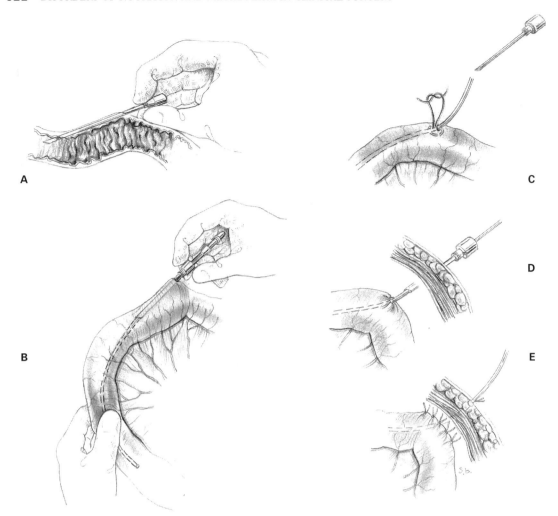

Fig. 9.5 Technique of fine needle catheter jejunostomy. **A** A needle is tunnelled in the submucosal layer of the proximal jejunum. **B** A fine plastic catheter is inserted through the needle into the lumen of the jejunum. **C** The needle is removed and the catheter is firmly anchored to the jejunal wall with an absorbable suture. **D** The remaining catheter is now passed through the abdominal wall. **E** Most important of all is the attachment of the jejunum with absorbable sutures to the parieties. The jejunum must lie in a smooth arc and kinking of the bowel at this point must be avoided.

it is important to look and ensure that excessive tension is not being applied to the tube and if this is present it is necessary to release the collar to compensate for the underlying expansion of the abdominal wall. Feedings are begun in the morning following the procedure.

The push technique. The principle here is for the placement of a guidewire through the abdominal wall into the stomach and out through the oesophagus and mouth which then allows a specially modified firm gastrostomy tube with a tapered end to be pushed down over the guidewire and out through the abdominal wall. There seems to be little difference in the results or difficulty in insertion between the 'pull' and 'push' techniques (Hogan et al 1986).

The introducer technique. The introducer technique is similar in concept to that used during the insertion of a subclavian catheter. The gastroscope is introduced as above and the appropriate site for puncture is identified. A needle is thrust into the stomach through the identified site and a guidewire is passed through the lumen of the needle. The needle is then withdrawn. An

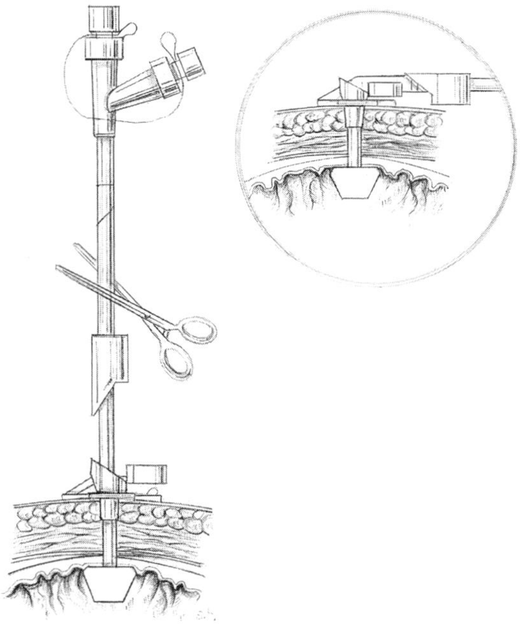

Fig. 9.6 Bower PEG polyurethane tube after placement in the stomach. Note the retention balloon, the tube fixation device at the skin level and the Y adaptor which allows irrigation of the tube without disconnection of the feeding portal. The pointed proximal end has been cut off after it has penetrated the gastric wall and abdominal wall.

introducer with a peel away sheath around is then passed over the guidewire and into the stomach. Once the introducer and the sheath are in place, the introducer is removed and a Foley catheter is inserted through the sheath. Once the balloon is inflated the sheath is peeled away leaving the Foley catheter lying in the stomach.

These endoscopic procedures although considerably less traumatic than the surgical techniques (Jones et al 1990), are still not without danger. Septic complications are the most common problems with necrotising fasciitis having been described (Person & Brower 1986). This is relatively rare although minor infections around the tube are fairly common. It is encouraging to know, however, that those who perform PEG regularly have reported a marked dimunition in their complication rate with increasing experience. They also cite the use of prophylactic antibiotics and very great care over the pressure which is applied to the tube as being especially important. The surgeon should not be too concerned if pneumoperitoneum is seen after this procedure for it appears to be of no clinical consequence (Stassen et al 1986).

If a jejunal tube is required as well as a gastrostomy tube then a special combination tube is inserted. This allows the passage of a fine bore jejunal tube through a side arm of the gastrostomy tube down through the pylorus into the upper jejunum. One PEJ technique is described in which two tubes are inserted, a 16 french rubber gastric tube and an 8 french polyurethane jejunal tube (Figure 9.7). The combination gastrostomy/jejunal tube is now the most popular form of jejunostomy allowing direct jejunal feeding whilst at the same time allowing gastric aspiration if required.

Radiological techniques. Tubes may also be placed percutaneously under radiological guidance, thereby avoiding endoscopy altogether. A polyurethane tube which is both a combined jejunostomy and gastrostomy tube which is passed percutaneously and transpylorically with fluoroscopic not endoscopic guidance is now available.

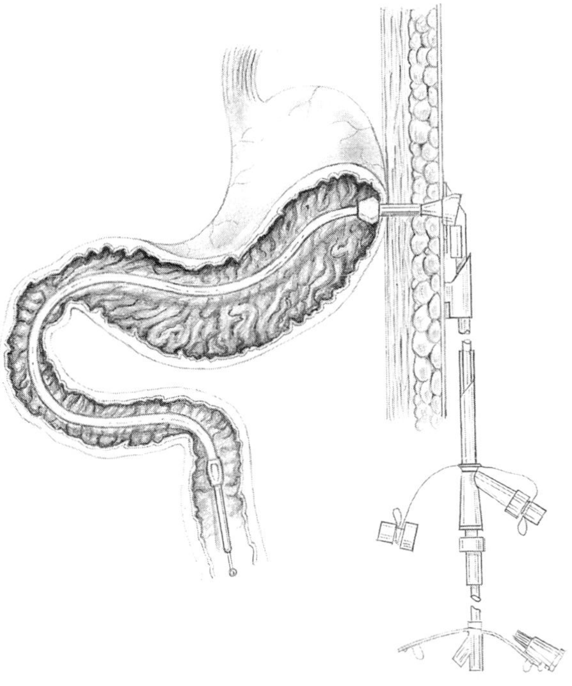

Fig. 9.7 A 'Silk' jejunostomy tube is placed through the Bower gastrostomy tube into the upper jejunum. This can be done by either spontaneous passage, fluoroscopy or endoscopy.

Technical points concerning siting of tube in the stomach

- It must be near the antrum. Since one of the main reasons for the gastrostomy tube is decompression its placement in the stomach is critical. The antral mill is mainly responsible for gastric emptying and it is therefore best to place the gastrostomy tube in or just proximal to the antrum. When there has been a previous Billroth I gastrectomy the tube should be as near to the anastomosis as possible.
- The tube should be placed opposite the incisura to avoid sharp angulation of the stomach. Impaired gastric emptying will occur if, when the gastric wall and the parieties are apposed, the stomach is sharply angulated. If that portion of the stomach near the greater curve opposite the incisura is used this is unlikely to happen.
- It is important to avoid perforating the left lobe of the liver or the transverse colon during insertion of the tube. If these structures intervene between the stomach wall and the parieties clear translumination of the stomach through the abdominal wall is not possible. Furthermore when the technique of digitally indenting the stomach wall is used a localised indentation is not seen when the transverse colon or a large left lobe of the liver intervenes between the two structures.

COMPLICATIONS OF PEG AND PEJ

- Perforation of the upper gastrointestinal tract during placement or aspiration may occur while the patient is sedated. Transient bacteraemias and local sepsis have been described. Quite nasty abdominal wall infections have been associated with these techniques.
- Jejunal tube malposition. The jejunal tube that is placed via the stomach has an annoying problem of migrating back into the stomach in perhaps 20% of cases. Although it may be repositioned endoscopically or fluoroscopically it sometimes proves to be an insuperable recurrent problem.
- Obstruction of the tube. The smaller tubes may block when an incompletely blenderised diet is used or there is excessive administration of phosphate or calcium, or the injection of medication down the tube without subsequent flushing. Blockage can usually be prevented by regular flushing of the tube with 20 ml of saline every 6 hours or so. If medications are passed into the tube it is important for the nurse to follow this with another irrigation of 20 ml of saline.
- Post-removal fistula. After removal of either a gastroscope or jejunal tube an enterocutaneous fistula may develop. If the nutritional state of the patient is good, underlying sepsis is controlled and there is no distal obstruction, then the fistula will invariably close.

SECTION III
ADMINISTRATION OF TUBE DIETS

INFUSION RATE

With fine bore tubes, continuous infusion of nutrients is preferable because nursing care is easier and there is less diarrhoea and fewer problems with nausea and vomiting. Although 3 L of nutrient solution can quite easily be administered by gravity feeding over a 24-hour period, the use of a pump enables a more constant infusion to be maintained. Feeding should be commenced gradually usually at full strength at around 25 ml per hour, increasing by 10 ml per hour every 6 hours as tolerated until full intake is reached. Feeding into the duodenum is initially half strength but at the same rate. By the third or fourth day it is usually possible to give full strength formula. Poor tolerance is noted clinically by the presence of vomiting, severe intestinal colic, increased abdominal distension, and worsening diarrhoea.

MONITORING

As with all forms of nutritional therapy there is need for careful monitoring of the patient with regard to fluid and electrolytes, watching for fluid retention, hyperglycaemia and electrolyte imbalances. A standard protocol should be used to ensure uniformity of care, nutritional goals are met and complications kept to a minimum (Table 9.3).

COMPLICATIONS

These are gastrointestinal (mainly diarrhoea), mechanical (mainly blockages), metabolic (similar to those with parenteral nutrition) and infections (infected diet). *Diarrhoea* which is a common complication is usually corrected by slowing the rate of delivery and by reducing the osmotic load. After ensuring that this is not infectious diarrhoea we begin by reducing the rate of infusion to 20 ml/h and then if diarrhoea continues reduce the osmotic load by diluting the nutrient solution by half. If diarrhoea still persists 30 ml of kaolin–pectin is injected down the tube followed by a 20 ml saline irrigation. If after 36 hours, during which kaolin–pectin has been administered every 4 hours, diarrhoea is still a problem loperamide (2–4 mg b.d.) is used.

It is not clear whether patients with hypoalbuminaemia have impaired absorption of the nutrient solution or not but many clinicians feel that diarrhoea is more common in hypoalbuminaemic patients (Brinson et al 1987, Edes et al 1990). One just needs to examine a small bowel radiological study in such a patient to realise the gross mucosal swelling and oedema that accompanies low levels of plasma albumin and it defies the imagination to believe that absorption from its lumen is not impaired. We therefore return albumin levels to the normal range before commencing enteral nutrition. There is also considerable debate over the efficiency of fibre-containing enteral formulas in preventing or controlling diarrhoea (Dobb & Towler 1990). To date there are no clear data that show unquestionably that fibre-containing enteral formulas are of value in this setting (Scheppach et al 1990). Sometimes all efforts to control enteral diet induced diarrhoea are of no avail and the patient must be fed by the parenteral route.

Table 9.3 Protocol for enteral nutrition

- Ensure tube is in correct position
- If the tube is in the stomach elevate head of the bed 45°
- Check volume, concentration, and duration and rate of infusion of the liquid formula
- Formula should not hang for longer than 8 hours
- Aspirate stomach every 4 hours — if there is more than 50% of ordered volume stop feeding for 4 hours. If problem persists, inform medical staff
- Weigh patient Monday, Wednesday and Friday; if more than 0.3 kg has been gained on more than two occasions inform medical staff
- Record intake and output of fluid daily
- Change administration set daily
- If blockages occur irrigate tube with 20 ml saline every 6 hours
- Plasma electrolytes on Monday and Friday
- If tube is blocked irrigate with 20 ml of carbonated drink

SECTION IV
TYPES OF ENTERAL DIETS

Before enteral nutrition can be started the most appropriate diet must be selected. The help of an experienced dietitian is most valuable here for there has been a proliferation of commercially produced enteral diets and at this time of writing over 100 are commercially available. The surgeon must work out the patient's requirements for protein, energy, fluid, electrolytes and vitamins and explain to the dietitian the type of disease and the likely effects of it on the ability of the patient to absorb or retain the administered nutrients. The ideal formula for normal nutritional needs should have about 1000 kcal/L with the nitrogen/calorie ratio of about 1/200. Broadly speaking, formulas can be classified into 5 groups, that is *meal replacements, supplements, feeding components* and *elemental diets*, and *disease specific* diets. Table 9.4 describes these broad categories and lists their most appropriate uses. A comprehensive list of available enteral nutrients is given in Appendix II.

Table 9.4 Enteral nutrition formulae (a complete list is given in Appendix II)

Classification	Constituents	Use	Examples	Composition
Meal replacements	Balanced proportions of protein, carbohydrate and fat with electrolytes	Provide complete and balanced meals	Ensure, Isocal, Osmolite, Clinifeed	1 kcal/ml; 30–50 g protein/L
Supplements	Proportions of protein, carbohydrate and fat with particular emphasis on either protein or carbohydrates	Added to regular meals to provide extra calories or protein	Sustacal-HC (extra calories) Replete (extra protein)	1.5 kcal/ml 62 g protein/L
Feeding components	Only one or two components	Used to make up specific diets for specific purposes	Polycose (carbohydrate) MCT oil (fat) Casec (protein)	Glucose polymers 2 kcal/ml 8.3 kcal/g 95% protein
Elemental diets	No-residue balanced diets with protein components reduced to basic elements (amino acids, simple sugars)	Suggested for malabsorption pancreatic insufficiency	Travasorb Vivonex	1 kcal/ml 30 g AA/L 1 kcal/ml 44 g AA/L
Disease specific diets	Basic nutrients in monomeric form. Contains amino acids in different proportions and higher concentrations of carbohydrate	Stress	Vivonex TEN Traum-Aid HBC	33% branched-chain amino acids 50% branched-chain amino acids
		Hepatic encephalopathy	Hepatic-Aid Travasorb hepatic diet	Increased branched-chain amino acids, decreased aromatic amino acids
		Renal failure	Travasorb renal diet	Contains all essential amino acids but no nonessential amino acids

SECTION V
DISEASE SPECIFIC ENTERAL DIETS

HYPERCATABOLIC STATES

Formulas enriched with branched-chain amino acids (BCAA) are proposed for patients with hypercatabolic states. Major trauma and sepsis are particular examples. Up to 40–50% of the total amino acids are supplied as BCAA (leucine, isoleucine and valine) and it is argued that their administration improves nitrogen balance by serving as precursors of muscle protein in stressed patients (Brennan 1986). To date no clinical benefit has yet been shown for these so called 'stress formulas'.

LIVER FAILURE

Formulas designed for hypercatabolic patients with hepatic encephalopathy contain increased amounts of BCAAs and decreased quantities of aromatic amino acids (i.e. phenylalanine, tyrosine and tryptophan) and of the sulphur-containing amino acid methionine. Studies suggest that such solutions improve mental recovery from high grade encephalopathy but some suggest caution because of the potential for increased mortality. The conclusion of a recent meta-analysis of trials to date suggest that further trials are required before such solutions should be widely used (Berlin & Chalmers 1989).

RENAL FAILURE

Formulas containing all essential amino acids but lacking in nonessential amino acids are designed for patients with renal failure who do not need dialysis or who are receiving broad spectrum antibiotics which reduce urea recycling by colonic bacteria. These formulas promote the re-use of the nitrogen contained in urea and may have a place in this setting. This complex subject is reviewed in depth by Steffe & Anderson (1984).

For further discussion on disease specific diets see Chapter 10.

10. Parenteral nutrition

INTRODUCTION — A NEW DEVELOPMENT AND NEW INSIGHTS

Total parenteral nutrition is the provision of all nutrient requirements intravenously without use of the gastrointestinal tract. The development of total parenteral nutrition (TPN) as a practical clinical proposition came in the 1960s when safe techniques were found for the administration of hypertonic nutrient solutions into the superior vena cava (Dudrick et al 1968). The clinical use of TPN led to exciting advances in surgical practice with a growing appreciation of the problems of malnutrition in surgical patients and new insights into complex surgical disease and how particularly difficult surgical problems might be successfully managed (Wilmore & Dudrick 1968).

SECTION I
INDICATIONS FOR TOTAL PARENTERAL NUTRITION

THE GEORGETOWN FORUM

The Programme on Technology and Health Care of the Georgetown University School of Medicine convened an invited forum to establish practice guidelines for health professionals on the technique of total parenteral nutrition (Pillar & Perry 1990). Their final report pointed out that TPN is used in a number of specialties, such as surgery, paediatrics, gastroenterology, oncology and critical care, and although hard evidence of its efficacy was not always available, there are many in those specialities who find it an indispensible part of modern day treatment.

The Georgetown forum suggested that the primary indication for the use of TPN is dysfunction of the gastrointestinal tract. It is particularly applicable to the following situations in general surgery:

- *Preoperatively,* to improve surgical outcome (see Chs 11 & 18)
- *Postoperatively,* for patients with ileus or wound infection, or in whom gastrointestinal function is not adequate for a prolonged period (see Chs 15 & 18)
- *For inflammatory bowel disease* (Ch. 13), pancreatitis (Ch. 20) and massive enterectomy (Ch. 14)
- *For patients with protein energy malnutrition* who have organ failure, major sepsis, some malignancies and trauma (see Chs 12 & 19 to 22).

INDICATIONS FOR TPN IN GENERAL SURGICAL PRACTICE

As surgeons, we find it easier to divide the indications according to the condition of the alimentary tract, namely:

When the alimentary tract is obstructed

Patients with oesophageal, gastric or upper intestinal malignancies who need preoperative nutritional therapy and in whom the enteral route can not be used are prime examples.

When the alimentary tract is too short

This includes those patients who have had a massive enterectomy. Generally speaking, when less than 3 metres of small bowel remain, a number of serious metabolic and nutritional abnormalities occur, although these can usually be treated by dietary means. When 2 metres or less of small bowel remain most patients require a period of TPN but eventually may be weaned from it. On the other hand those patients with less than 1 metre of small bowel remaining need TPN at home on an indefinite basis.

When the alimentary tract is fistulated

Enterocutaneous fistulas, particularly in the upper small intestine, are particular examples of the value of TPN in modern surgical practice.

When the alimentary tract is inflamed

The perioperative care of patients with Crohn's disease and ulcerative colitis are prime examples of the use of TPN in this setting.

When the alimentary tract cannot cope

Such patients include those with an ileus secondary to major intraabdominal sepsis or inflammatory processes such as pancreatitis.

SECTION II
METHODS USED FOR PARENTERAL NUTRITION

There are three forms of parenteral nutritional support that are being used in general surgery. While each has a place in the nutritional support of patients, total parenteral nutrition through the central venous route remains the standard method of providing balanced nutrition for surgical patients.

PROTEIN SPARING THERAPY

Dextrose free amino acid solutions given via a peripheral vein have been shown to have a nitrogen sparing effect. The concept is to promote low glucose and low insulin concentrations in plasma which in turn allow mobilisation of endogenous fat stores that satisfy the energy deficit by ketogenesis (Blackburn et al 1973). It has been shown that, if additional glucose is given in situations such as this, nitrogen sparing is less and that elevation of insulin impairs visceral protein synthesis. After a short period of enthusiastic use it is now clear that this form of therapy has a very small place in clinical surgery. There is no doubt that amino acids alone are protein sparing, they can be given via peripheral veins and are associated with fewer side effects than when full TPN is given. Nevertheless in a major prospective study of 30 patients undergoing rectal excision (Young & Hill 1980) we showed that the postoperative provision of the patient's energy requirements together with the amino acids has marked clinical and metabolic advantages compared with amino acids alone. In this study body composition, plasma proteins and plasma amino acids were compared in each of three groups of patients (n=10) before and 15 days after rectal excision: group 1 — received no TPN, group 2 — received amino acids alone for 14 days postoperatively, group 3 — received full TPN for 14 days postoperatively. Infusion of amino acids alone spared body protein (Fig. 10.1) but branched-chain amino acids were increased well above normal values and plasma proteins did not increase. In contrast TPN spared more body protein and fat and restored plasma proteins (Fig. 10.2) and amino acids and was associated with a better clinical outcome (Fig. 10.3). This study convinced us that there are very few indications for the use of isotonic dextrose free amino acid solutions in surgical practice.

PERIPHERAL PARENTERAL NUTRITION (PPN)

The standard solution used for total parenteral nutrition through the central venous route contains nearly 2000 mOsmol/L. The physical properties of such solutions encourage thrombosis of peripheral veins and it was not until catheterisation of the superior vena cava became practical and safe that such hyperosmolar

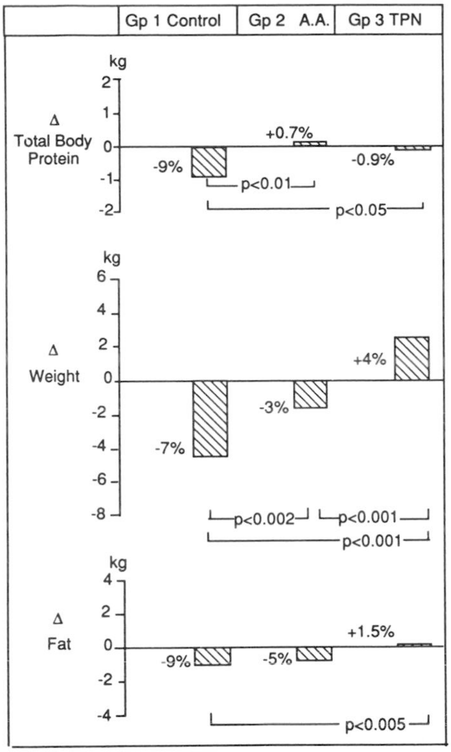

Fig. 10.1 Changes in body composition over 15 postoperative days in controls (group 1), patients treated with amino acids alone (group 2) and patients given a full course of TPN (group 3). It can be seen that both peripheral amino acid therapy and full TPN spared body protein. (Redrawn from Young G A, Hill G L 1980 Ann Surg 192: 183, by permission of the publisher, J B Lippincot Company.)

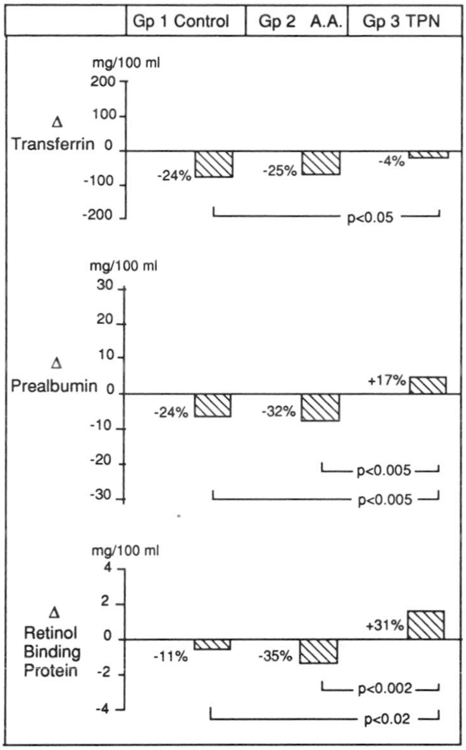

Fig. 10.2 Changes in plasma proteins over 15 postoperative days in controls (group 1), patients treated with amino acids alone (group 2), and patients given a full course of TPN (Group 3). It can be seen that only full TPN restored plasma proteins to normal. (Redrawn from Young G A, Hill G L 1980 Ann Surg 192: 183, by permission of the publisher, J B Lippincot Company.)

solutions could be given for any length of time to surgical patients. Nutrient solutions which are only slightly hypertonic (somewhere between 600 and 900 mOsmol/L) can be prepared by mixing appropriate proportions of amino acid and dextrose solutions and fat emulsions. With large volumes of fluid such solutions can be administered through peripheral veins for short periods (about a week or so). These nutrient mixtures have a low caloric density (about half that of standard parenteral nutrition) providing only about 1500 kcal in 3 L of solution (Freeman & Fairful-Smith 1983).

Technique for PPN

Catheter care

We use the protocol recommended by Hessov et al (1977) and used successfully in a large number of patients (142 patients for a total of 700 days) by Nordenstrom et al (1991).

The largest possible arm vein is used, the veins on the back of the hands are avoided and thin (1.0 mm diameter) short plastic cannulae are used. The daily nutritional programme is completed within 12 hours. After completing the infusion, the catheter is immediately removed. The following day when the infusion is recommenced the contralateral arm is used. At the end of the infusion period it is not necessary to take precautions against rebound hypoglycaemia.

Intravenous nutrients

The PPN mixture we use contains 1 L of Synthamin 9 (with electrolytes), 1 L of 10%

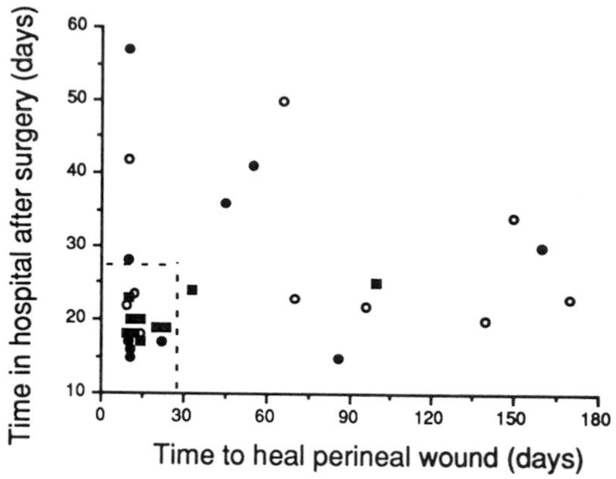

Fig. 10.3 Clinical results of a controlled study of dextrose free amino acids and total parenteral nutrition after excision of the rectum. The postoperative hospital stay and time taken for perineal wound healing in 30 patients are shown. Patients at home with healed perineal wounds within 4 weeks of surgery are enclosed by the broken lines. It can be seen that 8 out of the 10 patients who received TPN were home with healed perineal wounds within 4 weeks. This is significantly better than either of the other two groups ($p < 0.05$). Key: controls = ●; dextrose free amino acids = ○; total parenteral nutrition = ■ (Redrawn from Collins J P, Oxby C B, Hill G L 1978 Lancet 1: 788, with permission.)

Intralipid and 1 L of 18% dextrose. This gives 9 g of N and 1620 non protein kcals with an osmolality of 680 mOsmol/L. The electrolyte content is 70 mmol of Na, 60 mmol of K, 5 mmol of Mg, 70 mmol of Cl, 30 mmol of PO_4 and 100 mmol of acetate. It has a shelf life of 1 month.

Clinical results of PPN

In our own study in which we compared the effect of nutritional therapy in 9 patients who received PPN with 21 patients receiving TPN we found that PPN was as effective as TPN. There was a significant improvement in grip strength and Peak Expiratory Flow Rate over 5 days in both groups (Stokes 1991). Nordenstrom et al (1991) using similarly compounded nutrient solutions found an incidence of phlebitis of 18%, and 75% of their patients were fed successfully by PPN until resumption of oral nutrition. This incidence of phlebitis is similar to that found by others receiving isotonic glucose solutions or various other non-nutritional solutions (Falchuk et al 1985).

In our practice the place of peripheral total parenteral nutrition is limited to:

- supplementing enteral nutrition which cannot meet requirements because of continuing gastrointestinal dysfunction
- providing basal requirements in non-depleted patients who can tolerate 3 L of water per day
- patients in whom a central line is contraindicated.

CENTRAL TOTAL PARENTERAL NUTRITION (TPN)

The development of central venous catheterisation has enabled the safe delivery of hypertonic solutions. The glucose, fat and amino acid admixture is given through a central venous line with its tip in the superior vena cava. The solutions used for central venous nutrient infusion (TPN) usually contain 1 kcal/ml, and water and electrolyte requirements are prescribed to meet the individual patient's requirements. The key to successful TPN is in the insertion and care of the central venous cannula.

Insertion of central venous cannula

The Dudrick technique. A 20-cm-long 16 gauge radio-opaque silicone catheter passed into the subclavian vein and on into the superior vena cava through a 5 cm 14 gauge needle under strict aseptic conditions is the technique described by Stanley Dudrick which has gained wide acceptance because it is associated with the fewest number of problems. With practice there is almost no occasion on which this route cannot be used (Dudrick & Copeland 1973).

The initial step is to place the patient on his back with the foot of the bed elevated to 15°. A small pad is placed between the shoulder blades to allow the shoulders to drop backwards. The skin is prepared with betadine solution in the same manner as for a surgical operation. The drapes are placed carefully and the operator who is scrubbed up wears gown, gloves and a hat. Local anaesthetic is infiltrated into the skin, subcutaneous tissue and periosteum at the inferior

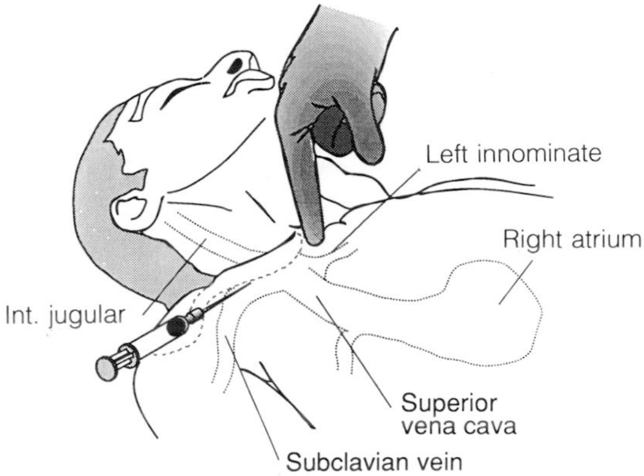

Fig. 10.4 A 14 gauge needle is inserted just lateral to the midpoint of the clavicle and directed toward the suprasternal notch. Puncture of the subclavian vein is indicated by a flush of blood into the syringe. (From Dudrick S J, Copeland E M 1973 Surgery annual, by permission of the publisher, Appleton-Century-Crofts.)

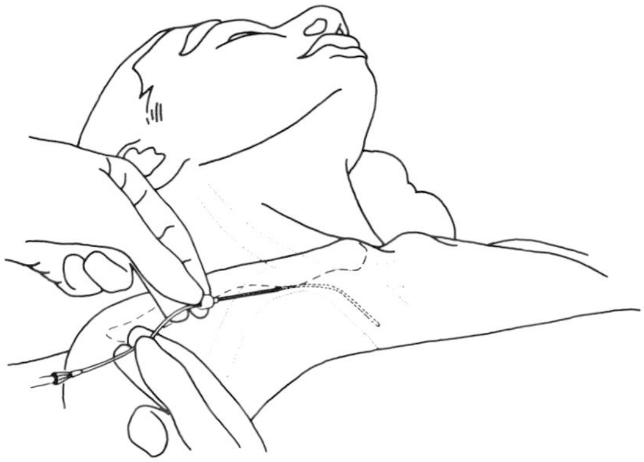

Fig. 10.5 A 16 gauge catheter is advanced into the vein to lie in the superior vena cava. (From Dudrick S J, Copeland E M 1973 Surgery annual, by permission of the publisher, Appleton-Century-Crofts.)

border just lateral to the mid point of the clavicle. The needle, attached to a small syringe, is advanced towards the tip of the finger which is placed firmly in the suprasternal notch (Fig. 10.4). The needle should be very close to the inferior surface of the clavicle and penetration of the subclavian vein is signalled by a rush of blood into the syringe. The needle is advanced a few millimeters more to ensure that it is entirely within the vein. The patient is then asked to perform a Valsalva manoeuvre and the thumb is held over the needle hub as the syringe is removed. The radio-opaque catheter is then introduced through the needle and threaded into the superior vena cava (Fig. 10.5). The needle is then withdrawn from the patient and a small plastic cuff is fitted over the junction of the catheter and needle tip. The catheter is then connected to an intravenous administration set and a slow infusion of normal saline is begun while the catheter is sewn to the skin (Fig. 10.6). Antiseptic ointment is applied around the entrance of the catheter into the skin and a dressing is applied over it including the junction of the intravenous tubing and the hub of the catheter (Fig. 10.7). Confirmation that the catheter is in the correct place is obtained firstly by lowering the saline and seeing blood return up the tubing and secondly by a chest X-ray. If the catheter tip is in the right atrium or ventricle the catheter should be pulled back an appropriate distance so that the tip is positioned in the superior vena cava. If the catheter tip is in the contralateral subclavian vein or directed upwards into veins in the neck attempts are made to reposition it under fluoroscopic control and image intensification.

The Seldinger technique. Central venous catheterisation by the Seldinger technique has now an established place in clinical nutrition (Bonadimani et al 1987). The first step in this approach is to insert a small diameter needle into the vein (the same way as described above),

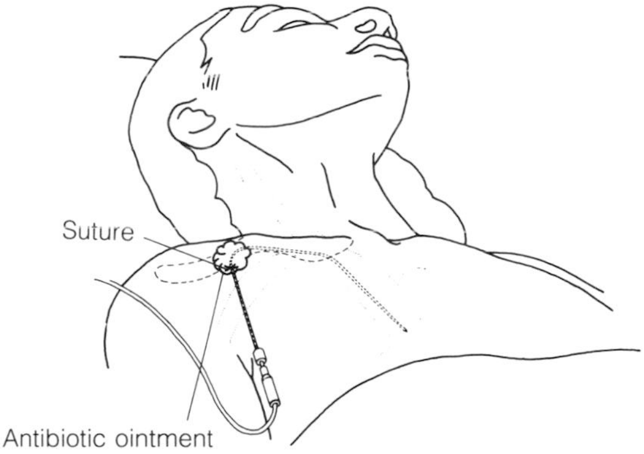

Fig. 10.6 The catheter is sutured to the skin and antiseptic ointment is placed around the catheter at the skin entrance site. (From Dudrick S J, Copeland E M 1973 Surgery annual, by permission of the publisher, Appleton-Century-Crofts.)

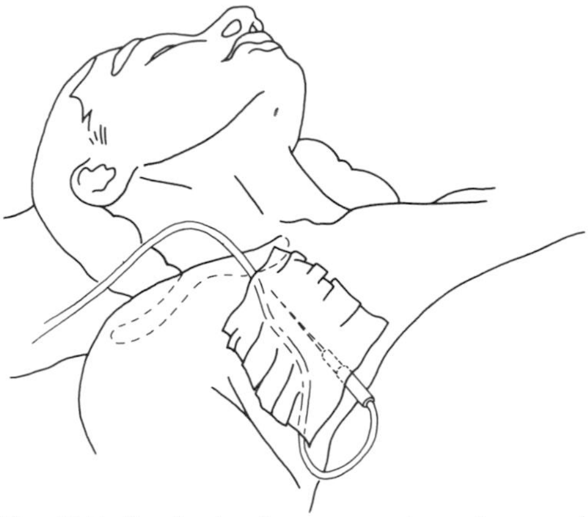

Fig. 10.7 Sterile dressing secures the catheter and tubing in place. The site is cleansed every Monday, Wednesday and Friday and the infusion tubing is changed. (From Dudrick S J, Copeland E M 1973 Surgery annual, by permission of the publisher, Appleton-Century-Crofts.)

remove the syringe and then direct a flexible guidewire through the needle into the vein. The needle is then removed and a dilator is passed over the wire to create a track, and finally the catheter is threaded over the wire into the superior vena cava. The technique is probably safer than the one mentioned above but *all of the time-honoured principles of the approach described by Dudrick still apply.*

Other methods and types of catheter to use. The internal and external jugular veins, the cephalic veins and the basilic veins are alternative sites for catheter insertion. They provide access for TPN in patients who have undergone head and neck surgery or who have infected tracheostomies. Polyvinyl, teflon, polyurethane or silicone rubber catheters can be used: silicone rubber is the most popular and seems to be associated with the lowest incidence of thrombosis.

Care of the central venous cannula: golden rules

The catheter is used exclusively for the nutrient solution. Once positioned the catheter is used exclusively for the administration of the nutrient solution. Drawing blood, monitoring central venous pressure, administering medications and the use of this catheter for nutrient administration postoperatively are prohibited. Triple lumen central venous catheters are now available and if one of the ports is devoted entirely to nutrient administration and the rules above are adhered to reports suggest that the rates of catheter sepsis are the same as when a single lumen catheter is used (Gil et al 1989). We, like others (Apelgren 1987), feel that at the present time this is not proven but in the critical care situation if strict protocols are maintained to ensure that the one lumen is dedicated to nutrient infusion and the other lumens are handled safely and that the catheters are removed as soon as they are no longer required, it is a reasonable practice.

Strict rules of asepsis must apply. High standards of maintenance of the catheter are critical for achieving success for TPN (Murphy & Lipman 1987). The dressing over the catheter insertion site should be removed each Monday, Wednesday and Friday. At this time the skin around the catheter exit site should be cleansed with ether and acetone and the skin painted again with betadine solution. Antiseptic ointment should be placed around the catheter exit site and after the tubing is changed a sterile dressing is reapplied (Petrosino et al 1988).

Catheter related sepsis

This is the most dangerous part of patient treatment with TPN and is defined by:

- clinical evidence of bloodstream infection i.e fever and a high white cell count
- no clinical evidence of another source of the septicaemia and
- isolation of the same organism from the catheter tip and from the peripheral blood.

Definition of catheter contamination. Catheter contamination is present when there is isolation of an organism from the catheter tip but not from the peripheral blood. The problem clinically is that patients who may have catheter related sepsis on clinical grounds frequently have only catheter contamination which is probably of no clinical significance. Catheter removal in these circumstances may be an unnecessary and expensive waste of time.

Protocol when catheter related sepsis is suspected. Failure to recognise catheter related sepsis and to remove the catheter promptly may prove to be life-threatening to the patient. There are two ways of handling the dilemma that the catheter may not be the cause of the sepsis.

1. In the patient suspected of having catheter-related sepsis the catheter is removed over a guidewire and replaced by a new one. The catheter tip and peripheral blood are cultured and if, when the results are available, both the catheter tip and the peripheral blood are growing the same bacteria the diagnosis of catheter related sepsis is confirmed and the catheter is removed. This is a technique we have been using safely and successfully for some time (Pettigrew et al 1985).
2. The catheter is left in place but blood is taken simultaneously through a peripheral vein and through the suspected central venous catheter and quantitative blood cultures are obtained. Around 16 hours later the results are available and a central venous catheter blood colony count 5 times (or more) higher than the peripheral vein colony count can be considered as indicating catheter related sepsis and the catheter is removed. This technique is used successfully by Meguid and his colleagues (Mosca et al 1987).

Whichever of these two methods is used the results depend on the local availability of the appropriate microbiological techniques but both are now established and safe procedures. In one study over 90% of catheters removed for suspected sepsis were not the cause of catheter related sepsis (Pettigrew et al 1985) and in another, of 28 catheters suspected as a source of sepsis, 18 were proven not to be the source (Mosca et al 1987).

Treatment of established catheter related sepsis. Most patients with catheter related sepsis respond promptly and favourably to removal of the catheter. A favourable response is defined as that which occurs when the temperature and white blood count return to normal and local signs of inflammation at the catheter insertion site resolve within the 24-hour period. No other treatment is necessary and a new catheter can be inserted on the other side when all signs of sepsis have subsided. If the patient continues to show clinical signs of bacteraemia after removal, a brief course of antibiotics is indicated and particularly so if the catheter tip culture reveals a large number of colonies of *Staph. aureus*.

The nutrient solution

The role of the surgeon and the role of the pharmacist. Once the intensity and type of malnutrition has been assessed and the nutritional goal has been set the patient's requirements are calculated. *The daily quantities of energy, protein, water, electrolytes, vitamins and trace metals are prescribed by the surgeon and the pharmacist formulates an appropriate nutrient solution.* Some surgeons prefer to prescribe precise types and concentrations of amino acid, dextrose and fat solutions but modern pharmacists are better equipped than their surgical counterparts to choose and mix the detailed ingredients to meet the patient's prescribed nutrient needs.

Generally speaking, the pharmacist formulates a solution from commonly available combinations of 70% dextrose, 10% amino acid solutions and 20% fat emulsions to which electrolytes, vitamins and trace elements are added. All the nutrients are mixed together in a 3 L bag and the entire contents of the bag are infused over the 24-hour period. There is an automated mixing device available which allows the pharmacist to manufacture a variety of nutrient combinations from these components and at the same time generate a label for the bag which allows its precise contents to be known.

It is important for the surgeon not only to prescribe exactly the quantities of energy, protein and water to be given but also to state precisely the quantities of cations and anions required to be added to the base formula.

Sodium and potassium are added as the chloride or acetate salts, depending on the patient's requirements. Generally there should be equal quantities of chloride and acetate. If there are increased gastric losses, however, the salts should all be in chloride form, all the time remembering that excessive chloride administration can lead to the potentially fatal problem of hyperchloraemic metabolic acidosis. Acetate is used whenever extra base is required. Sodium bicarbonate cannot be incorporated into nutrient solutions and acetate which is metabolised to bicarbonate, is used instead.

Phosphate which is essential in patients receiving high glucose intakes, is usually given as the potassium salt; when potassium is contraindicated it is supplied as the sodium salt.

Reference to Chapter 8 and Appendix II shows that some amino acid mixtures already contain sodium, potassium, chloride, acetate and phosphate so it is only if quantities over and above these are required that additional electrolytes are added. Fat emulsions also contain phosphate.

Commonly available preparations of vitamins and trace elements are also added to the 3 L bag (Bradley et al 1978).

Berocca Parenteral Nutrition (Roche) and MVI-12 (Armour) provide fat- and water-soluble vitamins to meet recommended daily requirements. Very depleted patients should receive loading doses of i.m. vitamin B12, folate and vitamin K before the commencement of feeding.

Patramin-6A (Pentcal) is designed to provide recommended daily requirements of zinc, copper, manganese, iron, chromium and selenium.

EXAMPLE

An example of how the nutrient requirements are prescribed and how the nutrient solution is formulated is given in Tables 10.1 and 10.2.

Special additions to and deletions from the nutrient solution

Albumin. Severe hypoalbuminaemia, that is plasma albumin 30 g/L or less, is best treated at the commencement and throughout the course of TPN. 25–50 g per day of salt-poor albumin given during the first few days of replenishment may restore the colloid osmotic pressure and gastrointestinal function in patients where sepsis has been eliminated or controlled (Reid et al 1988). It probably is wasteful to give albumin in critically ill patients suffering from continuing sepsis (Foley et al 1990).

Potassium and phosphorus. It is important to remember that the need for potassium and phosphorus may be quite high in very debilitated patients. In order to achieve positive nitrogen balance and tissue synthesis not only must adequate calories and sufficient nitrogen be provided but also potassium and phosphorus must be supplied in sufficient quantities to support cellular growth without causing hypokalaemia or hypophosphataemia (Hill et al 1979a). The recommended daily doses of potassium and phosphorus may be insufficient in severely depleted patients and the exact requirement can best be controlled according to daily plasma levels.

Sodium. Wasted patients with hypoalbuminaemia usually have an expanded extracellular water space and require little or no sodium in the nutrient solution until body hydration is normalised.

Insulin. This is added in sufficient quantities to the nutrient solution to keep the blood sugar within the normal range.

Table 10.1 Prescription for the maintenance of the nutritional state of a 56–year-old man who weighed 71 kg. His 24-hour nutritional requirements were calculated and prescribed as follows:

Energy	2866 kcal/day (40 kcal/kg/day)
Protein	106 g/day (1.5 g/kg/day)
Water	2500 (35 ml/kg/day)
Na	75 mEq
K	75 mEq
P	37.5 mmol
Mg	12.5 mEq
Calcium	11.8 mEq
Chloride	125 mEq
Acetate	175 mEq
1 ampoule of MVI–12	
1 ampoule of trace element solution.	

Note: Please supply approximately 30% of non protein energy as fat

Table 10.2 In the pharmacy the nutrient admixture was formulated as follows:

	Volume	Content	Energy
Amino acids (10%)	1000 ml	100 g	400 kcal
Dextrose (70%)	700 ml	490 g	1666 kcal
Fat emulsion (20%)	400 ml	800 g	800 kcal
Free water	400 ml		

Total:
Volume 2500 ml
Protein 100 g
Energy 2866 kcal
To this were added electrolytes, vitamins and trace metals as specified in Table 10.1

Other medications that are commonly added to the nutrient solution include the H_2 blockers, ranitidine and cimetidine.

Administration of nutrient solution

Great care must be taken in delivering the nutrient solution which is usually given over a 24-hour period. Some authorities use cyclical parenteral feeding but in ordinary surgical practice it is simpler to continue feeding at a constant rate throughout the day and night using a volumetric infusion pump. It is usual to give 1–1.5 litres in the first 24-hour period, followed by the administration of a further litre every 12 hours for the next 48-hour period or until requirements are met. Supplemental water, sodium and potassium are given separately as indicated from balance studies and plasma levels. This careful administration of moderate increments avoids hyperosmolarity problems and gives the pancreas time to adapt with increased insulin output in response to the glucose load. Within 2 or 3 days, most patients cope well with their full requirement.

Monitoring

This is not the sort of treatment that can be given casually. The patient should be weighed daily and an accurate intake and output record should be kept. Each time the patient passes urine it should be tested for glucosuria. If this is present blood glucose should be monitored until the situation is under control, either by reducing intake or giving added insulin.

A monitoring schedule that is used widely is shown in Table 10.3.

Complications

Numerous complications may occur during the administration of parenteral nutrition (Table 10.4) but with experience and proper management most of these can be avoided or, if they happen, be detected early and treated properly and successfully.

Before patients undergo surgical procedures TPN should be tapered and during the operation itself the line kept open with a 10% dextrose

Table 10.3 Monitoring patients on TPN

Measurement	**Frequency Required**	
	First week	Thereafter if patient is stable
Body Weight	Daily	Daily
Volume of infusate	Daily	Daily
Oral intake	Daily	Daily
Urine output	Daily	Daily
Plasma electrolytes	Daily	3× per week
Plasma albumin	3× per week	3× per week
Blood glucose	Daily	3× per week
Haemoglobin	3× per week	Weekly
Calcium	3× per week	Weekly
Magnesium	3× per week	Weekly
Triglycerides	3× per week	Weekly
Urine		
Glucose	4–6× daily	2× daily
Sodium	As indicated	As indicated
Potassium	As indicated	As indicated

Table 10.4 Common metabolic complications of TPN

	Usual cause	Treatment
Hyperglycaemia	Too rapid infusion, developing sepsis	Slow rate, add insulin, treat sepsis
Hypoglycaemia	Rapid cessation of nutrient infusion	When nutrient infusion is stopped give 10% dextrose solution for 8 hours or so
Hypertriglyceridaemia	Too much fat being administered	Discontinue fat infusion
Hyperchloraemic metabolic acidosis	Too much chloride	$Na^+ + K^+$ administered as acetate salts
Prerenal azotaemia	Excessive amino acid infusion	Reduce intake or increase free water
Hypophosphataemia	Insufficient phosphorus in infusate	Stop infusion and ensure that 20 mmol of phosphate are being given for every 1000 kcal
Hypokalaemia	Very depleted patient with insufficient K^+ in infusate	Slow administration and add more K^+
Hyperkalaemia	Metabolic acidosis, renal failure	Stop all K^+ intake, treat cause

solution. Before commencing TPN again when the patient is stable after surgery it is necessary to change the catheter over a guideline because catheter related sepsis occurs frequently if that is not done.

Special conditions

There are several conditions encountered in general surgical practice which sometimes require modification of the nutrient regimen.

Hepatic failure. In patients with fulminant hepatic failure administration of conventional amino acid solutions may worsen the encephalopathy. Hepatic encephalopathy has been related to the high levels of aromatic amino acids (phenylalanine, tyrosine and tryptophan) in the plasma acting as precursors of false neurotransmitter amines in the central and peripheral nervous systems. Administration of branched-chain amino acid solutions (enriched with leucine, isoleucine, and valine) will normalise the plasma aminogram and possibly reverse the coma in patients with chronic encephalopathy. Glucose should be used as the energy source in hepatic failure but it needs careful monitoring. Blood levels may fluctuate widely because carbohydrate tolerance is impaired as a result of peripheral insulin resistance. Intravenous lipid infusions are contraindicated as they have a synergistic effect in producing coma particularly with ammonia and they may exacerbate coma by displacing tryptophan from plasma protein binding sites. Patients with chronic hepatic failure should also receive increased amounts of vitamins. In spite of several trials, which together show that such solutions do indeed improve encephalopathy there continues to be concern over the possibility that they may be associated with an increased mortality (Berlin & Chalmers 1989).

Renal failure. Patients with acute renal failure are usually hypercatabolic and have increased requirements for energy and nitrogen. They have a high mortality. Generally they suffer from serious surgical problems and/or major trauma and are often unable to eat. They frequently need TPN. Because of limited fluid volumes and the increased blood urea from protein administration, modified nutritional regimens have been suggested for such patients. However, with the early use of dialysis many of these problems can be overcome and a full nutritional regimen prescribed. It has been suggested that the use of essential amino acids alone may improve survival as well as improve blood urea levels (Able et al 1973). Others have shown that the administration of adequate amounts of protein and energy with haemodialysis is more important in improving survival than the use of essential or nonessential amino acids (Feinstein et al 1981, Mirtallo et al 1982). In fact there are some data to suggest that recovery of renal function is enhanced when the amino acid load is reduced (Zager & Venkatachalam 1983). Careful monitoring of potassium, phosphate, hydrogen, magnesium and calcium ions in patients with renal failure on TPN is essential. Thus the composition of nutrient solution used in patients with acute renal failure should take into account the patient's nutritional status and ability to tolerate amino acids, fluids and electrolytes.

Respiratory failure. Administration of high doses of glucose to patients with borderline respiratory function may increase their carbon dioxide production to the point of compromising respiratory function. Such patients in intensive care may benefit from the replacement of some glucose energy intake with fat. High rates of infusion of amino acids may increase respiratory drive in some patients; this may be important therapeutically (see Ch. 6).

Cardiac failure. The goals of TPN in patients with cardiac failure are to provide adequate nutritional requirements in a concentrated form and with lower sodium intakes than usual.

Major injury or sepsis. Branched-chain amino acids (leucine, isoleucine, valine) are essential amino acids that may be used primarily as fuel for skeletal muscle. Leucine in particular stimulates protein synthesis and inhibits protein breakdown in muscle. It has therefore been proposed that amino acid solutions for stressed patients should be fortified with leucine, isoleucine and valine. Such solutions are now available and are used to enrich standard solutions up to 46%. Some clinical studies have noted improved nitrogen retention with such solutions but no major effect on outcome has been demonstrable.

Short chain peptides in TPN. The very low solubility of cysteine and tyrosine and the instability of cysteine and glutamine in aqueous solutions prevent addition of these amino acids to nutrient solutions. A way has now been found of supplementing commonly available synthetic amino acid solutions with synthetic dipeptides. For instance the synthetic dipeptide L-alanyl-L-glutamine can be used as a safe and efficient source of free glutamine as part of a commercial solution (Furst et al 1989, Albers et al 1989).

Glutamine dipeptides in TPN. Glutamine, apart from its use as a 'gut fuel', has potential as a general anabolic mediator (Wilmore 1991) and in the future it will be a standard component of parenteral nutrient solutions (Hammarquist et al 1989).

Growth factors and parenteral nutrition

Growth hormone has anabolic, lipolytic and diabetogenic properties. Early studies with pituitary extracts showed its anabolic effects in convalescent patients (Roe & Kinney 1962) and those with burns (Liljedahl et al 1961), but, until the production of growth hormone by recombinant-DNA methods began, the small supply of pituitary derived human growth hormone limited its use to the treatment of children with growth hormone deficiency. The wide availability of synthetic human growth hormone has raised the question as to its role in clinical nutrition. Low-dose growth hormone and hypocaloric nutrition (20 kcal/kg/day, 1 g protein/kg/day) has been found to attenuate the loss of protein after elective gastrointestinal surgery (Jiang Z-M et al 1989). This effect of growth hormone was achieved through increased protein synthesis and was also associated with increased muscular strength.

As we have seen, patients with sepsis and/or trauma continue to lose body protein in spite of TPN. The administration of recombinant human growth hormone increases whole body protein synthesis and the net loss of protein is decreased (Douglas et al 1990).

More comprehensive studies are now underway both with growth hormone and its mediator (insulin-like growth factor-1) to see if the combined effect of using them with hypocaloric feeding can reduce morbidity and length of hospital stay for surgical patients (Wilmore 1991).

11. Management of surgical patients with protein energy malnutrition — principles and clinical examples

INTRODUCTION — SIX PRINCIPLES OF NUTRITIONAL MANAGEMENT

In Chapters 7 and 8 we learnt how the assessment of the nutritional status and nutrient requirements of a patient may be made. We have also learnt how best to select the most appropriate route for nutritional support and how it then may be administered and monitored (Chs 9 & 10). Putting it all together therefore it might be said that for the nutritional management of a particular patient the surgeon needs to be able to answer the following questions:

- Is the intensity of the malnutrition sufficient to require nutritional support, i.e. is the PEM causing (or will do so soon) clinically obvious physiological impairment?
- Of the three types of PEM which one is this? Marasmic kwashiorkor and kwashiorkor have a worse prognosis than marasmus as they are associated with an expanded extracellular space and immune incompetence.
- Is there evidence of metabolic stress (i.e. is the RME raised)? If the patient has a raised metabolic rate it is not likely that body protein stores can be repleted.
- What are the nutritional/metabolic goals for this patient? Is the goal protein and fat accretion, maintenance of protein and fat or is it short term improvement of physiological function recognising that protein and fat stores cannot be repleted within the time frame available?
- What are the nutrient requirements necessary to achieve this goal? These include requirements for energy, protein, water, electrolytes, vitamins, and trace metals.
- How might these nutrient requirements best be given (i.e. orally, enterally or parenterally)?

In this chapter we set out in some detail the nutritional and surgical care of four patients who each illustrate aspects of the management of PEM in situations which are not uncommonly encountered in surgical practice.

SECTION I
MARASMUS

The surgeon usually encounters this type of PEM in patients with weight loss who are awaiting a major surgical procedure. Their management, which brings up the whole question of pre- and postoperative nutrition, is on the basis of an understanding of the defects in body composition, metabolism and physiological function.

EXAMPLE: A PATIENT REQUIRING PERIOPERATIVE NUTRITION

HISTORY

The management of the marasmic patient awaiting a major operation can be explained by considering a 54-year-old man who had been admitted to hospital with the diagnosis of adenocarcinoma of the gastric fundus. There was no evidence of metastatic disease and a total gastrectomy was planned.

He had lost 18% of his body weight over a

2-month period. He had been a fit architect who had enjoyed walking and trout fishing. He was troubled by dysphagia for all but liquid food and had not been walking or participating in his hobby preferring to sit around the house increasingly over the previous month or so. He felt tired and listless.

CLINICAL ASSESSMENT OF NUTRITIONAL STATE

The patient had not been eating properly and the 18% weight loss was consistent with that. His appearance was that of a person who clearly had lost weight with lax subcutaneous tissue over his upper arms and buttocks in particular. Palpation of fat and protein stores revealed considerable wasting. There was no evidence of any specific vitamin deficiency. Tests of grip strength and other muscle strengths and respiratory function all showed reduced values. Plasma albumin was normal and there was no ankle or sacral oedema. He had no fever and no evidence of metastases in the neck, liver, peritoneum or pelvis.

MALNUTRITION CATEGORY

With this degree of weight loss, wasting of fat and muscle and clear evidence of physiological impairment he was categorised as suffering from moderate–severe PEM. With no evidence of present or recent sepsis or injury, a normal plasma albumin and no oedema this was classified as *nutritional marasmus without metabolic stress.*

OBJECTIVE TESTS OF NUTRITIONAL/METABOLIC STATUS

Body composition

Table 11.1 shows that he had lost 11 kg of body weight comprising 4.1 kg of fat, 3.5 kg of protein and the rest was water. The percentage of the fat free body that was extracellular water, normally 35%, had changed little, being measured at 37%. Although there was a slight increase in plasma volume consistent with the small increase in extracellular water, there had been a fall in red cell volume of the same order of magnitude as the fall in total body protein. The plasma albumin was within the normal range although there were modest falls in both plasma transferrin and plasma prealbumin indicating reduced energy intake.

Physiological and metabolic stress

It was physiological function which was particularly affected by the loss of body protein. The table shows that grip strength and all the respiratory function tests were depressed by the same order of magnitude as the loss of total body protein. The stress index which is a measure of his resting metabolic expenditure compared with his estimated metabolic expenditure was not raised, confirming the clinical impression that he was not septic or suffering from advanced metastatic disease.

Energy metabolism

Indirect calorimetry and an estimate of his total energy expenditure confirmed the clinical history which showed his activity level had fallen appreciably. This was the main cause for the reduced total energy expenditure. It can be calculated that the caloric equivalent of the loss of fat and protein over the 2-month period comes to about 850 kcal per day (4.1 kg fat = 36 900 kcal; 3.5 kg protein = 14 000 kcal) showing that the liquid intake he was able to consume was only about half of that required. TEE was assessed as 1664 kcal/day at this level of physical activity. Metabolically he was behaving as a subject suffering from prolonged starvation with most of his energy requirements coming from fat.

Wound healing

A measurement of his wound healing response using the subcutaneous Goretex implant technique showed after 7 days the response was just below the normal range. Red cell folate was 110 nanograms per ml (normal 250 nanograms per ml) and white cell vitamin C was 8 micrograms per 10^8 (normal 20 micrograms per 10^8). Though there was no clinical evidence of vitamin deficiency it is clear that this level of white cell vitamin C deficiency may contribute to the impairment of wound healing.

Table 11.1 A patient requiring perioperative nutrition — *male 54 years, adenocarcinoma of the gastric fundus, awaiting total gastrectomy. Study on admission to hospital prior to gastrectomy*

	Estimated value when well	Measured value	Change measured	Change %
Body composition				
Body weight (kg)	63.0	52.0	11.0	−18
Total body fat (kg)	14.8	10.7	4.1	−28
Total body protein (kg)	9.8	6.3	3.5	−36
Total body water (L)	34.5	30.6	3.9	−11
Extracellular water (L)	17.0	15.3	1.7	−10
ECW/FFM	0.35	0.37	0.2	+6
Intravascular phase				
Plasma volume (L)	2.5	2.6	0.1	+4
Red cell volume (L)	1.9	1.5	0.4	−21
Blood volume (L)	4.4	4.0	0.4	−9
Haematocrit (%)	44	36	4	−9
Plasma albumin (g/L)	38	36	2	−5
Transferrin (mg/dl)	230	176	54	−23
Prealbumin (mg/dl)	22	15.7	6.3	−29
Physiological function				
Grip strength (kg)	36	28	8	−22
Forced expiratory volume$_{1\ sec}$ (L)	3.6	3.2	0.4	−11
Vital capacity (L)	4.3	3.6	0.7	−17
Peak expiratory flow (L/min)	513	385	128	−55
Metabolic expenditure				
Resting metabolic expenditure (kcal/24 h)	1209	1140	69	−6
Activity energy expenditure (kcal/24 h)	1059	542	1011	−34
Total energy expenditure (kcal/24 h)	2268	1664	1080	−21
Stress index	1.00	1.02	0.02	+2

Immune function

Although skin tests were not performed on this patient they might have been expected to be normal or show only partial anergy.

INTERPRETATION

Overall this man was not a major risk for the surgeon provided it was understood that there was an impairment of a number of important physiological functions and that the patient's wound healing was impaired. Body composition, apart from reduced stores of fat and protein showed only marginal overhydration. Nevertheless, physiological impairments such as these affect respiratory function in particular and patients with this degree of weight loss who have evidence of physiological impairment have been shown to have a longer hospital stay and an increased probability of major complications, particularly postoperative pneumonia. The presence of tiredness and fatigue before surgery and the diminished stores of body protein and total body fat together with the known diagnosis of adenocarcinoma of the upper stomach ensure that he would suffer for a prolonged period postoperatively (more than 6 months) from tiredness and fatigue.

MANAGEMENT AND NUTRITIONAL/METABOLIC GOALS

This patient could be expected to gain about 0.5 kg (8%) of total body protein with 2 weeks of nutritional repletion. Depleted patients without raised metabolic rate behave as growing children and accumulate protein avidly. It would be difficult to prove, however, that this gain in total body protein would improve his prognosis over and above that which occurs as the result of the improvement in physiological status that would occur after only a few days of nutritional therapy. At best it would be unlikely to be cost effective. The nutritional/metabolic goal here was to repair vitamin and trace metal deficiencies and improve physiological function in order to prepare the patient for the very major procedure of total gastrectomy. Thus energy requirements were calculated at TEE × 1.2 and protein requirements at 1.5 g/kg/day.

There was no necessity for blood or albumin transfusions

The patient was slightly hypoproteinaemic and anaemic but not of sufficient degree to consider preoperative transfusion. The plasma albumin was still in the normal range although it had probably fallen a few points. This was of doubtful significance and probably would not impact in any way on his postoperative course. The haematocrit level of 36% suggested mild anaemia but there was no evidence that this degree of anaemia would impair postoperative recovery in any way. Although there is a guideline which indicates that a haemoglobin value of less than 10 g/dl or a haematocrit of less than 30% indicates a need for perioperative red cell transfusion, the evidence to support this practice is not available. No single measure can replace good clinical judgement as the basis for decisions regarding perioperative transfusion, and common sense suggests that otherwise healthy patients with haematocrit values of 30 or greater rarely require preoperative transfusion. Wound healing is not impaired by this degree of anaemia and there is no evidence to suggest that the frequency or severity of postoperative infections is increased. On the other hand there are immediate and long term risks of red cell transfusion. Human hepatitis viruses, human immunodeficiency virus, cytomegalovirus, human T cell lymphotropic viruses, and, on rare occasions, other microbial agents including parvoviruses, plasmodia, Epstein–Barr virus, and *Babesia* may cause infection and disease.

Water and salt must be administered cautiously

The patient had cancer of the upper stomach, he had lost nearly 20% of his body weight, and he had a low plasma sodium concentration (129 mmol/L). It could be argued that he had a salt deficit causing significant hypotonicity and this could have led to his being given intravenous salt. The data though suggested quite the opposite. The administration of salt-containing solutions to patients like this promotes fluid overload and oedema. This patient already had a modestly expanded extracellular water space and was in a salt retaining, water retaining phase. He was given as little water and salt as possible until operation and then the minimum required to maintain an adequate urine output.

A short course of nutritional therapy improves physiological function

Within the time frame available it was not possible to significantly restore body stores of fat or protein. Vitamin and trace metal deficiencies may, however, be repaired quickly and a significant improvement in physiological function could be expected within 3–4 days with a calorie rich, protein rich, vitamin rich diet. This could be given either via a fine nasogastric tube or intravenously. In this patient it was possible to pass a fine bore nasogastric tube past the obstruction to lie in the distal stomach and 25 ml/h of full strength Osmolite was administered for a period of 6 hours and then increased by 10 ml/6 h until a total of 2000 kcal/day (1664 × 1.2) were being received together with 74 g of protein (1.4 g/kg/day). By the fourth day a measurable improvement in grip strength and respiratory function was observed. The wound healing response and white cell vitamin C levels also improved, and a small increase in the short half life plasma proteins was seen.

Mobilisation and physiotherapy is an essential part of the preoperative preparation

Over the few days in hospital prior to surgery during which time this intensive preparation was underway the patient was encouraged to be up and about the ward, wearing graduated compression stockings to avoid deep venous thrombosis, and was under the tutelage of the physiotherapist who taught him good habits of breathing, coughing and leg exercises.

The operation — gentleness and careful replacement to minimise the metabolic assault

The operation was a radical R2/R3 total gastrectomy with distal oesophagectomy performed through a left thoracoabdominal incision. Meticulous technique was essential in this patient to avoid a major metabolic assault and to minimise the risk of postoperative complications. The reconstruction was a stapled Roux-en-Y oesophagojejunostomy with a Hunt–Lawrence pouch. Leaks from the anastomosis at the time of surgery were looked for by the instillation of diluted Betadine into the new stomach via a nasogastric tube. There was quantitative replacement of red cells and plasma during the operation and for the first 2 days postoperatively. The anaesthetist was careful not to oversalt the patient during the procedure being content to have a urinary hourly volume of around 40 ml per hour.

Postoperative nutrition to prevent further protein loss during enforced starvation

The same principles of avoidance of excessive water and salt applied during the first postoperative day. On the second postoperative day, the patient was stable and total parenteral nutrition was commenced through a central venous line. For this patient 1600 kcal and 75 g of protein together with appropriate vitamins and trace metals were required each 24 hours to preserve nutritional state. 50–75 mmol of sodium per day helped prevent further hyponatraemia and made up for the small losses through the nasogastric tube and urine. When the water intake was insufficient to maintain urine output at 40 ml per hour, more was given until this volume increased. Because of the extensive anastomoses the patient received nothing by mouth until the tenth postoperative day when they were tested radiologically and found to be secure. The patient then commenced oral intake and when the dietitian confirmed that he was taking at least 1000 kcal/day spread over 3 separate meals the TPN was stopped and he was discharged from hospital. Then the patient started his long uphill climb to return to health hampered by the highly variable digestive effects of total gastrectomy. He was encouraged to take his food at 3 or 4 distinct times each day and avoid frequent small meals. In this way the new stomach was utilised fully right from the start and prevented from contracting down.

Long term recovery — failure to regain normal body composition after total gastrectomy

After 3–4 weeks the patient was eating sufficient energy and protein to meet his requirements. 3 to 6 months from the time of surgery he acquired his definitive body composition.

After total gastrectomy it is unlikely that he would ever return to his normal body weight or normal body protein, although his body composition and particularly the components within the fat free body would be in normal proportions and ratios. One would expect also that his physiological function would return to something like normal. Postoperative fatigue, however, would be long and prolonged, lasting perhaps as long as 6 months. It would not be influenced by pre- or postoperative feeding. Because abnormalities of vitamin D, folate, and calcium metabolism and iron deficiency have all been demonstrated after gastrectomy appropriate supplementation was required. Since a curative resection had been performed vitamin B_{12} injections were given every 2 months or so (see Ch. 17).

SECTION II
MARASMIC KWASHIORKOR

The surgeon encounters this type of PEM in patients suffering from semistarvation or total starvation on top of which major injury and/or sepsis has supervened. Management depends on whether this metabolic stress is continuing or has abated.

EXAMPLE 1: MARASMIC KWASHIORKOR IN A PATIENT WITH CONTINUING SEPSIS

HISTORY

The management of this problem may be illustrated by the case of a 30-year-old woman with a 10-year history of ulcerative colitis. Until 3 weeks prior to admission to hospital she had been coping well at home on 5–10 mg prednisone per day and having 3–5 normal coloured bowel movements daily. Then the number of bowel movements increased markedly over a few days and in spite of increasing the prednisone dosage to 40 mg per day, she was having 12–15 bowel movements, containing blood and pus, per 24 hours. She suffered from deep aching pain in the suprapubic area and felt nauseous whenever she tried to eat. After 3 weeks, feeling increasingly sick, tired and listless and with no evidence of remission she was admitted to hospital. After a full assessment and colonoscopic biopsies, she was commenced on TPN and the prednisone dose was raised to 60 mg per day.

CLINICAL ASSESSMENT OF NUTRITIONAL STATE

She had lost 16% of her body weight over 3 weeks confirming her very low food intake. She looked pale and exhausted, her face was thin and her eyes were sunken. Although wasting of soft tissues was not prominent around the shoulder girdle it was marked in the region of the buttocks which were thin and flat. There was slight pitting oedema at the ankles. Palpation of body fat stores revealed no gross abnormality but palpation of the biceps, triceps and shoulder girdle muscles all showed depletion. There was no evidence of a specific vitamin deficiency or any evidence of unhealed cuts or wounds. Plasma albumin had fallen to 30 g/L. Clinical tests of physiological function revealed an overall weakness of muscle power. Her respiratory function, however, seemed normal. She had a fever of 38.7°C. Flexible sigmoidoscopy revealed severe inflammation of the rectum which extended above the range of the instrument.

MALNUTRITION CATEGORY

She was, on the basis of this clinical examination, classified as having moderate PEM (weight loss, tissue loss, physiological impairment). This was of the marasmic-kwashiorkor type (hypoalbuminaemia, oedema) with ongoing metabolic stress (fever, colorectal inflammation).

OBJECTIVE TESTS OF NUTRITIONAL/METABOLIC STATUS

Body composition

Table 11.2 shows that she had lost 9.1 kg of weight prior to admission to hospital. This was composed of 4.1 kg fat, 1.3 kg protein and 3.7 kg of water. Red cell volume had decreased by nearly 30% although there was an over-expansion of the plasma volume. This was consistent with a raised extracellular water content of the fat free body from 36% to 43%. As expected, the protein loss from the inflamed colon combined with the continuing systemic effects of the sepsis have led to a fall in plasma albumin as well as falls in the levels of plasma transferrin and prealbumin.

Physiology and metabolic stress

Again the loss of total body protein was associated with objective evidence of widespread defects in skeletal muscle and respiratory muscle function. The stress index was 1.34 (i.e. RME 34% above predicted) indicating a high degree of continuing stress from the colitis.

Table 11.2 Marasmic-kwashiorkor in a patient with continuing sepsis — *female 30 years, acute attack of severe ulcerative colitis. Study on admission to hospital 21 days after onset of attack, at commencement of a course of TPN. The measurements were repeated 14 days later.*

	Estimated value when well	On admission day 0	After 14 days of TPN
Body composition			
Body weight (kg)	58.3	49.2	49.1
Total body fat (kg)	13.2	9.1	9.3
Total body protein (kg)	8.6	7.3	7.5
Total body water (L)	33.8	30.1	29.6
Extracellular water (L)	16.8	17.2	15.5
ECW/FFM	0.36	0.43	0.39
Intravascular space			
Plasma volume (L)	2.3	2.4	—
Red cell volume (L)	1.8	1.3	—
Blood volume (L)	4.1	3.7	—
Haematocrit (%)	43	29	38
Albumin (g/L)	40	28	31
Transferrin (mg/dl)	291	150	210
Prealbumin (mg/dl)	28.0	13.0	22.2
Physiological function			
Grip strength (kg)	34	26	30
Respiratory muscle strength (cm H_2O)	90	65	76
Forced expiratory volume$_{1\ sec}$ (L)	3.4	3.0	3.3
Vital capacity (L)	4.1	3.6	3.8
Peak expiratory flow rate (L/min)	479	428	462
Maximum voluntary ventilation (L/min)	203	162	197
Metabolic expenditure			
Resting metabolic expenditure (kcal/24 h)	1166	1472	1483
Activity energy expenditure (kcal/24 h)	1166	594	579
Total energy expenditure (kcal/24 h)	2332	2066	2062
Stress index	1.0	1.34	1.26

Energy metabolism

Although the resting metabolic rate was markedly increased at 1472 kcal/day compared with the predicted rate of 1166 kcal/day, total energy expenditure was less (2066 kcal/day) because of her very low activity level. The daily energy deficit can be calculated from the combined loss of protein and fat and amounts to about 2000 kcal per day. This shows just how little food she had been eating.

Wound healing, immune function and vitamin status

These were not measured but wound healing would probably be impaired as would immune function, and vitamin status would be expected to be low.

INTERPRETATION

The patient had come into hospital in the hope that the acute attack of colitis would settle. It is a surgical rule that if some indication of remission is not apparent after a few days surgery is indicated. In the meantime, this patient, already with moderate PEM, and with continuing sepsis was commenced on TPN to prevent further functional deterioration. Although she did show signs of settling (reduced number of blood stained bowel movements, no signs of dilatation) by the fifth day in hospital, TPN was continued for a further 9 days (total of 14 days) by which time her prednizone dosage had been reduced to 35 mg per day and she was eating 1200 kcals each day. On the other hand, if she had not settled and surgery had been required it can be seen from Table 11.2 that the nutritional therapy had been beneficial, for further nutritional deterioration had been prevented and a number of physiological functions had markedly improved.

MANAGEMENT AND NUTRITIONAL/ METABOLIC GOAL

The patient was septic, starved and passing blood and protein rich fluid in her stools. Her dietary intake was minimal and very major surgery was possibly indicated in the near future. Clearly nutritional support was required to prevent further loss of protein and fat and to improve body hydration and physiological function. The nutritional/metabolic goal was to limit further protein loss and to improve body hydration and physiological function while waiting for the clinical course to declare itself. The goal was achieved by providing daily energy and protein requirements while at the same time giving only sufficient sodium to maintain plasma osmolality in the near normal range.

Total parenteral nutrition rather than enteral nutrition was used here because she was:

- hypoalbuminaemic
- had an expanded extracellular space and
- had continuing severe diarrhoea.

Although not all agree, most nutritionists feel that diarrhoea is made worse when hypoalbuminaemic patients are fed enterally and this may indicate impaired intestinal absorption. Furthermore, it is difficult (but not impossible) to supply a balanced enteral diet in which the sodium concentration is very low. Lastly it is not easy to manage a patient with severe diarrhoea on an enteral diet which may in itself cause diarrhoea. It is for these reasons that we use, in patients like this, total parenteral nutrition.

TPN was commenced after red cells, vitamins and trace metals had been repleted. The nutritional goal was to prevent further deterioration and she received 2100 kcal per day and 2.0 g protein/kg/day — the increased protein because of the increased stool losses. Patients with colitis may lose a further 60 or 100 g of protein in the stools daily. It cannot be expected that this patient would gain total body protein but further loss could be prevented. The TPN solution, which contained less than 30 mmol Na^+ per day enabled the overhydrated fat free body to resume a near normal state. As can be seen from Table 11.2, skeletal muscle function, respiratory function and wound healing all improved in a few days. Immune function did not improve whilst sepsis continued.

Blood, albumin and vitamins were replaced empirically

The patient was anaemic and hypoproteinaemic and red cells and albumin were given. It is difficult to justify this practice on solid science but as a general principle we endeavour to restore these components back to normal. Thus, before the first bag of TPN was given, the patient was given red cells and albumin, vitamin B_{12}, folate, and vitamin K together with a bolus of trace metals.

Nutritional therapy will prevent further tissue loss, reduce overhydration and improve physiological function

It cannot be expected to restore lost reserves of protein in a septic patient such as this, but TPN will prevent further loss of protein and be associated with marked clinical improvement. The patient is better to receive nothing by mouth until the abdominal pain has settled and be encouraged to be up and around the ward. Table 11.2 shows that the TPN achieved the desired result. As expected, the total body protein change was insignificant but the relative overexpansion of the extracellular water was diminished. Physiological function improved significantly.

Long term recovery

Although the patient was only in hospital 21 days, return to her former state of health was a prolonged affair. When measurements were taken again 200 days later the patient was in remission, off prednisone and back at work. Body composition results were very similar to those that were estimated for her preillness state.

EXAMPLE 2: MARASMIC KWASHIORKOR IN A PATIENT NOW FREE OF SEPSIS

HISTORY

The problem of management of marasmic kwashiorkor, developing as a consequence of a severe septic episode but present now in a patient free of sepsis, is typified by the example shown in Table 11.3. He is a man of 52 years who $3\frac{1}{2}$ weeks before this assessment was admitted to hospital for excision of a diverticular stricture. The operation had been more difficult than expected, multiple adhesions had been found and the colorectal anastomosis proved to be difficult. On the fourth day following surgery the patient complained of severe low abdominal pain, developed a fever of 39°C and had frank signs of peritonism. This was treated conservatively at first and over the next week he continued on a stormy course and a CT scan demonstrated a large collection in the right flank. This was percutaneously drained with some improvement in his condition but 4 days later he developed a high swinging fever again and a further CT scan showed that there was now another collection in the left flank which was also drained percutaneously. Though there was no frank bowel content in either of the drains, 4 days later the abdominal incision became red and inflamed and, after removal of the sutures, intestinal contents appeared. A further CT scan showed that the two previous collections had disappeared, but there was a further one under the right diaphragm. Further CT guided drainage was established successfully and the patient's fever settled but because of excessive nausea and vomiting his inability to eat continued. He was referred to our department for further management. Soon after admission the vomiting settled. There was no nasogastric aspiration and the fistula output was measured at 200 ml/day.

CLINICAL ASSESSMENT OF NUTRITIONAL STATE

This patient had had nothing to eat for over 3 weeks, he appeared exhausted, cachectic, pale and dehydrated. Fat folds and muscle bellies both were shrunken, grip strength was weak and he was breathless on movement. A small wound on his left ankle was unhealed and lay open and gaping. Plasma albumin was 29 g/L. He had both sacral and ankle oedema.

MALNUTRITION CATEGORY

Weight loss, combined with clinical evidence of fat and protein depletion, and functional defects in muscle strength and wound healing made the diagnosis of moderate to severe PEM relatively simple. Because of the low plasma albumin and oedema this was categorised as *marasmic kwashiorkor* without ongoing metabolic stress.

OBJECTIVE TESTS OF NUTRITIONAL/METABOLIC STATUS

Body composition

The initial data are shown in Table 11.3. He had lost 20% of his body weight, a loss composed of nearly 5 kg of fat, 3.5 kg of protein and 5.7 kg of water. He had hypoalbuminaemia and low levels of transferrin and prealbumin. Like the previous patient and in contrast to the patient with marasmus, who was not hypoalbuminaemic and had not been septic, this patient had a marked expansion of extracellular water. The normal hydration ratio of 0.35 had risen to 0.43 and the patient was clearly oversalted and overwatered.

Table 11.3 Example: Moderate–severe PEM — no stress. *Male, 53 years, 3 weeks after establishment of enterocutaneous fistula. Now free of sepsis. Study at commencement of course of TPN and again 3 weeks later*

	Estimated value when well	Day 0 TPN	After 21 days of TPN
Body composition			
Body weight (kg)	70.1	56.6	56.7
Total body fat (kg)	16.0	11.1	11.3
Total body protein (kg)	10.0	6.5	7.6
Total body water (L)	40.1	34.4	33.2
Extracellular water (L)	19	19.6	17.4
ECW/FFM	0.35	0.43	0.38
Plasma proteins			
Albumin (g/L)	39	29	33.0
Transferrin (mg/dl)	240	110	180
Prealbumin (mg/dl)	26.3	7.6	19.8
Physiological function			
Grip strength (kg)	40	26	35
Respiratory muscle strength (cm H_2O)	104	65	84
Forced expiratory volume$_{1\ sec}$ (L)	4.0	3.0	3.6
Vital capacity (L)	4.8	3.6	4.1
Peak expiratory flow rate (L/min)	576	428	490
Metabolic expenditure			
Resting metabolic expenditure (kcal/24 h)	1289	1277	1469
Activity energy expenditure (kcal/24 h)	1515	500	940
Total energy expenditure (kcal/24 h)	2804	1777	2408
Stress index	1.00	1.09	1.25

Physiology and metabolic stress

As might be expected following sepsis, there were deficits in skeletal muscle function and respiratory function as a consequence of the protein depletion. It can be seen that the stress index, that is the measured resting metabolic expenditure compared with the predicted resting metabolic expenditure, was not significantly raised confirming that his sepsis was now under control at the time and he was no longer metabolically stressed.

Energy metabolism

Table 11.3 shows that his total energy expenditure had fallen markedly due to his reduced activity. It was 1777 kcal/day. The patient, over the 3 weeks prior to admission to our unit, had a daily loss of 170 g of protein or nearly 2% of his body protein per day. Although, he was free of sepsis at the time of nutritional assessment and conserving body protein, there had been a massive and rapid erosion of his tissue reserves during the septic episodes, leaving him very depleted.

Wound healing, immune function and vitamin status

With this combination of starvation and sepsis, impairments of the wound healing response and immune function would be expected.

INTERPRETATION

'Septic starvation takes its toll quickly and leaves in its wake an exhausted, cachectic avitaminotic patient who cannot tolerate any additional trauma or broncho pulmonary trauma.' This statement from Dr F D Moore (1959b) aptly describes this patient. The metabolic/nutritional goals were to replete this patient of his deficits and restore vital physiological function to enable healing of the fistula. This required repletion of plasma albumin, restoration of red cell mass and the provision of vitamins and trace metals. Zinc in particular is likely to be depleted in a patient such as this and an extra 10 mg/day was provided until plasma levels returned to normal. Requirements for energy were calculated at 2000 kcal/day (TEE × 1.2) and 1.5 g protein/kg/day. Water requirements were calculated as 2000 ml/day (35 ml/kg + 200 for fistula loss) and sodium as 80 mmol (60 + 20 from fistula).

MANAGEMENT

There was no time constraint because a conservative approach had to be taken to see if spontaneous healing of the fistula would occur (see Ch. 15). The proper treatment of a postoperative enterocutaneous fistula, after sepsis is controlled, is to commence TPN, forbid all oral intake and control intestinal secretions with somatostatin. 50% of patients treated in this way will experience spontaneous fistula closure and the others will require definitive surgery which because of the obliterative peritonitis present cannot be carried out until it has subsided. Thus surgery is usually undertaken after a period of 6–8 weeks when all signs of sepsis have disappeared and the patient is in a sound nutritional state. Interest lies therefore not only in the immediate physiological response to TPN but whether appreciable gains can be made in total body protein with substantive improvement in skeletal muscle function, respiratory function, wound healing and immune function. Like the marasmic patient who was also severely protein depleted he was expected to gain protein avidly with proper nutritional therapy. Before commencing TPN, plasma albumin and red cells were given in sufficient quantity to restore normal values and he also required in addition 2 units of plasma to normalise peripheral perfusion and restore urine output to 50 ml/h. Measurements again 3 weeks after commencement of TPN (Table 11.3) show that he had gained considerably from this treatment. It can be seen that although body weight had not risen, more than 1 kg of total body protein had been gained and the overexpanded extracellular water had reduced by 2 litres or so. The latter was the result of careful limitation of sodium intake in the TPN fluids. All the plasma proteins had risen and there were substantial improvements in physiological function. The wound healing response, also, had returned to normal. Although immune function was not measured it would be expected that after

3–4 weeks of TPN the patient would react once again to routine skin tests.

SURGERY AND POSTOPERATIVE CARE

This patient after 6 weeks of TPN gave no indication that there would be spontaneous fistula closure. Radiology revealed that there was a fistula of the mid-jejunum kept open by a distal obstruction somewhere near the terminal ileum. Thus surgery was planned. At surgery, the entire small intestine was dissected and a mass of adhesions was found near the terminal ileum, causing the obstruction. The ileum was dissected free, the area of jejunum containing the fistula was excised and an end to end anastomosis performed in an area of intestine free of oedema and friability. The patient withstood this procedure well and required 2 units of red cells, 1 L of plasma and 3.5 L of crystalloid during the operation. On the second postoperative day the patient was commenced on TPN to avoid further loss of total body protein. 7 days later after an uncomplicated postoperative course the patient was commenced on a fluid diet and after a further 3 to 4 days a normal diet was commenced. By the middle of the second postoperative week, the patient was taking a light diet comprising 1200 kcal a day and 50 g of protein per day. The TPN was then stopped and the patient was discharged from hospital on the 14th postoperative day. It would be expected that full restoration of body composition would take a further 6 months. He would then be found to be fully restored to normal but fat stores would be a kg or so more than those present when well. Hydration of the fat free body would be within normal limits.

This case study illustrates a patient with marasmic kwashiorkor who had been septic but was now free of sepsis. The fundamental difference between this patient and the patient with marasmus is the overexpanded extracellular water compartment secondary to the recently resolved sepsis. Failure to recognise that patients can be oversalted and overwatered to this degree has led many patients to receive excessive sodium intakes with consequent oedema of the tissues (making suturing difficult) and interstitium of the lung. Thus sodium content in the TPN solution, if present at all, must only be sufficient to maintain normal serum osmolality. Because the metabolic stress had subsided, this depleted patient gained protein avidly with substantial improvements in a range of physiological functions. The clinical setting allowed a prolonged period of nutritional repletion with considerable advantage to the patient's recovery.

SECTION III
KWASHIORKOR

Mild stress, such as that which accompanies routine surgery, causes disturbances of protein metabolism which have little clinical impact. Major injury or serious sepsis by markedly increasing whole body breakdown of protein causes massive losses from body protein stores with important effects on physiological function. Very quickly a state of protein depletion and overhydration occurs and a condition resembling childhood kwashiorkor is seen.

EXAMPLE: A PREVIOUSLY WELL PATIENT WITH PERFORATED TOXIC MEGACOLON WHO RAPIDLY BECAME PROTEIN DEPLETED

HISTORY

The patient, a 58-year-old car salesman became acutely unwell, with frequent bloody stools, fever and joint pains. 3 days later he was admitted to hospital where, for the first 2 days, he was treated for suspected infectious diarrhoea. On the sixth day he deteriorated markedly with abdominal distension, peritonitis, fever, and developing septic shock. The haematocrit was 32 and plasma albumin 21 g/L. Sigmoidoscopy showed severe inflammation of the rectal mucosa which extended above the level of the sigmoidoscope. Plain abdominal X-ray showed massive dilatation of the colon. Urgent surgery was advised. At surgery he had a total colitis, megacolon and a localised perforation with abscess at the splenic flexure. Total colectomy, right iliac fossa end ileostomy and oversewing of the rectal stump were performed. The patient went to the critical care unit postoperatively for artificial ventilation, and haemodynamic support. Here he had intermittent positive pressure ventilation, positive end expiratory pressure, colloid and crystalloid resuscitation fluids, haemodynamic monitoring, inotrope infusions and appropriate broad spectrum antibiotics.

By the second postoperative day he was haemodynamically stable and needed no more colloid infusion. The first body composition measurement was carried out at this time just before commencement of TPN. The second measurement was carried out 10 days later.

CLINICAL ASSESSMENT OF NUTRITIONAL STATE

The patient was a fit and well man up until 8 days before this assessment. He was heavily muscled and had major truncal obesity. Resuscitation from this overwhelming sepsis had required 14 L of crystalloid and colloid and as a consequence he was swollen and oedematous. Although he had not been eating or receiving any calories during the illness and was clearly in negative protein and energy balance there were no physical signs of PEM. Fat folds, because of the tissue oedema, made proper assessment of fat stores impossible and being normally a heavily muscled man his limb muscles were still hard and bulky. Because he was on the ventilator and relaxed it was not possible to assess respiratory muscle function. Although plasma albumin just prior to emergency surgery was 21 g/L, it was 31 g/L at this assessment, which was carried out on the second postoperative day, due more to the 250 g of plasma protein that had been administered than to an improvement in albumin production.

MALNUTRITION CATEGORY

This was kwashiorkor. Some authorities call this condition *hypoalbuminaemic malnutrition*, recognising that the predominant clinical finding so soon after the onset of this catastrophic illness is hypoalbuminaemia. Nevertheless there was already an expanded extracellular fluid space and major losses of body protein would soon be observed (Table 11.4). It is for this reason that we prefer to call this condition kwashiorkor or protein-malnutrition-kwashiorkor like.

Table 11.4 Protein malnutrition-kwashiorkor like. *Male, 58 years, developed bloody diarrhoea and then toxic megacolon with perforation. Well, until 8 days prior to measurement 1*

	Estimated value when well	Measurement 1 just before commencing TPN on 2nd postoperative day	Measurement 2 after 10 days of TPN when patient was on road to recovery
Body composition			
Body weight (kg)	82.3	90.1	83.9
Total body fat (kg)	19.0	16.5	18.7
Total body protein (kg)	13.8	12.9	11.4
Total body water (L)	45.6	55.9	49.1
TBW/FFM	0.72	0.76	0.75
Plasma proteins			
Albumin (g/L)	39	31.4	34.6
Transferrin (mg/dl)	240	160	150
Prealbumin (mg/dl)	27	12	11.0
Metabolic expenditure			
Resting metabolic expenditure (kcal/24 h)	1414	1800	1850
Total energy expenditure (kcal/24 h)	3312	1825	2027
Stress index	1.00	1.3	1.3

OBJECTIVE TESTS OF NUTRITIONAL/METABOLIC STATUS

Body composition

Table 11.4 shows that over the 8-day period since the onset of his illness he had gained 7.8 kg of body weight, in spite of losing 2.5 kg of fat and 0.9 kg of protein. Resuscitation of this seriously septic patient, involving both crystalloids and colloids, had resulted in a net gain of total body water of 11.1 L over the 8 days since his illness had commenced. The percentage of the fat free body that was water had as a consequence risen from its normal level of 72% to 76%. Although extracellular water measurements were not made in this patient it would be expected that this gain would be mostly composed of extracellular water.

Physiology and metabolic stress

No assessments of muscle function or stress were made at this stage of his illness. Resting metabolic expenditure was measured at 1800 kcal/24 h, about 30% more than predicted.

Energy metabolism

Total energy expenditure was not directly measured during his acute illness and subsequent major surgery. Over the 8 days of illness he had burnt 22 500 kcal of fat and 3600 kcal of protein, i.e. a total daily energy consumption of nearly 3300 kcal.

Wound healing

A Goretex tube was inserted at the commencement of the TPN and showed markedly reduced accumulation of collagen.

Immune function

It would be expected that the patient would have no reaction to delayed hypersensitivity skin tests at the time of the first assessment.

INTERPRETATION

Here is a typical example of massive and rapid fluid accumulation and protein depletion in a very ill surgical patient. Severe peritoneal sepsis is the usual cause but complicated trauma and severe pancreatitis may cause a similar picture. Tissue loss was rapid and profound. Although there was an increased rate of lipolysis (2.5 kg of fat were lost in 8 days) the physiological impact of losing about 1% of body protein each day was much greater. Continuing losses of this magnitude quickly impact on respiratory and skeletal muscle function. The massive expansion of extracellular water was accentuated here by the manner of resuscitation but this phenomenon, to a greater or lesser extent, is always seen when rapid protein loss secondary to sepsis or trauma is observed.

The important point is that protein malnutrition like this, mirrors the acute kwashiorkor syndromes of children but, because PEM is not obvious on physical examination, the severity of the illness and the potential dangers may be underestimated.

MANAGEMENT AND NUTRITIONAL/METABOLIC GOAL

The goal here, after control of sepsis, was to limit protein loss, encourage diuresis and to resume oral intake as soon as practical. His requirements were taken as 40 kcal/kg/day, because we had no measurement of RME, and 2 g protein/kg/day — the higher figure being used because of the period of severe diarrhoea. Body weight was taken as that given to us as being his normal weight prior to the acute illness. Water and sodium requirements were kept at a level which kept plasma osmolality and renal function within normal limits. The patient was commenced on TPN on the third postoperative day. For the first 5 days of the 10-day course of TPN he was ventilator dependent but did not require inotropes. By the end of the course of TPN he was back in the ward, with a normal functioning ileostomy and beginning to take a soft diet.

TPN reduced but did not prevent massive protein losses

He received 2 g/protein/kg/day and 40 kcal/kg/day together with appropriate trace metals and vitamins. In spite of this he continued to lose 150 g of protein per day. Kinetic studies have shown that TPN increases protein synthesis but the sepsis-induced whole body protein catabolism continues unabated. Thus the TPN reduced losses from body protein stores but did not abolish them. On the other hand the patient was clearly in positive energy balance for there was a gain of 2.2 kg of fat (and/or glycogen) over the 10-day period. This patient received half his calories as fat and half as glucose. Net fat gain is associated with a raised respiratory quotient which may be counterproductive in a patient such as this in whom early ventilator weaning was required. Clearly the prescription of 40 kcal/kg/day was far too high. His RME was only 1800 kcal and he therefore received about 1400 kcal/day in excess of requirement. This illustrates the difficulty of estimating energy requirements in critically ill patients and the problem of overprescription in obese or oedematous patients.

Salt was not given and water was only given in sufficient quantities to keep serum osmolality normal

He had more than 11 L of excess extracellular water. With his sepsis in decline restriction of salt and water intake allowed this to be unloaded. No diuretic was given for on the second day of TPN the ileostomy started to produce copious amounts of ileostomy fluid — up to 2 L per day. No sodium was given in the TPN fluids and only sufficient water to maintain serum osmolality within the normal range. With this regimen he lost all evidence of tissue oedema, oxygenation rapidly improved and he was weaned from the respirator on the fifth day. Over the 10 days between the two body composition measurements he lost nearly 7 L of extracellular water.

Oral intake was commenced as soon as possible

In patients like this it is essential that oral nutrition is commenced as soon as the gastrointestinal tract can cope. By the eighth day of TPN he started on oral fluids and by the end of the tenth day he was commencing a soft diet. Although a high protein diet would be the ideal, the patient preferred a carbohydrate rich diet for a further few days before fairly normal food was taken.

Long term management

Post traumatic obesity. Body composition measurements performed at 1 month, 3 months, 6 months and 12 months postoperatively showed that he did not return to his normal state until somewhere between the sixth and twelfth month postoperatively. 1 year after his illness he weighed 81.5 kg, with a total body protein of 13.1 kg, a normally hydrated fat free body and an excess of body fat (20.5 kg compared with estimated well value of 19.0 kg). This is the phenomenon of postoperative obesity that is almost universal in surgical patients many months after a devastating illness. Calorie intake is more than calorie output; the solution lies in redressing this imbalance.

Control of ileostomy output and sodium balance. Patients with end ileostomies have, when well, outputs of salt and water in proportion to their body weight. In the early postoperative period this patient had high outputs of 2–3 L (200–300 mmol Na^+) per 24 hours. These fell quickly and by the second postoperative week, when all signs of peritoneal inflammation had disappeared, his output settled to 600–700 ml per day. With a liberal salt intake to accompany his meals he was able to maintain positive sodium balance. A larger output, such as 1200–1500 ml per day would result in ileostomy losses of between 100–200 mmol of sodium each day and a negative sodium balance would have been likely. A patient in negative sodium balance cannot gain protein. Control of sodium output by decreasing ileostomy output (loperamide) and increasing salt intake must occur before nutritional repletion can take place.

PART 3

Metabolism and Nutrition in Surgery of the Alimentary Tract

Part 3 Contents

Prevention of protein energy malnutrition after surgery
— Nasogastric decompression with jejunal feeding
— Fine needle catheter jejunostomy
— Total parenteral nutrition
— Enteral nutrition versus parenteral nutrition

Section III Cost effectiveness of perioperative nutrition

12. Alimentary tract — obstruction

SECTION I
OESOPHAGEAL OBSTRUCTION

INTRODUCTION

Oesophageal obstruction causes dysphagia necessitating a change to a soft or liquid diet but sooner or later there is weight loss. Most commonly the obstruction is due to a carcinoma; it is usually a squamous carcinoma when it arises in the upper two thirds of the oesophagus and an adenocarcinoma when it arises in the lower third. Of all the malignancies of the gastrointestinal tract these have the worst prognosis. Curative surgery for oesophageal cancer is only a reality for a small proportion of patients and palliation remains the realistic objective for the majority. The aims of palliation are to achieve trouble free swallowing and freedom from aspiration of saliva. When resection is not possible either due to the nature of the tumour or to the condition of the patient intubation is used. Whatever the treatment, the majority of patients with oesophageal malignancy die within 1 year or 18 months.

Less commonly, benign lesions such as peptic strictures or achalasia cause dysphagia and may be associated with weight loss. Treatment which may involve dilatation or surgery is usually successful.

OESOPHAGEAL CANCER

Protein energy malnutrition (PEM) in patients with oesophageal cancer

Prevalence. In a prospective study of nutritional and immunologic indices in more than 200 patients with carcinoma of the oesophagus Fekete & Belghiti (1988) found there was evidence of PEM and/or immunodeficiency in 40%. Most importantly they found that there was a strong relationship between malnutrition and resectability. In the 60% who had no evidence of PEM or immunodeficiency the tumour was resectable in 75%. In those patients with greater than 15% weight loss, plasma albumin less that 30 g/L, and skin test anergy, resectability was less than 20%.

Aetiology. Fekete & Belghiti (1988) also looked at the causes of malnutrition in this large series of patients. They performed a prospective nutritional assessment, including objective measurements and a nutritional interview, in 50 patients with carcinoma of the oesophagus who had severe dysphagia. Two groups of patients were defined, patients with dysphagia and anorexia (n = 21) and patients with dysphagia but no evidence of anorexia (n = 29). They found that anorexia was significantly correlated with the percentage weight loss. There was also a relationship between resectability rate of the tumour and anorexia. They found that anorexic patients were more likely to be malnourished and were also more likely to have disseminated malignancy and concluded that anorexia should be carefully assessed in patients with oesophageal carcinoma and when present the possibility of widespread disease should be entertained.

Protein metabolism. Using tracer methodology, Shaw & Wolfe (1988b) found that patients with advanced oesophageal cancer awaiting palliative surgery had a higher rate of protein breakdown than either volunteers or another group of patients with localised colon tumours.

Table 12.1 Nutritional assessment of 6 patients awaiting palliative treatment for malignant oesophageal obstruction

	Estimated value when well	Measured value	% change
Body composition			
Body weight (kg)	69.3 ± 9.1	52.7 ± 9.0	–24
Total body fat (kg)	16.5 ± 5.4	9.7 ± 6.2	–41
Total body protein (kg)	9.9 ± 2.7	6.6 ± 1.5	–33
Total body water (L)	38.5 ± 6.5	37.0 ± 14.6	–3.9
TBW:FFM	0.73 ± 0.02	0.76 ± 0.02	+4.1
Plasma proteins			
Plasma albumin g/L	35–48	31.8 ± 3.8	—
Metabolic expenditure			
Resting metabolic expenditure (kcal/d)	1126 ± 150	1216 ± 229	+8

They showed also that there was an elevated rate of gluconeogenesis from amino acids but this was not suppressible by glucose infusion and that the high rate of protein breakdown could not be reduced by 4 days of total parenteral nutrition. Their study suggests that *the usual response of a marasmic patient to gain protein with TPN could not be expected in most patients with oesophageal carcinoma.*

The type of protein energy malnutrition. Table 12.1 shows a study of the nutritional state of a group of patients (n = 6) awaiting palliative treatment for advanced carcinoma of the oesophagus. The picture is that of marasmic kwashiorkor — gross deficits in fat and protein, albumin below the normal range and an expanded hydration of the fat free body. This is the end point of the kinetic effects described above and demonstrates the effects of the advanced cancer over and above the effects of the PEM itself.

It should be noted, however, that patients without bulky tumours in whom no metastases can be found have a different metabolic response than this. In Table 12.1 where the patients studied had large tumours the cancer is a metabolic stress and the patient's metabolism is like that of a patient with sepsis. In cancer of the oesophagus at an earlier stage and of the type where extirpative surgery is possible, the metabolic changes are similar to those of simple starvation (see Ch. 3).

Immune competence. These patients are almost always immunocompromised. In a very interesting study Fekete & Belghiti (1988) hypothesised that PEM was an association rather than a cause of skin test anergy. In order to evaluate the cause of immunodeficiency they compared one group of 18 patients with oesophageal cancer and a group of 15 patients with benign stricture with the same degree of PEM as assessed by anthropometric and biologic factors. Immunodeficiency was significantly less in patients with benign strictures suggesting that pure protein and energy deprivation might not be the cause of the impaired skin reactivity. This study confirms again that advanced cancer, causing PEM of the marasmic kwashiorkor type rather than pure marasmus, is associated with immunodepression.

Clinical significance of PEM in patients with oesophageal cancer

Mortality and the incidence of anastomotic breakdown is high. Fekete & Belghiti (1988) were able to show that their patients with abnormal nutritional status had higher mortality and fistula rates, although the numbers were too small to achieve statistical significance. Surprisingly, in view of the study of Windsor & Hill (1988c) which showed that malnourished patients had a higher incidence of postoperative pneumonia, this was not so apparent in Fekete & Belghiti's study perhaps because of the high overall incidence (30%) of pneumonia in their patients.

Some patients need preoperative nutritional support. We will discuss this matter in depth in Chapter 18 but generally speaking we can do no better than take the approach advocated by Fekete & Belghiti:

- *Where moderate to severe protein energy malnutrition is not present,* preoperative nutrition is not required. A strong effort must be made to improve respiratory status in order to limit postoperative pneumonia and attention must be given to technical details in order to avoid an anastomotic leakage.
- *Where moderate to severe PEM is present* every effort is made to exclude widespread disease. If there is a realistic expectation that the tumour is resectable then nutritional support should be instituted.

Preoperative metabolic preparation

Although the route for preoperative nutritional support has not been studied in a carefully controlled way most oesophageal surgeons believe that TPN is more liable to achieve nutritional repletion than any form of enteral nutrition (Lim et al 1981, Moghissi et al 1977). In our view it would be difficult to show that scientifically, and it is our practice to use nasogastric feeding whenever a fine tube can be passed beyond the tumour. A 5–7-day period of metabolic preparation is recommended for those in whom a major resection is contemplated. Such a programme would be along these lines:

Day 1
Admission to hospital. Clinical assessment of nutritional status and calculation of nutritional requirements. Administration of vitamins and red cells if required.

Day 2
Restore albumin to normal range over a period of 3 days. Commence nutritional support with low sodium initially and aiming to give 30–35 kcal/kg/day and 1.5 g protein/kg/day.

Day 3
Continue nutritional support. Vigorous physiotherapy and mobilise.

Day 6
Assess response to nutritional support in terms of increased grip strength, and vigour and improved respiratory function. Haematocrit should be 35 or more and plasma albumin in the normal range. If improvements are seen and patient is up and about the ward with clear lung bases then proceed to surgery on Day 7.

Postoperative nutrition

Once the patients is stable postoperatively we recommence nutritional support. If a jejunostomy tube can be placed without putting tension on the anastomosis we use this as the route for the administration of a balanced liquid diet. If not, TPN is used and continued until it has been demonstrated that the anastomosis is intact and the patient has a voluntary food intake of 1000 kcal/day.

BENIGN OESOPHAGEAL OBSTRUCTION

Most of these patients are treated long before severe malnutrition develops but when it does it is of the pure marasmic type, i.e. the hydration of the fat free mass is normal, hypoalbuminaemia is not present and the patients react normally to delayed hypersensitivity skin testing. If there has been reduced dietary intake over the weeks prior to assessment the wound healing response will be impaired (Windsor et al 1988). Patients who are severely malnourished will have an increased risk of postoperative complications and it might be expected that a short course of metabolic and nutritional therapy will not only improve physiological function but also result in an increase in total body protein stores. Since most of the operations required for relief of peptic strictures (dilatation) or achalasia (balloon dilatation or oesophagomyotomy) are not large procedures nutritional therapy is rarely required.

SECTION II
GASTRIC OUTLET OBSTRUCTION

INTRODUCTION

There has been a marked reduction in the number of cases presenting with gastric outlet obstruction in recent years. There are two reasons for this. Firstly gastric outlet obstruction secondary to duodenal ulceration has declined, probably as a result of the widespread use of H_2-receptor antagonists and secondly there is a changing location of gastric adenocarcinoma away from the distal stomach towards the proximal stomach. *In the past, most gastric outlet obstructions were due to peptic ulceration, today they are more likely to be malignant* (Johnson & Ellis 1990).

GASTRIC OUTLET OBSTRUCTION DUE TO MALIGNANCY

Patients with malignant gastric outlet obstruction usually have an increasing problem with regurgitation of food and intermittent vomiting. This is associated with weight loss, increasing tiredness and, as the malignancy increases in size, deep pain in the epigastrium. As distinct from gastric outlet obstruction due to duodenal ulcer there is no alkalosis and the effect of the disease on the patient is to cause protein energy malnutrition associated with anaemia, tiredness and fatigue.

Principles of metabolism and nutrition

The main problem is the effect of lack of food often over a period of some months. The patient will have lost 10–20% of his/her body weight, be anaemic and if the malignancy is advanced suffer from hypoalbuminaemia. The low or absent acid in the stomach associated with a large fungating ulcer, leads to overgrowth of bacteria with the effects of low grade sepsis. There are often vitamin B_{12}, vitamin C and folate deficiencies.

Weight losing gastric cancer is associated with metabolic effects, the most important of which is increased protein breakdown which is unresponsive to infusions of glucose or TPN (Shaw & Wolfe 1987c). Although TPN causes an increase in protein synthesis it is unlikely to make the patient anabolic unless the cancer is small. Body composition studies show gross wasting of fat and protein with increased hydration of the fat free body particularly so if the patient is hypoalbuminaemic. Almost always there are physiological impairments, diminished or absent wound healing responses and skin test anergy. In common with the general protein depletion red cell mass is diminished. This is marasmic kwashiorkor and if the cancer has widely metastasised the RME will be raised as well.

Management

General plan. The nutritional management is dependent on the magnitude of the planned operative procedure: in advanced disease a simple bypass may be all that is required and the sooner the surgeon gets on with it the better. If, however, a resection is required and particularly if that is a curative one involving a radical lymphadenectomy then a complete programme of metabolic and nutritional restoration is required.

Detailed plan

- *Assessment of operability.* The clinical examination is focused on the presence or absence of metastatic disease. Abdominal examination may reveal an enlarged liver and a palpable epigastric mass and these together with deep abdominal pain usually mean irresectability. The surgeon should look for Virchow's node, a rectal shelf or ovarian metastases for the same reason. Ultrasound or CT scan may help to determine less obvious degrees of metastases and the presence of ascites. If the situation is beyond surgical help clearly metabolic and nutritional care are not a consideration and palliative treatment is the prime objective.
- *Assessment of the metabolic problem.* The acid base disorder is minor compared with that encountered in the high acid stomach associated with peptic obstruction. Alkalosis, if present, will be mild although hypokalaemia may be present usually arising on the basis of the vomiting of sodium rich fluid leading to retention of sodium at the renal tubule and the excretion of excessive potassium. If one encounters a patient with a large distended stomach who has been vomiting a lot, has hypokalaemia and yet no evidence of alkalosis then the diagnosis of malignant gastric outlet obstruction is very likely. Clinical examination reveals whether there is extracellular fluid loss with poor tissue turgor, a dry tongue, sunken eyes and low urine output. If the ratio of sodium to potassium in the urine is measured, severe salt depletion is revealed by that ratio being less than one.

- *Assessment of the nutritional problem.* A history of weight loss, poor dietary intake and physical signs of decreased fat and protein stores suggest protein energy malnutrition of the marasmic type. If weight loss is greater then 10% and/or there is evidence of increasing tiredness, impaired respiratory and skeletal muscle function, or unhealed wounds or scratches then there is significant malnutrition which increases the likelihood of postoperative difficulties should major surgery be necessary. Hypoalbuminaemia usually suggests advanced disease.
- *Correction of metabolic disorder.* If there is extracellular fluid volume depletion which is evident both clinically and by demonstration of decreased sodium in the urine then the cautious administration of sodium chloride is indicated. Red cells are unnecessary unless the haematocrit is below 30–35 after the patient has been rehydrated. Patients with achlorhydria may well have vitamin B_{12} deficiency as well as vitamin C deficiency and both of these vitamins should be replaced generously. Since plasma albumin deficits are associated with postoperative gastric emptying problems and stomal oedema it is necessary to restore plasma albumin above 35 g/L with infusions of concentrated albumin. Simple metabolic repair such as this is all that is necessary for patients undergoing palliative gastrectomy or gastroenterostomy.
- *Preoperative nutrition is only for those in whom a major curative resection is planned.* Those patients who have severe protein energy malnutrition with clinically obvious impairments of physiological function have an increased incidence of postoperative complications after major resectional surgery (Windsor & Hill 1988d). It is this group, in whom major curative resection is planned, who should receive preoperative nutritional therapy. It has been shown by Lim et al (1981) that it can be expected that positive nitrogen balance can be achieved with a 7–10 day course of TPN. In any event the labile protein pool will be replenished, vitamin, trace metals and plasma protein levels returned to normal and there will be objective improvements in skeletal muscle function, respiratory function and the wound healing response–these effects will be seen after 4–7 days TPN.

An example of patient management

The preparation for this sort of surgery is very similar to that which was outlined in Chapter 11 for the management of the patient with marasmus. Preoperative preparation can safely be achieved over a 7-day period.

Day 1
Full history, assessment of operability and nutritional state. CT scan if curative surgery is a strong possibility. Calculate nutritional requirements.

Day 2
Treatment starts with repair of the metabolic defects of water and salt, vitamin B_{12}, vitamin C and albumin. If it is clear that the patient has advanced disease and palliative surgery is indicated, operation should proceed the next day. If major curative surgery, however, is anticipated, and there is moderate to severe marasmus with physiological impairments, a 7-day course of TPN is begun with sufficient energy and protein to meet daily requirements. This should be preceded, however, by replacement of red cells if the haematocrit is below 30. Red cells should be given in sufficient volume on this day to return the haematocrit to 35.

Days 3–7
Continue TPN. Patient receives vigorous physiotherapy and is encouraged to be up and about around the ward.

Day 8
If the metabolic defects are repaired and there is clinical improvement in physiological function, clear lung bases and the patient is moving freely around the ward, operation is planned for the next day. Gastric lavage, with antibiotic solution to lower the bacterial count, physiotherapy instruction and bowel preparation are then proceeded with.

Intraoperative management

The anaesthetist is careful to replace red cells and extracellular fluid loss accurately. The patient's urine output should be in the region of 50 ml per hour. Plasma should also be given if the procedure takes longer than 2 hours.

Postoperative management

This proceeds as follows:

Day 1
The patient's response to the volume infusion received perioperatively and in the immediate postoperative period is assessed initially in terms of peripheral perfusion, pulse rate, blood pressure and urine output. 1.5–2.0 L of 5% dextrose, and 500 ml normal saline usually suffice to maintain perfusion and keep the urine output at 40–50 ml per hour. If, however, the operative dissection has been large, up to 200 ml of fluid may be lost (third space effect) every hour or so for about 12 hours postoperatively and this should be replaced, half as plasma and half as Ringer's lactate. This is over and above maintenance fluids. The haematocrit should be measured and red cells are given if the haematocrit is less than 30%. Fit patients can usually be safely maintained with haematocrits of 30%, for the low haematocrit, providing vascular volume is accurately replaced, is compensated for by a rise in cardiac output. Patients with diseased coronary arteries should have red cells sufficient to bring the haematocrit up to 35%.

Day 2
If the nasogastric aspirate is small the tube can be removed and the patient encouraged to sip a small amount of water by mouth. Most patients who received TPN preoperatively should continue with this during the postoperative period to prevent further weight and protein loss (see Table 12.2).

Day 4
By this stage one would expect the bowel sounds to have returned, the patient beginning to take a soft diet and mobilising well around the ward. If there is any question of postoperative sepsis or an intraabdominal complication developing, TPN, if not already started, should be instituted to avoid further losses of body protein. Many patients, however, very quickly recover from this sort of surgery and normal eating patterns are restored by the eighth or ninth postoperative day; as soon as 1000 kcals per day are being consumed orally TPN is stopped.

Table 12.2 Changes in body composition that occurred in 6 patients after total gastrectomy. Measurements were made on postoperative day 2 at the commencement of a course of total parenteral nutrition and again 14 days later, at which time the total parenteral nutrition was stopped. It can be seen that the usual postoperative losses of body weight, fat and protein were prevented by the nutritional therapy. Values are mean ± s.e.m.

	Postoperative day 2	Postoperative day 16	p
Body weight (kg)	62.3 ± 8.9	63.0 ± 7.6	NS
Total body fat (kg)	17.0 ± 5.8	17.6 ± 6.1	NS
Total body protein (kg)	7.8 ± 1.1	8.0 ± 1.2	NS
Total body water (L)	33.9 ± 3.8	33.7 ± 4.1	NS

GASTRIC OUTLET OBSTRUCTION DUE TO PEPTIC ULCER

Gastric outlet obstruction caused by a peptic ulcer is almost always due to a chronic cicatrising duodenal ulcer with the stenosis being in the first part of the duodenum. Uncommonly, the ulcer may be in the pyloric canal or even in the distal stomach. Since the introduction of the H_2 receptor antagonists peptic obstruction is much less common. The problem comes about because of developing fibrosis around a chronic ulcer but is usually precipitated by an enlargement or flare up of an ulcer with surrounding oedema. A patient presenting with projectile vomiting, especially of food identified as having been eaten the previous day, a gastric splash heard 3 to 4 hours after the last meal, visible gastric peristalsis or a palpably distended hypertrophied stomach has peptic obstruction until proved otherwise. If this is accompanied by metabolic alkalosis, then one can be almost assured of the diagnosis and know that the patient needs admission to hospital and surgery soon thereafter.

Principles of metabolism and nutrition

The patient with peptic ulcer induced gastric outlet obstruction is almost always thin, exhausted and depleted of extracellular fluid. In advanced cases, tetany may be induced by tapping over the facial nerve. The blood picture shows a high haematocrit, with serum sodium, potassium chloride and calcium low. The pH, plasma bicarbonate and urea are raised. The urine will be small in volume and in advanced cases may have a low pH.

Gastric juice from patients with pyloric stenosis contains around 100 mmols of chloride,

50 mmols of sodium and 15 mmols of potassium. An excess of chloride over sodium is lost in the vomit, the excess being in the form of hydrochloric acid. Normally, in the unobstructed stomach, as hydrogen ion is secreted into the stomach bicarbonate passes into the plasma and neither hydrogen nor chloride is lost from the body. In pyloric obstruction both are lost and this is reflected in the plasma which shows a low plasma chloride and a high bicarbonate. In the beginning this alkalosis is compensated by an increased urinary excretion of sodium bicarbonate. If the vomiting continues sodium and water are depleted as well and the kidney defends the extracellular fluid volume by avidly retaining sodium at the expense of potassium. The bicarbonate then is accompanied, not by sodium but by potassium and, to a lesser extent, hydrogen ion. It is at this stage that the well known paradox of an alkalotic patient passing acid urine may be found. *The patient therefore has an increasing metabolic alkalosis with hypokalaemia and hypochloraemia.* Another change that accompanies the metabolic alkalosis is that ionised calcium changes to its unionised form predisposing the patient to tetany. The loss of extracellular fluid results in a decreased urea clearance and a rising blood urea.

Management

Overall plan. There are four general principles:

- decompress the stomach
- control activity of the ulcer
- correct acid base abnormality and restore extracellular fluid volume
- improve the general condition of the patient.

These objectives can usually be realized quite quickly and the surgeon should plan for these sequential but overlapping phases to be accomplished within 4 or 5 days and aim to have the patient ready for surgery within this time frame.

Detailed management. The treatment of established pyloric stenosis caused by duodenal ulceration is surgical but it must be preceded by a period of careful preparation along these lines.

Decompression of the stomach. A wide bore tube is passed into the stomach and the gastric residue is aspirated and measured. The stomach is then washed out with 0.9% saline. This procedure is carried out twice a day but once the residue has fallen to 300 ml or so it can be reduced to once a day. Once the gastric residue is clear and is clearly falling, the patient may drink a defined formula diet and have free fluids as desired. We use the balanced diet Osmolite in these patients, because of its isotonicity.

Control activity of the ulcer. H_2 blockers are given; ranitidine, 150 mg twice a day, is commenced. Within a few days the ulcer will begin to heal and the adjacent tissue becomes less inflamed. This contributes to the lessening of the degree of obstruction and better toleration of the liquid feeds.

The alkalosis is corrected and extracellular fluid restored. Nearly always the hypokalaemic, hypochloraemic metabolic alkalosis can be corrected by the administration of 0.9% saline. If there are clear signs of extracellular fluid depletion then 3–4 L of normal saline are given during the first day. As soon as urine flow has been established at around 50 ml per hour, potassium chloride is added to give a total of about 120–200 mmols of K^+ during the first day. The patient is placed on water soluble parenteral vitamins and vitamin K. Under such treatment plasma albumin and the haematocrit should return to normal but it takes longer for the potassium concentration to rise to normal. By the end of 3 or 4 days the alkalosis should have resolved and the chloride concentration will be rising towards 100 mmols per litre.

Exceptionally severe hypokalaemic, hypochloraemic metabolic alkalosis may be refractory to treatment with 0.9% saline and potassium. Although infusion of ammonium chloride was advised in the past, ammonia toxicity has been recorded and it is no longer used. 0.1 N hydrochloric acid is an effective treatment and Abouna et al (1974) have advised the following method of administration. A preparation of an isotonic solution is made by the addition of 150 ml of 1 N hydrochloric acid to one litre of sterile water. This gives 150 mmols of hydrogen and 150 mmols of chloride. The hydrochloric acid will then be added to a litre of 0.9% saline and the infusion should be administered over a 24-hour period with measurements of pH, $P\text{CO}_2$, and serum electrolytes every 6 hours. Usually 1 or 2 L of this solution over a period of 24 hours is sufficient.

Improve general condition of the patient. Vitamins are replaced; ascorbic acid is given by injection, for the long period of dietary restriction makes severe depletion possible. Vitamin K is given by the intramuscular route. Haematocrit and albumin, if very low, are returned to normal by infusion of red cells and concentrated albumin. Hypoalbuminaemic patients, in particular, may have difficulties with gastric emptying.

If, after 4 or 5 days, but occasionally longer, the patient has acid base status returning to normal, plasma potassium within the normal range, chloride, haematocrit and albumin normal, is up and about around the ward and has dry lung bases, the time has come for surgery.

Surgery–operation of choice. Although a number of procedures including gastric resection, gastroenterostomy alone, proximal gastric vagotomy with dilatation, proximal gastric vagotomy and pyloroplasty have been described as successful treatments for this condition the *gold standard is truncal vagotomy with either pyloroplasty or gastrojejunostomy.* Ellis (1986) has reported a large series of patients treated in this way, the results of which are uniformly satisfactory apart from one patient who developed stomal ulceration on the jejunal side of the gastrojejunostomy.

Postoperative course. The nasogastric tube is removed the morning after operation, oral feeding with small amounts of liquids is begun and, as soon as the patient shows that these have been accepted and is passing wind freely, active feeding is commenced. Discharge is usually at the end of the first week after surgery.

SECTION III
SMALL BOWEL OBSTRUCTION

INTRODUCTION — CHOOSING THE TIME TO OPERATE

Small bowel obstruction is the cause of about 5% of all surgical emergencies. In developed countries 60% of the obstructions are caused by adhesions (mainly postoperative), 15% by hernias and the rest are due to neoplasms, inflammatory lesions, vascular occlusions and intraluminal blockages.

The most important decision the surgeon has to make is when to operate. In most cases this should be early, certainly within 1 or 2 days of admission to hospital. Early surgery is advised because of the difficulty in identifying those patients with strangulating obstruction. A number of authors (Silen 1962, Saar et al 1983) have shown that clinical indications of strangulation are often misleading, and even the judgement of experienced surgeons is often incorrect. It is because of this that non-operative treatment can be hazardous.

There are, however, a few patients in whom a conservative approach is the wisest course unless there is very clear evidence of strangulation. These include patients who have had multiple operations for adhesive obstructions in the past, many patients with postoperative mechanical obstruction, and some patients with advanced malignant obstruction where it is known that the abdomen is full of metastatic disease.

PATTERNS OF PRESENTATION

There are two patterns of presentation of patients with small bowel obstruction and the metabolic care of each is quite different. There may be those patients who present within a few hours of onset whose metabolic disturbance is little and, after diagnosis and correction of that, surgery can be proceeded with safely and rapidly. Other patients present, sometimes after many days, with gross distension of the abdomen and severely disturbed metabolism. Early surgery in these patients can be hazardous unless the surgeon understands clearly the metabolic process going on and has made substantive attempts to correct it.

THE METABOLIC PROBLEM IN SMALL BOWEL OBSTRUCTION

The fundamental problem is that of extracellular fluid depletion which can sometimes be massive.

This is due to the pumping of water and salt into the lumen of the small intestine where it becomes unavailable for metabolic interchange. Acid base balance can be either way. Where there has been much vomiting there may be a metabolic alkalosis but if there has been loss of bicarbonate into the intestinal lumen metabolic acidosis may become apparent.

It took surgeons a long time to understand that the cause of death in patients with long standing small bowel obstruction was shock secondary to loss of extracellular fluid in the gut. Hartwell & Hoguet (1912) demonstrated this when they showed that dogs with complete obstruction in the lower duodenum lived only a few days. However, if they injected subcutaneously a quantity of saline solution slightly in excess of the combined loss of urine and vomitus the dogs survived for 3 or more weeks.

Shields (1965) showed how extracellular fluid was lost in increasing amounts into the lumen of the obstructed bowel of the dog as time progressed. Using isotopically labelled sodium and water, he showed that within 12 hours of the onset of the obstruction there was decreased absorption from the intestinal lumen into the blood stream and after 36 hours this was accompanied by an increased secretion resulting in net accumulation of water and electrolytes within the bowel lumen. After 60 hours he showed that an obstructed ileal segment with a surface area of 100 cm^2 secreted 14 ml of water and 2 mmols of sodium every 10 minutes. As the obstructed state persisted, fluid accumulated not only within the lumen but also within the wall of the bowel. Transudation of fluid eventually took place from the oedematous bowel wall leading to the accumulation of free (and infected) peritoneal fluid.

The small intestinal contents also become feculent following luminal obstruction. There is gross bacterial overgrowth above the obstruction even in patients with acute obstruction although there is a return to a normal microflora within 4 or 5 days after the obstruction is relieved. When strangulation occurs there is loss of blood, death of tissue, transudation of toxic materials and sometimes frank perforation of the necrotic segment into the peritoneal cavity. The exudate from the strangulated bowel when injected into dogs has proven to be lethal.

The amounts of extracellular fluid lost into the lumen of the gut can be quite massive. In early obstruction 2 or 3 litres only may be lost but in long standing obstruction where there is massive dilatation of the bowel and the patient is shocked 7 or 8 litres may be lost. The accumulated gut fluid comes initially from the compartment of the greatest reserve, that is interstitial fluid, with initial protection of the circulating plasma volume. One sees a loss of tissue turgor, a dry tongue and the patient is thirsty. As the capacity of the interstitial compartment diminishes, changes in circulating plasma volume occur with compensatory tachycardia and vasoconstriction. In severe extracellular fluid depletion shock occurs. The signs and symptoms of extracellular surgical dehydration are shown in Table 12.3.

MANAGEMENT OF EARLY OBSTRUCTION OF THE SMALL BOWEL

The surgeon faced with a patient with bowel obstruction needs to find out:

- what is obstructed
- what is the magnitude of the extracellular fluid loss

Table 12.3 Signs and symptoms of extracellular fluid deficit

Deficit	Mild (1–2 L ECF)*	Moderate (2–4 L ECF)*	Severe (5–9 L ECF)*
Symptoms	Gives history of recent loss of ECF	Apathy, anorexia, tachycardia, collapsed veins	Stupor or coma, ileus, pale, hypotensive, cold extremities, absent pulses
Signs	Usually no signs	↓ blood pressure, narrow pulse pressure, ↓ tissue turgor, dry tongue	↓↓ blood pressure, ↓↓ tissue turgor, sunken eyes

* Calculated for 70 kg subject with normal body fat stores. In a fat patient of this body weight the deficits would be less. In a very thin patient the deficits would be correspondingly greater.

- whether the blood supply of the intestine is intact.

Overall plan

Management of early small bowel obstruction follows an orderly course which includes confirmation of the diagnosis, drainage of the stomach with a nasogastric tube, replacement of the extracellular fluid deficit and restoration of the urine output before proceeding with surgery to relieve the obstruction.

Confirm diagnosis, drain stomach and insert urinary catheter. Soon after the patient has been admitted to hospital an intravenous line is set up and an infusion of a crystalloid solution is commenced. Blood is taken for urea, haematocrit, haemoglobin and serum sodium, potassium and chloride. If there is any concern about acid base balance arterial blood is taken for blood gases. A nasogastric tube is inserted into the stomach and aspirated, a urinary catheter is passed in order that urine output can be closely followed. Plain X-rays of the abdomen are taken: an erect or decubitus film to confirm clinical diagnosis (fluid levels) and a supine film to demonstrate the site (ileum is featureless).

Assess intensity of depletion and replace rapidly. The degree of extracellular fluid depletion is calculated. This may be done by classifying the intensity of depletion using the mild, moderate or severe system as shown in Table 12.3. Other surgeons use the 4, 6, 8 rule. Thus a mildly dehydrated patient has lost 4% of his total body weight as extracellular fluid, and a patient with severe dehydration has lost 8%. Once calculated, this deficit is replaced rapidly over a period of 2–4 hours and as soon as an adequate urinary output is obtained, unless blood chemistry shows some unexpected distortion, the patient can proceed to surgery. The replacement fluid will usually be Ringer's lactate but if there has been much vomiting 0.9% saline is used.

Proceed to surgery. The surgery in these patients should be carried out under general anaesthesia under the cover of prophylactic antibiotics. The anaesthetist should be particularly aware of the possibility of aspiration during endotracheal intubation and needs to ensure that further extracellular fluid losses are replaced during the procedure. If bowel distension is gross, the small bowel can be emptied by the surgeon by gently milking the contents in a proximal direction up to the duodenojejunal flexure and with gentle pressure the contents are advanced through the duodenal loop into the stomach which is emptied by the anaesthetist applying intermittent suction to a wide bore stomach tube. The surgeon lifts the distended small bowel tracing it carefully loop by loop down to the point of obstruction. This is clearly indicated when the bowel below is collapsed. A band or adhesive kink is the most likely finding. The postoperative course is straightforward providing the surgeon ensures the extracellular fluid volume is properly replaced and urine volume is about 50 ml/h. It is not long before these patients are eating well and feeling normal again.

In the majority of patients with adhesive small bowel obstruction this is the end of their problems although some continue to have recurrences. Krook (1947) followed 309 patients after adhesiolysis and found that 14% required a later laparotomy for recurrent small bowel obstruction and 15% of that group suffered a third adhesiolysis.

MANAGEMENT OF LATE OBSTRUCTION OF THE SMALL BOWEL

Compared with early obstruction the history is usually much longer, the dilatation of the small bowel is much greater and by the time the patient presents, a complex metabolic picture is present. The changes have taken place over some days and there are massive compensations which will take 2 or 3 days to repair. These patients are brittle and if handled incorrectly may quickly become gravely ill.

Overall plan

The patient needs:

- a quick diagnosis, with an assessment of whether the bowel is strangulated
- an assessment of the severity of his or her metabolic distortion

- gentle repair of the metabolic deficit
- surgery when the metabolic deficit is returning towards normal.

Diagnosis, nasogastric tube and urinary catheter. After a thorough physical examination and plain abdominal X-rays confirming the obstruction a nasogastric tube is passed, and a urinary catheter and an intravenous line are inserted. In most patients a central venous pressure monitor is set up. Blood will already have been taken for urea, haematocrit, haemoglobin and serum sodium, potassium and chloride. Arterial blood is taken for acid base status and urine is sent for estimation of osmolality. A chest X-ray and an ECG are required and in some very ill patients pulmonary artery wedge pressure is monitored.

Assessment of severity of metabolic disturbance. If there is peritonitis, perforation or clear evidence of dead gut there is only time for very rapid repair of the metabolic defect and this should follow the lines as for early obstruction. The real problems in such patients will arise postoperatively and will be discussed in Chapter 22. Many of these patients have lost 5 or more litres of extracellular water into the gut lumen and may well have a moderate to severe disturbance in acid base balance as well. Some will be shocked, suffer from metabolic acidosis, have low blood pressure and increasing pulse, an elevated haematocrit, a markedly elevated blood urea with early clinical signs of uraemia, severe hyponatraemia, oliguria and the appearance of a patient who is both acutely and chronically ill. Clearly such people can not withstand surgery until proper repair has been carried out.

Gentle repair of metabolic defect. If peripheral perfusion is impaired, and the patient's blood pressure is low and the pulse rapid, initial attention should be paid to plasma volume replacement. Plasma or a plasma substitute should be given, initially 1 or 2 litres over the first hour, and this should produce rapid restoration of the patient's vital signs towards normal. The pulse will trend downwards and blood pressure and urinary volume upwards. This is followed with restoration of interstitial volume using Ringer's lactate. Based on the calculated deficit the aim should be to provide daily maintenance requirements together with the total repair to be accomplished over a period of 48 hours or so. Usually the acidosis present responds to treatment with Ringer's lactate alone and bicarbonate is not required. These patients often have a slightly elevated plasma potassium concentration at the outset which falls very rapidly as the extracellular fluid volume is replaced. Potassium must then be given in increasing quantities. As extracellular fluid volume returns towards normal a low plasma albumin level may be uncovered. This should be returned to normal, for hypoalbuminaemia is associated with extreme sensitivity to excessive salt administration with consequent swelling of the gut wall, often to a degree that makes suturing hazardous.

Surgery. When blood volume and interstitial volume have been returned to normal and the metabolic deficits described above are returning towards normal then surgery can safely be undertaken. Preparation for operation should also include physiotherapy to ensure clear lung bases, stockings on the legs to prevent deep venous thrombosis and prophylactic antibiotics. The operative procedure would most likely consist of release of an adhesive band obstruction, the unwinding of a volvulus or the reduction of bowel from within a hernial sac and resection if necessary.

Postoperative care. Postoperatively, one seeks to advance the patient as quickly as possible and, as soon as nasogastric aspirate drops off and wind is passed, the patient starts sipping fluids and moves on to a soft diet. Unfortunately return of effective peristalsis is often slow in patients after longstanding obstruction and it is important to ensure that during this postoperative phase plasma osmolality and serum sodium and potassium are kept within the normal range. Sometimes the whole illness becomes rather extended with the patient refusing to take food (or vomiting) and a period of TPN is required to get over the first week or two postoperatively, giving time for the bowel to decompress properly and regain its tone again before attempting to cope with food. We set a time. If the patient is not eating by the fifth postoperative day we commence TPN. It should be remembered that gastric emptying is not going to be normal if plasma albumin is low.

DIFFICULT PROBLEMS WITH SMALL BOWEL OBSTRUCTION

Postoperative adhesions

Patients recovering from major surgery sometimes follow a slow course. When normal bowel activity has not returned by the fifth postoperative day and there is increasing distension it is clear that there is an obstruction which needs further investigation. Generally speaking such obstructions are caused by adhesions and/or sepsis; they are often incomplete and they rarely strangulate. *Thus many settle on conservative therapy, although it needs to be stressed that if the obstruction is complete and distension is increasing in a deteriorating patient laparotomy is essential.* If this can be carried out before the end of the second postoperative week it is possible to break down the soft adhesions by gentle digital pressure but if surgery is necessary after that time the surgeon may encounter a degree of obliterative peritonitis that makes surgery hazardous if not impossible. Not a few patients with postoperative obstruction have been made worse by untimely or injudicious surgery.

Thus, as a general rule, when a patient after a large operation develops postoperative small bowel obstruction our practice is to commence a course of TPN. A nasogastric tube is inserted and all intake by mouth is stopped, the patient is encouraged to mobilise and every effort is made to ride out the situation in this way. In the vast majority of the cases surgery will not prove to be necessary and the problem settles within 2 or 3 weeks.

Paralytic ileus

Paralytic ileus is a symptom not a diagnosis and the surgeon needs to find out the cause of the paralysed bowel. Causes of paralytic ileus include peritoneal sepsis, infarcted gut, intraperitoneal blood, pancreatitis, biliary or renal colic, major fracture, major chest disease such as myocardial infarction or pneumonia, or electrolyte problems particularly hypokalaemia and hypomagnesaemia. Metabolic alkalosis, uraemia or diabetes may also cause paralytic ileus. Anticholinergics, narcotics and ganglion blocking agents are sometimes the cause of paralytic ileus. It is doubtful if idiopathic paralytic ileus occurs. The surgeon sees distension of all parts of the bowel from stomach to rectum although the stomach and colon are more greatly affected than the small bowel. The patient will experience anorexia and nausea from gastric stasis and will vomit if oral fluids or food are given. Colonic stasis results in uncomfortable distension of the abdomen and constipation. Infrequent bowel sounds may be heard. The management of paralytic ileus involves nasogastric decompression, intravenous correction of fluid and electrolyte deficiencies and correction of the underlying cause.

The patient with multiple episodes of adhesive obstruction

As mentioned earlier, some patients continue to have multiple episodes of adhesive small bowel obstruction and in some surgery may be helpful. Knowing that laparotomy will reveal massive adhesions and that the obstruction may be very difficult to relieve, surgeons are understandably reluctant to reopen these patients. Nevertheless, the problem may become so intransigent that a definitive procedure is required. Our practice is, after excluding by thorough barium studies and a CT scan any pathology other than adhesions, to reopen the patient and perform a very thorough and painstaking separation of the adhesions enabling the entire small intestine to be unravelled from duodenojejunal flexure to the ileocaecal valve. We use blunt nose scissors, dividing every adhesion and releasing completely the whole length of the small intestine. Then some 20 cm distal to the duodenojejunal flexure a small enterotomy is made on the antemesenteric border of the intestine and a Baker's tube (18 FG) is passed. The balloon is blown up so that it lies comfortably in the jejunum without distending it and the balloon is milked through the intestine. If a stricture is encountered then it is divided longitudinally and resutured transversely. The tube then continues throughout the length of small intestine until the ileocaecal valve is reached. The balloon must then be deflated to allow its passage through the valve, but once through into the caecum it is blown up again. The attachment of the jejunostomy to the abdominal wall is made so that the jejunum lies in a smooth arc without kinking because it is possible for this to form another site of adhesion. Following the procedure the patient is commenced on a 3-week course of total gut rest with TPN. At the end of that time, the balloon is deflated and under sedation the tube is slowly removed over a period of a few hours. The results of intraoperative intubation of small bowel for chronic adhesive obstruction have been reviewed by Jones (1987). Of 109 patients who had intraoperative small bowel intubation for recurrence of adhesive obstruction after one or more operations, only 1 suffered a recurrent episode over a reasonable follow up time of 2–5 years.

SECTION IV
LARGE BOWEL OBSTRUCTION

Large bowel obstruction differs considerably from that of the small bowel. Acute complete obstruction is much less common while chronic or subacute obstructive symptoms usually due to cancer or less commonly diverticular disease are much more frequent. The metabolic deficit suffered by patients with obstruction of the large bowel is slight. Distension of the large bowel does not cause hypersecretion and loss of extracellular fluid in any great quantity into the lumen. The large bowel responds to dilatation while maintaining its tone and blood supply until very late in the process and it thus becomes gas filled and filled with liquid faeces even though there is little evidence of major extracellular fluid loss. If the ileocaecal valve is incompetent, reflux of liquid faeces into the small bowel may be quite considerable and in this situation more fluid is lost because the small bowel also becomes distended. The general plan in large bowel obstruction is for the surgeon to decide first if the obstruction is complete and if the patient needs emergency surgery, and that usually is not so. Thus he is able to wait, to decompress the bowel and ensure that the patient comes to surgery in as sound a state as possible. A nasogastric tube to permit some drainage should be introduced as soon as the patient with acute large bowel obstruction appears in the ward and in all cases prior to surgery. The primary purpose is to empty the stomach, to prevent vomiting and aspiration during anaesthesia and reduce the chance of postoperative ileus. It is left in place until peristalsis returns in the postoperative period. Parenteral fluids and electrolytes are usually only required to make up the small deficits and to maintain the patient.

13. Alimentary tract – inflammation

SECTION I
INFLAMMATORY BOWEL DISEASE IN GENERAL

Inflammatory bowel disease describes a continuous spectrum of non-specific inflammation of the intestine, the clearest examples of which are ulcerative colitis and Crohn's disease.

ULCERATIVE COLITIS

Clinical patterns

The metabolic and nutritional management of patients with ulcerative colitis is based on an understanding of the natural history of the disease. Ulcerative colitis is a chronic large bowel disorder causing rectal bleeding and diarrhoea. The most common form of ulcerative colitis is associated with recurrent attacks of bloody diarrhoea with complete freedom from symptoms in between. This is called the *intermittent type* of ulcerative colitis. A much less common form of the disease occurs when the symptoms, having begun, persist indefinitely although fluctuating in severity. This is called the *chronic continuous type* of disease. There are a few patients who have a *single severe* attack of chronic ulcerative colitis and then are free of disease for many years. They almost always, however, have another attack.

Onset

The onset of ulcerative colitis may be gradual or sudden. A gradual onset is more common, the first symptom often being the passage of a small amount of blood, which then becomes bloody diarrhoea. Less common is a sudden onset of bloody diarrhoea and in the worst cases the patient may become gravely ill in just a few days.

Severity

Many patients with ulcerative colitis have it in a *mild* form and are never admitted to hospital. They are not constitutionally upset, an acute attack for them is to have up to 4 bowel movements each day with only small amounts of macroscopic blood in the stool. The outcome of an attack like this is nearly always good. On the other hand, patients may present with a *severe* attack, with 6 or more motions a day, macroscopic blood in the stool and constitutional upset. Patients with severe attacks should be hospitalised early and, if a quick response to maximum medical therapy is not obtained, total colectomy is indicated. The mortality has been dramatically reduced by resorting more readily to surgery. Of every 10 patients who are hospitalised with a severe attack of ulcerative colitis between 4 and 6 will require surgery during that admission. *Moderate* disease, that is intermediate between mild and severe, can, like mild disease, usually be treated satisfactorily on an outpatient basis. If a response does not occur promptly the patient should be admitted and treated as for severe disease.

CROHN'S DISEASE

Crohn's disease is a distinct entity of inflammatory bowel disease, characterised by transmural involvement, severe perianal involvement and the fact that, unlike ulcerative colitis which is confined to the colon, the small intestine is frequently involved. In ulcerative colitis, surgery can cure the patient but in Crohn's disease, where surgery is frequently needed, recurrences may follow. It occurs predominantly in young people, it is chronic and recurrent and its treatment is unpredictable and is often suboptimal.

Clinical patterns

In nearly half the patients with Crohn's disease the inflammatory process affects the terminal ileum and the ascending colon, in a third it involves the jejunum and ileum, in most of the remainder it involves the colon and, in a very small number, the whole of the intestine may be involved. The most common indication for surgical treatment in a patient with small intestinal Crohn's disease is obstruction and for those with ileocolic disease a combination of perforation with abscess and/or obstruction is the most common indication for surgery. In those with colonic Crohn's disease the indications for surgery are diverse with perianal manifestations being the most frequent and chronic illness with diarrhoea failing to respond to medical therapy another factor. Enterocutaneous (or enterovaginal or enterovesical) fistulas occurring either spontaneously or postoperatively also form an absolute indication for surgery in Crohn's disease.

Onset

The majority of patients with Crohn's disease present with diarrhoea, abdominal pain and weight loss, and many present with perianal sepsis, fissures and fistulas. The disease may remain undiagnosed for up to 5 years before it is clear that Crohn's disease is present.

Severity

Like ulcerative colitis the disease is subject to periods of increased activity. Unlike ulcerative colitis a simple mild, moderate and severe classification cannot be used and a number of activity indices have been used to quantify the disease severity. Although none is entirely satisfactory, in this book we have used the activity index of Best et al (1976) because of its widespread use (Table 13.1). Active Crohn's disease is said to be present when the Best score is greater than 150.

MALNUTRITION IN INFLAMMATORY BOWEL DISEASE

PEM is associated with active disease

The overall prevalence of protein energy malnutrition in patients with inflammatory bowel disease is not known for it has only been properly studied in patients who have been admitted to hospital (Hill et al 1977a). Figure 13.1 shows that significant protein deficits, that is a 20% or more deficit of body protein, are a feature of patients with active ulcerative colitis or Crohn's disease. When the ulcerative colitis is in remission, or the Crohn's disease is inactive, total body protein, although not normal, is usually not sufficiently depleted to affect physiologic function.

PEM is of the marasmic kwashiorkor type

Most patients who are admitted to hospital with active Crohn's disease or an acute attack of ulcerative colitis suffer to a greater or lesser extent from *marasmic kwashiorkor*. This is caused by a combination of factors which include decreased oral intake, increased whole body protein breakdown and increased losses of protein via the

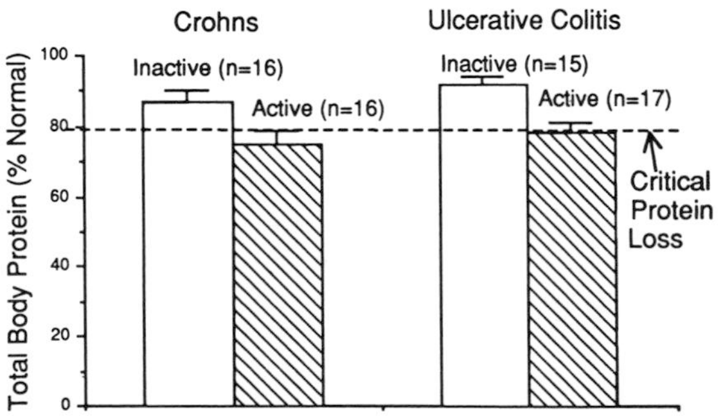

Fig. 13.1 Total body protein deficits in inflammatory bowel disease. Critical protein loss (i.e. when physiological impairments occur) is when there is more than a 20% deficit of total body protein. (Mean ± S.D.)

Table 13.1 Format for calculation of Crohn's disease activity index (from Best W R, Becktel J M, Singleton J E et al 1976 Gastroenterology 70: 439, by permission of the publishers, W B Saunders Company)

		Days 1 2 3 4 5 6 7	Sum	× Factor	=	Subtotal
1	Number of liquid or very soft stools			× 2	=	
2	Abdominal pain rating (0 = none, 1 = mild, 2 = moderate, 3 = severe)			× 5	=	
3	General wellbeing (0 = gen1 well, 1 = sl under par, 2 = poor, 3 = v poor, 4 = terrible)			× 7	=	
4	Number of 6 listed categories patient now has Underline the specific items 1 Arthritis/arthralgia 2 Iritis//uveitis 3 Erythema nodosum/pyoderma gangrenosum/aphthous stomatitis 4 Anal fissure 5 Other fistula 6 Fever over 100°F during past week			× 20	=	
5	Taking Lomotil/opiates for diarrhoea 0 = no, 1 = yes)			× 30	=	
6	Abdominal mass (0 = none, 2 = questionable, 5 = definite)			× 10	=	
7	Haematocrit	Males (47 − crit) Subtotal: Females (42 − crit) ______		× 6	=	
8	Body weight	Standard weight				
	Indicate units (1 = lbs, 2 = kg)					
	Percent below standard weight (nomogram):			× 1	=	
	Add (underweight) or subtract (overweight) by sign, to give Crohn's Disease Activity Index, CDAI				=	

bowel. Absorption of nutrients may be decreased because of decreased absorptive capacity, rapid transit time and excessive fluid and electrolyte losses via the anus or stoma. Protein, blood, bile salts and trace elements can be lost in similar ways. Examination shows that these patients have lost weight, skinfold thickness is diminished and muscle wasting is apparent. They are often tired and exhausted. Many are febrile, hypoalbuminaemic and suffer from vitamin deficiencies. If not present at admission to hospital it soon happens that the intensity of the malnutrition is sufficient to impair physiological function, the wound healing response and the response to delayed hypersensitivity skin testing.

Figure 13.2 shows the results of a protein turnover study in a patient with a severe attack of ulcerative colitis and compares it with a similar study of a depleted patient with inactive Crohn's disease. It is clear that the patient with severe colitis has increased protein breakdown, on the other hand, the patient with inactive Crohn's disease is similar metabolically to one who is starving with only a small net loss from body protein stores. The increased whole body breakdown of protein in severe inflammatory bowel disease results in a picture of marasmic kwashiorkor with hypoalbuminaemia and body protein deficits of 20–40% (Table 13.2).

Table 13.2 shows the body composition and

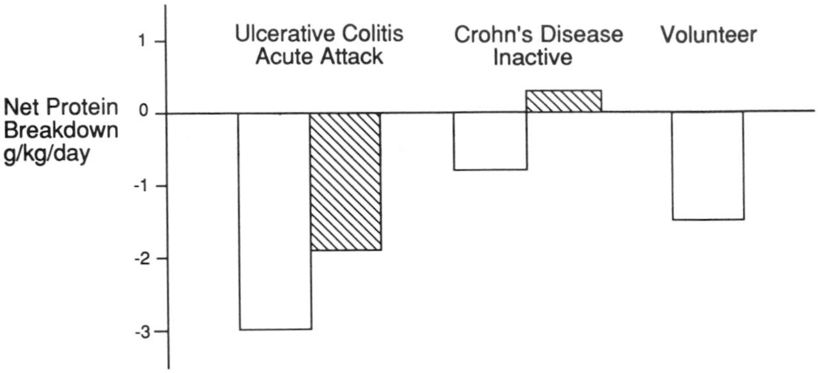

Fig. 13.2 Protein turnover in two patients with inflammatory bowel disease. The patient with inactive Crohn's disease has net protein breakdown similar to a normal subject. The patient with acute ulcerative colitis has a marked increase in net protein breakdown. TPN reduces the loss of body protein but does not eliminate it (data supplied by Dr J Shaw). Key: □ = basal □ = TPN

metabolic data which we obtained on the day of admission of a young woman with a severe attack of acute ulcerative colitis. Her picture is typical of such patients and shows the classical picture of marasmic kwashiorkor. Besides severe protein deficiencies there are also decreased fat stores due to the oxidation of fat for energy, an enlarged extracellular water, and a shrunken red cell mass consistent with the loss of body protein. Functionally there is impaired skeletal muscle function, impaired respiratory function together with mental and physical exhaustion, poor wound healing and anergy.

Rapid deterioration occurs during acute attack which increases risk if surgery is required

In most patients with inflammatory bowel disease which is in remission the intensity of PEM is mild. A few with the chronic continuous form of ulcerative colitis or panintestinal Crohn's disease suffer chronic continuing septic starvation and bravely contend with a less than optimal existence. Such malnutrition, if unresponsive to outpatient medical and nutritional therapy, may be a relative indication for excisional surgery. The problem of moderate to severe marasmic kwashiorkor, however, is usually one that accompanies and worsens during acute attacks which are of sufficient severity to require hospitalisation. The combination of sepsis, steroids, continuing protein loss and the inability to eat properly leads to rapid deterioration during an acute attack of either Crohn's disease or ulcerative colitis (Hill et al 1988). The patient may lose 1 to 2% of his/her protein stores each day. As we can see in Table 13.2, this results in the rapid development of marasmic kwashiorkor. This type of PEM is known to be associated with increased complications in the postoperative period with a longer hospital stay, a longer period of postoperative fatigue and prolonged convalescence (Windsor & Hill 1988d). Nutritional support is thus one of the key elements of the medical care of patients hospitalised with acute inflammatory bowel disease, about half of whom will require major surgery during their time in hospital (Dickinson et al 1980).

Micronutrient deficiencies

Apart from negative balances of sodium, and water that may occur because of excessive losses of small bowel fluid (usually from fistulas or stomas) a number of trace metal and vitamin deficiencies may occur in patients with inflammatory bowel disease (Driscoll & Rosenberg 1978) and these include *hypocalcaemia* which occurs particularly in Crohn's disease due to decreased

Table 13.2 Marasmic kwashiorkor in a 30-year-old female with an acute attack of severe ulcerative colitis. This study was performed on admission to hospital 21 days after the onset of the attack.

	Estimated value when well	Measured value on admission	% Change
Body composition			
Body weight (kg)	58.3	49.2	−16
Total body fat (kg)	13.2	9.1	−31
Total body protein (kg)	8.6	7.3	−15
Total body water (L)	33.8	30.1	−11
Extracellular water (L)	16.0	17.2	+8
ECW/FFM	0.36	0.43	+19
Intravascular space			
Plasma volume (L)	2.3	2.4	+4
Red cell volume (L)	1.8	1.3	−27
Blood volume (L)	4.1	3.7	−10
Haematocrit (%)	43	29	−33
Albumin (g/L)	40	28	−30
Transferrin (mg/dl)	291	150	−48
Prealbumin (mg/dl)	28.0	13.0	−54
Physiological function			
Grip strength (kg)	34	26	−24
Respiratory muscle strength (cm H_2O)	90	65	−28
Forced expiratory volume$_{1\ sec}$ (L)	3.4	3.0	−12
Vital capacity (L)	4.1	3.6	−12
Peak expiratory flow rate (L/min)	479	428	−11
Maximum voluntary ventilation (L/min)	203	162	−20
Metabolic expenditure			
Resting metabolic expenditure (kcal/24 h)	1166	1472	+26
Activity energy expenditure (kcal/24 h)	1166	594	−49
Total energy expenditure (kcal/24 h)	2332	2066	−11
Stress index	1.0	1.34	+34

intake or absorption of calcium from secondary effects of vitamin D deficiency. *Magnesium deficiency* presenting as hypomagnesaemia with hypocalcaemia (low plasma magnesium reduces the ability of parathormone to mobilise bone calcium) usually occurs in combination with other fluid and electrolyte abnormalities and manifests itself with either pins and needles in the tips of the fingers and toes or as frank tetany. Deficiencies of *fat soluble vitamins* (A, D, E and K) may occur in any situation where steatorrhoea is present. The usual cause of steatorrhoea in patients with inflammatory bowel disease is ileal resection or dysfunction with a reduced intestinal bile salt concentration which causes impaired micelle formation. Deficiency of *water soluble vitamins*, especially vitamin C, vitamin B_{12} and folate may also occur in patients with inflammatory bowel disease. Whereas vitamin C deficiency is most commonly a result of decreased intake, vitamin B_{12} deficiency usually occurs as a result of extensive terminal ileal disease or ileal resection. Bacterial overgrowth which occurs above small bowel strictures or within blind loops also causes vitamin B_{12} and folate deficiency.

NUTRITIONAL/METABOLIC GOALS

The surgeon cannot always expect patients with active disease to gain body protein even when aggressive nutritional support is provided. Very depleted patients, even those in whom RME is raised 30% or more, may gain a small amount of protein with 2 weeks of TPN but this probably is only sufficient to replenish the circulating amino acid pool and encourage the synthesis of circulating plasma proteins (Hill et al 1991). Nevertheless all patients will have significant improvements in physiological function which are probably of sufficient magnitude to lessen postoperative risk should surgery become necessary. We recently studied 19 patients, all with marasmic kwashiorkor, who were admitted to hospital with acute attacks of inflammatory bowel disease and received a 2-week course of TPN. Table 13.3 shows that as a group they gained only 200 g of protein over the 2-week study period (a gain that was not statistically significant) and there were small rises in plasma transferrin and plasma prealbumin. Table 13.4 shows, however, that during the first week of TPN there were significant improvements in physiological function. Compared to a group of matched controls the patients had physiological impairments of 20–40%. After only 4 days of TPN there were improvements in all the physiological measurements (~12%). We have recently found that a similar effect accompanies the administration of enteral nutrition (see Ch. 6, Fig. 6.2). It is for these reasons that we suggest that *the nutritional/ metabolic goal for these patients is to prevent further loss of body tissue, improve physiological function and to limit overhydration of the body.*

Table 13.3 Changes in protein nutriture that occurred in 19 patients with acute attacks of inflammatory bowel disease (*on day 0 the patients were commenced on a 14-day course of TPN (44 kcal/kg/day–1.7 g protein/kg/day)*. Values are mean ± s.e.m. (From Christie P M & Hill G L 1990 Gastroenterology 99: 730, by permission of the publishers, W B Saunders Company)

	Day 0	Day 14	p^*
Weight (kg)	49.2 ± 2.1	49.1 ± 1.8	NS
Total body protein (kg)	7.3 ± 0.5	7.5 ± 0.5	NS
Plasma transferrin (mg/dl)	215 ± 12	253 ± 23	<0.05
Plasma prealbumin (mg/dl)	19.0 ± 2.0	27.5 ± 2.3	<0.05

* Paired t test

NUTRIENT REQUIREMENTS

Energy

There have been a number of studies looking at the energy expenditure of patients with inflammatory bowel disease and generally speaking total energy requirements are not raised appreciably (Barot et al 1981, Barot et al 1982). Using 24-hour whole body calorimetry, workers at the Dunn Clinical Nutrition Centre at Cambridge University (Pullicino et al 1991) measured energy expenditure in patients receiving TPN while in remission from Crohn's disease. TEE was not raised, DIT was 6.1% of the energy intake and AEE was 12.9% of TEE. Other studies have shown that resting metabolic expenditure is increased up to 30% in severe or very active disease; this is usually compensated for by reduced physical activity and the total energy expenditure is usually little over 2000 kcal per day.

Table 13.5 shows our own recent study of TEE and its components in patients with active Crohn's disease. It shows that TEE can be quite variable, with patients of the same weight and with the same disease activity having quite different values.

It is for this reason that we measure resting metabolic expenditure (RME) by indirect calorimetry whenever possible and calculate total energy requirements (TEE) directly by multiplying the measured value by 1.3.

Protein

It has been shown and discussed elsewhere that 1.5 g of protein per kg of body weight are sufficient for this type of patient and if more protein is given it is unlikely to be utilised. It is not known if severe colitics, in whom stool losses may reach 100 g of protein or more, should receive additional protein but it seems reasonable that they should do so and for that reason we give 2–2.5 g protein/kg/day in patients with heavy losses of mucus and pus in the stool.

Table 13.4 Changes in respiratory and skeletal muscle function over time in 19 patients with acute attacks of inflammatory bowel disease–2 weeks of TPN. (From Christie P M & Hill G L 1990 Gastroenterology 99: 730, by permission of the publishers, W B Saunders Company)

	Controls	Day 0	Day 7	Day 14	$p^{\dagger}$
Grip strength (kg)	40 ± 3*	26 ± 3	30 ± 3	30 ± 5	<0.005
Respiratory muscle strength (cm H_2O)	104 ± 10	65 ± 8	76 ± 9	78 ± 10	<0.005
Forced expiratory volume $_{1\ sec}$ (L)	4.0 ± 0.3	3.0 ± 0.2	3.2 ± 0.2	3.3 ± 0.27	<0.005
Vital capacity (L)	4.8 ± 0.3	3.6 ± 0.3	3.7 ± 0.2	3.8 ± 0.2	<0.01
Peak expiratory flow rate (L/min)	576 ± 23	428 ± 25	454 ± 22	462 ± 22	<0.01
Maximum voluntary ventilation (L/min)	268 ± 27	162 ± 12	195 ± 17	197 ± 18	<0.005

* Mean ± sem † paired t test

Table 13.5 Measurements of TEE and its components in 13 patients with active Crohn's disease (after Stokes 1991) – REE measured by indirect calorimetry, AEE calculated from tables. Key: SI = Small intestine; IC = Ileocolic; JIC = Jejuno-ileocolic; Cl = Colonic; CDAI = Crohn's disease activity index.

Sex	Age	Wt	Wt Loss	Site	CDAI	REE	AEE	TEE
F	51	51.7	28%	SI	240	1146	352	1498
M	63	44.6	26%	IC	308	1290	334	1594
F	34	41.4	17%	IC	268	1343	429	1772
F	51	58.0	27%	SI	197	1164	442	1606
F	35	63.9	12%	IC	225	1237	745	1982
F	45	72	5%	IC	289	1327	588	1915
F	27	56.5	0	JIC	145	1155	812	1967
M	21	69.5	1%	IC	181	1437	825	2262
M	27	60.9	3%	IC	162	1382	797	2125
F	18	51.4	11%	C1	302	1512	785	2297
M	15	32.1	20%	SI	256	1802	335	2137
F	21	44.4	6%	JIC	276	1079	282	1361
F	38	52.6	4%	C1	282	1373	503	1876

Salt and water

Most of these patients are on high dose steroids and have a tendency to retain salt and water with a greatly expanded extracellular water as a consequence. Body weight gains, more than 200 g per day in this setting, almost always suggest positive salt and water balance and should be treated by sodium restriction.

SECTION II
THE METABOLIC AND NUTRITIONAL CARE OF PATIENTS WITH CHRONIC ULCERATIVE COLITIS

Having set down the general principles of the nutritional and metabolic care of patients with inflammatory bowel disease we now need to discuss the detailed management of patients with ulcerative colitis and Crohn's disease separately.

TPN HAS NO PRIMARY THERAPEUTIC ROLE IN ULCERATIVE COLITIS

It has now been clearly established by two randomised prospective trials that total parenteral nutrition has no primary therapeutic effect at all in patients hospitalised with acute attacks of ulcerative colitis (Dickinson et al 1980, Mclntyre et al 1986). In our own controlled study of 27 patients with severe attacks of ulcerative colitis (Dickinson et al 1980), 14 were treated along conventional lines, 6 of them required surgery, and the other 8 settled in an average time of 24 days. The 13 patients who received TPN behaved in an almost identical manner. 7 came to surgery and 6 settled in an average time of 26 days.

OUTPATIENT NUTRITIONAL CARE

Total parenteral nutrition or enteral nutrition are not often required by patients between attacks although those with the chronic continuous type of ulcerative colitis need careful evaluation by a dietitian and clear instructions as to optimal eating habits. These are similar to those given to patients with Crohn's disease (see below). The trouble comes about when an acute attack develops at home, does not remit in a fairly short time and hospitalisation is required. It has been shown that such patients have already lost considerable amounts of body protein by the time they reach hospital (usually around 20%). Thus no time should be wasted before starting treatment to prevent further loss in case surgery is required. The fact that 40–60% of such patients will come to surgery during this admission to hospital should not be lost sight of.

NUTRITIONAL SUPPORT OF PATIENTS WITH SEVERE ATTACKS OF ULCERATIVE COLITIS

Patients with severe attacks of ulcerative colitis may be treated with enteral feeding through a fine bore nasogastric tube but we prefer TPN for most of these patients. We find it difficult to feed a hypoalbuminaemic patient, who already has severe diarrhoea, by the enteral route. Some patients, less ill, can, however, be fed enterally and with considerable benefit but for most TPN enables us to control requirements more closely. The day of admission is spent on nutritional assessment with restoration of red cells and albumin, trace metals and vitamins as required. TPN is commenced the next day, the goal being to preserve or to prevent further loss of body protein, improve physiological function and control and correct overhydration. Thus energy requirements are met by prescribing an amount equal to RME times 1.3 and protein requirements are met by giving up to 2.5 g protein/kg/day depending on excessive losses from the bowel. No sodium is given to patients who at admission are hypoalbuminaemic and water is given only in sufficient quantities to keep serum osmolality and renal function normal. After a few days when energy and protein requirements are being met and there are no signs of oedema sodium can be gradually introduced up to normal amounts.

Our longitudinal study of body protein stores in 10 patients with severe attacks of ulcerative colitis illustrates the real benefit of nutritional support in these patients (Fig. 13.3). After admission to hospital and a 7-day trial of conservative therapy each of the 10 patients came to surgery (either total colectomy or panproctocolectomy). After recovery from surgery and discharge from hospital they were followed until their convalescence was complete and they were back at work and feeling well — an average of 40 weeks. Figure 13.3 shows the changes in total

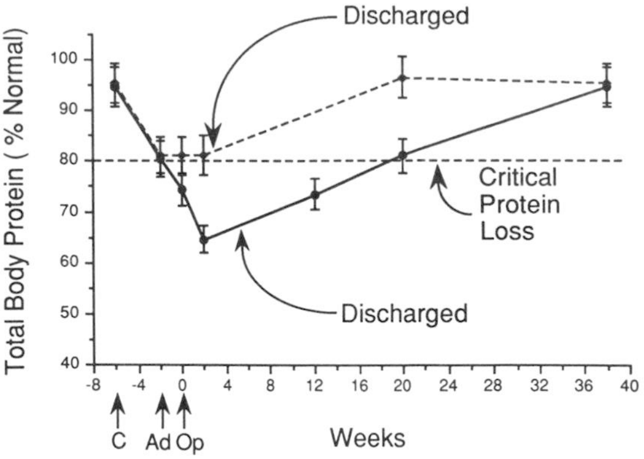

Fig. 13.3 Changes in total body protein that occurred in 5 matched pairs of patients with an acute attack of ulcerative colitis: the controls (solid black line, mean age 47.6 ± 12.1 yr, mean weight 59.4 ± 12.5 kg) received no extra nutritional support throughout their illness. The TPN patients (broken line, mean age 42.6 ± 10.2 yr, mean weight 60.8 ± 10.6 kg) received a full course of TPN which began on admission to hospital 3 weeks after onset of the acute attack and continued perioperatively until 14 days postoperation. The rapid loss of body protein that occurred during the 3-week period at home continued for the 2 weeks in hospital prior to surgery and increased after surgery for a further 2 weeks in the control patients. After commencement of TPN no further protein was lost either before surgery or in the postoperative period in the TPN group. Restoration to normal protein stores occurred about 18 weeks earlier in the TPN patients (mean ± s.e.m.). Key: C = Commencement of acute attack; Ad = admission to hospital; Op = total colectomy Discharged = discharged from hospital.

body protein that occurred from the time that they were at home before the attack occurred through their time in hospital including surgery up until 40 weeks postoperatively.

It can be seen that there was a rapid deterioration in total body protein stores over the 3 weeks prior to admission to hospital. 5 of the patients were commenced on TPN on admission to hospital and from then on further losses of total body protein were prevented. Normal body composition was measured in these 5 patients some 20 weeks after surgery. This beneficial effect of nutritional support whilst they were in hospital and beyond can be contrasted with the protein losses measured in the other 5 patients who were clinically very similar but who did not receive nutritional therapy during their hospital stay. 1% of their body protein was lost each day prior to surgery and even greater losses continued over the first postoperative week. Restoration of normal body composition took twice as long — 40 weeks (Fig 13.3).

In another study of 6 matched pairs of patients with ulcerative colitis who came to panproctocolectomy, the group who received postoperative TPN for the first 2 postoperative weeks were discharged from hospital earlier and had more rapid healing of the perineal wounds than those who received no added nutritional therapy (Collins et al 1978).

Whereas one must look at studies such as these with considerable caution because only a small number of patients have been included, there is enough here to suggest *a real clinical benefit for patients in whom continuing protein loss is prevented by appropriate nutritional therapy.*

ELECTIVE SURGERY — NUTRITIONAL THERAPY NOT USUALLY REQUIRED

In the past patients with ulcerative colitis not infrequently came for surgery in a parlous nutritional and metabolic state. These days with sphincter saving surgery patients are presenting earlier for surgery and malnutrition is not often a problem. In Table 13.6 are shown the results of a group of 16 patients who came to us for elective ileoanal J pouch surgery and received no

Table 13.6 Changes in body composition in 16 patients over 12 months after ileoanal J pouch surgery (mean ± 1 s.e.m.). Key: x = $p < 0.05$ xx = $p < 0.025$ xxx = $p < 0.01$ xxxx = $p < 0.005$ (From Christie P M & Hill G L 1990 Return to normal body composition after ileoanal J pouch anastomosis for ulcerative colitis. Dis Colon and Rectum 33: 584–586, by permission of the American Society of Colon and Rectal Surgeons)

	Estimated normal values	Before surgery	2 weeks after surgery	3 months after surgery	12 months after surgery
Body weight (kg)	71.4 ± 3.6	66.6 ± 3.4	63.05 ± 3.1	66.4 ± 3.3	70.8 ± 4.0
	. . . . .xx. . . .	. . . . .xxx. . . .	. . . . .xxx. . . .	. . . . .xx. . . .	
				xx	
			NS		
Total body protein (kg)	11.3 ± 0.8	9.2 ± 0.7	8.5 ± 0.8	9.1 ± 0.8	10.8 ± 0.7
	. . . . .xx. . . .	. . . . .xx. . . .	. . . . .NS. . . .	. . . . .xxx. . . .	
				xx	
			NS		
Total body fat (kg)	16.7 ± 1.0	17.1 ± 1.7	15.4 ± 1.4	16.9 ± 1.4	18.4 ± 2.1
	. . . . .NS. . . .	. . . . .xx. . . .	. . . . .x. . . .	. . . . .xx. . . .	
				xx	
			x		
Fat free mass (kg)	51.9 ± 3.0	49.9 ± 3.0	47.5 ± 3.0	49.8 ± 3.2	52.3 ± 3.0
	. . . . .xx. . . .	. . . . .xx. . . .	. . . . .xxx. . . .	. . . . .xx. . .	
				xx	
			NS		
Total body water (L)	37.2 ± 2.2	37.2 ± 2.0	34.8 ± 2.5	37.7 ± 2.4	38.7 ± 2.2
	. . . . .xx. . . .	. . . . .xxx. . . .	. . . . .xxx. . . .	. . . . .NS. . .	
				NS	
			NS		
Total body water fat free mass	0.73 ± 0.01	0.75 ± 0.01	0.74 ± 0.01	0.76 ± 0.01	0.74 ± 0.01
	. . . . .x. . . .	. . . . .NS. . . .	. . . . .xxx. . . .	. . . . .xx. . .	
				x	
			NS		

pre- or postoperative nutritional therapy. Only one of these patients developed postoperative complications. As a group their average time in hospital was 16 days and the data show that by the end of a 12-month period they all enjoyed normal body composition, had returned to work and were in good health.

SECTION III
THE METABOLIC AND NUTRITIONAL CARE OF PATIENTS WITH CROHN'S DISEASE

TPN HAS NO PRIMARY THERAPEUTIC ROLE IN CROHN'S DISEASE

Over the years there has been considerable debate about the value of gut rest and nutritional therapy in patients with Crohn's disease. A number of retrospective studies seemed to show that TPN in particular could be a real factor in avoiding surgery and restoring the patient back to normal life. Nevertheless two randomised prospective studies have been unable to confirm these impressions and it has to be concluded that gut rest and nutritional therapy does not induce a remission in patients with Crohn's disease (Greenberg at al 1988, Payne-James & Silk 1988).

OUTPATIENT NUTRITIONAL CARE

The surgeon who manages patients with Crohn's disease will realise that many of these patients are chronically unwell, continue to be underweight, are unable to eat adequately because of pain and suffer from a number of vitamin deficiencies. The combined effect of malabsorption, poor dietary intake, inability to eat protein compared with carbohydrate, the attacks of diarrhoea and the continuing sepsis make it a challenge to manage these patients on a day to day basis. The wise thing is to enlist the help of an expert dietitian with a special interest in patients with Crohn's disease. Such a person can work wonders and engender great confidence in these patients and make life a lot more tolerable for them. Some guidelines, produced by the dietitians at our hospital (L Gillanders & K Maher) specifically for the nutritional care of outpatients with Crohn's disease, are set out in Tables 13.7, 13.8 and 13.9.

NUTRITIONAL SUPPORT OF PATIENTS HOSPITALISED WITH CROHN'S DISEASE

Patients hospitalised with active Crohn's disease are usually admitted in the hope that intensive medical therapy will settle the disease down and surgery can be avoided. In spite of this, 1 in 4 patients who are admitted to hospital with a diagnosis of Crohn's disease come to surgery. It is therefore important that nutritional therapy is begun as soon as possible to avoid further deterioration of nutritional state. Many patients with Crohn's disease respond well to enteral

Table 13.7 Master food plan for patients with Crohn's disease

'A little of what you fancy' makes sense. Keep your food choices as close as possible to your normal meals but use the following groups as a guide.

Milk group — for protein, calcium and vitamins
2 servings daily
  milk, yoghurt, cheese, cottage cheese, milk products

Meat or meat substitute group — for protein, vitamins, iron and other minerals
2 servings daily
  beef, veal, lamb, pork, poultry, liver etc.
  fish, fresh or canned
  eggs, cheese, cottage cheese
  dried peas, beans and lentils
  nuts, peanut butter

Bread/cereal group — for energy, vitamins, minerals and fibre
3–5 servings daily
  bread — wholemeal or white, biscuits, cereals, breakfast cereals rice, macaroni, spaghetti, pastas

Fruit/vegetable group — for energy, vitamins, minerals and fibre
4–5 servings daily
  green and root vegetables, raw or cooked potatoes
  fruit, raw or cooked
  fruit or vegetable juices, especially citrus or tomato for extra vitamin C

Fat group — for energy, vitamins, and minerals
Usually added to the other groups
  butter, margarine, oils, vegetable fats
  cream
  peanut butter

Table 13.8 Food guidelines for patients with Crohn's disease complicated by partial obstruction

If you have lost weight and feel nauseated:
- eat small frequent meals rather than too much at any one time
- enjoy between meal snacks — simple hunger often prolongs nausea
- keep up your fluid intake — sip drinks slowly (6–8 cups/day)
- try ginger ale, lemonade (allow to go flat if you have an ostomy), fruitjuices, weak tea, marmite, vegemite, clear broths, iceblocks
- separate fluid intake from meals
- talk to your dietitian about using a supplement
- eat and drink slowly
- try foods which are quickly and easily digested — increase starchy foods e.g. cereals, bread, rice, pasta, root vegetables and decrease fatty foods and fried foods
- rest after eating
- relax before meals to reduce anxiety as worry affects appetite
- limit foods which fill you up and dull your appetite without being nutritious e.g. black coffee, sweets
- after periods of sleep or rest eat some dry crackers or crisp toast before activity
- choose foods which do not have a strong smell, cold meats, sandwiches, gelatin puddings, yoghurt, omelettes
- you may need a vitamin and mineral supplement

feeding and providing diarrhoea is not excessive and bowel obstruction is not present this is the feeding route of choice. Although Figure 13.4 shows that improved physiological function occurs whether the nutritional therapy is given parenterally or enterally, in severe marasmic kwashiorkor we prefer to use TPN. In a recent study we found difficulty in returning large extracellular water volumes to normal with an enteral

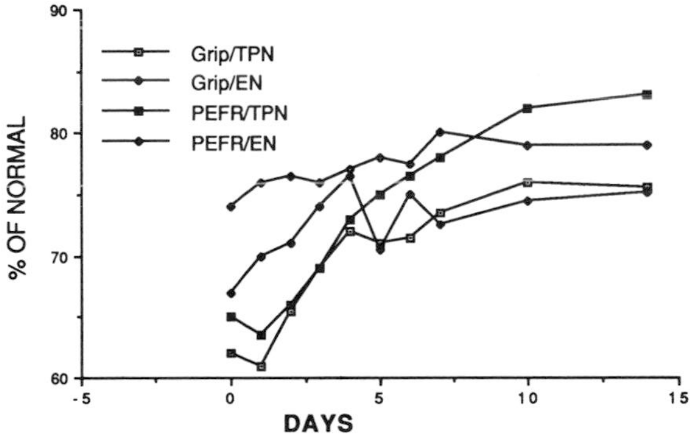

Fig. 13.4 The effect on physiological function of TPN (N = 21) and enteral nutrition (EN) (n = 11) is similar. PEFR = peak expiratory flow rate. (Data from Stokes 1991.)

Table 13.9 Food guidelines for patients with Crohn's disease complicated by diarrhoea

Diarrhoea
- Keep up your fluid intake between meals
- Reducing milk intake may be helpful — you may have an intolerance to lactose
- Avoid seeds, pips and skins, nuts, raw fruit and raw vegetables, whole grain cereals
- Avoid gas producing foods, e.g. cabbage, onions, cucumber, dried peas and baked beans

nutrition regimen compared with low sodium TPN (Stokes 1991).

Perioperative nutritional therapy in patients undergoing surgery for Crohn's disease

Surgery for Crohn's disease often involves operating on a patient with moderate to severe marasmic kwashiorkor. Knowing the difficulties involved with poor wound healing, impaired skeletal muscle function, expanded extracellular water, hypotonicity and avitaminosis it behoves the surgeon to carefully assess the patient's nutritional status and decide whether nutritional repair is required before embarking on what may prove to be a complex and difficult operation. It is of considerable advantage for the surgeon therefore to take some time over the metabolic and nutritional repair of Crohn's patients prior to surgery. If there is insufficient time to allow nutritional repair the surgeon is wise to restrict the magnitude of the surgery to dealing with the immediate problem, be it obstruction, abscess or fistula. Drain and defunction are the guiding rules here; if one strives to accomplish much more in patients who are metabolically and nutritionally depleted postoperative complications are a likely consequence. Postoperative TPN should be the rule after large procedures in malnourished patients with Crohn's disease. In this way anastomoses can be rested, further protein loss prevented and there can be a longer period of adaptation as diet is reintroduced in the recovery period. We use TPN rather than enteral nutrition in most Crohn's patients who require nutritional support postoperatively. This is because the extensive procedures often required have involved much handling, multiple anastomoses and long suture lines which taken together often result in a prolonged period of ileus.

SECTION IV
THE SPECIAL PROBLEMS OF PATIENTS WITH ENTEROCUTANEOUS FISTULAS ASSOCIATED WITH CROHN'S DISEASE

About 20% of patients with Crohn's disease of the small intestine develop fistulas. Roughly half of these are external fistulas which may develop either spontaneously or in the early postoperative period (Goligher 1984).

TYPES OF FISTULAS

In patients with enterocutaneous fistulas associated with Crohn's disease there are two clear patterns of presentation and subsequent behaviour.

Postoperative fistulas arising from the small intestine which is free of residual disease

These fistulas occur in patients with Crohn's disease and arise in the early postoperative period after an operation in which there have been extensive adhesions predisposing to inadvertent damage to the bowel or an anastomosis. These fistulas arise from the small intestine with no macroscopic evidence of Crohn's disease. They behave in a similar way to those that occur in patients without Crohn's disease (see Ch. 15).

Fistulas arising from diseased small intestine

In some patients, the fistula develops in the early *postoperative* period either from an anastomosis where some remnant of the disease remains or from another area of diseased bowel. In others the fistula develops *spontaneously* from an abscess which presents under the abdominal wall at an old drain site or through the site of a previous incision. These patients have macroscopic and/or microscopic evidence of Crohn's disease in the small intestine at the site of fistulation. While none of these fistulas close and stay closed with total gut rest and TPN, they sometimes close after a long period and remain so for a few weeks before discharge occurs again from the old site. The fistula may persist but be of nuisance value only.

Thus patients with Crohn's disease may develop enterocutaneous fistulas in two ways: a fistula from an apparently healthy bowel may arise in the early postoperative period after laparotomy or resection, or it may originate spontaneously from an area of residual disease. It is generally held that fistulas occurring immediately postoperatively may close spontaneously but that fistulas associated with residual Crohn's disease are refractory to all but surgical treatment.

GUIDELINES FOR THE MANAGEMENT OF PATIENTS WHO DEVELOP ENTEROCUTANEOUS FISTULAS IN CONNECTION WITH CROHN'S DISEASE

Like others we have learnt that the management of these patients is different depending on whether the fistula has arisen in the early post-operative period from damaged or sutured bowel or has originated in an area of diseased bowel (Irving 1983).

Management of postoperative fistulas arising from the small intestine apparently free of residual Crohn's disease

Generally speaking, the management of fistulas of this type in no way differs from that which we will describe later in Chapter 15 for postoperative fistulas in general. That is, it comprises four sequential but frequently overlapping stages, which include *control of the fistula output, drainage of sepsis, TPN and excision of the fistula* if there is no spontaneous closure. A special point about these patients is the severe intensity of the mal-nutrition which is present once the sepsis has

Table 13.10 Protein nutrition in 7 patients with Crohn's disease who developed postoperative fistulas (from Hill G L, Bourchier R G, Witney G B 1988 World J Surg 12: 191, by permission of the publishers)

	Estimated value when well	Measured value after resuscitation and drainage of sepsis	Change %
Total body protein (kg)	10.0	5.3	−47
Albumin (g/L)	39.2	35.4*	—
Transferrin (mg/dl)	260	194	−25
Prealbumin (mg/dl)	26.3	14.8	−44
Stress index†	1.0	1.2	+20

* Each patient had received albumin for resuscitation
† Measured RME/predicted RME

been brought under control. Table 13.10 shows the nutritional and metabolic status of 7 fistula patients with Crohn's disease and it shows the profound depletion of body protein stores that occurred as the result of postoperative sepsis. Each patient had developed a postoperative fistula and had peritonitis and intraabdominal collections as a consequence. These measurements were made just after the sepsis had been brought under control and immediately prior to the commencement of TPN. Since definitive surgery is often not technically possible for 6–8 weeks after all signs of sepsis have disappeared there is ample time for these severe defects in body protein to be restored. Provided the fistulas are not associated with a mass of Crohn's disease, one would expect to gain 150–250 g of protein each week with aggressive nutritional support and along with this would be substantial improvements in physiological function, wound healing and immune competence.

Fistulas arising from the small intestine containing Crohn's disease

We have shown, as have others, that there are really two types of fistulas within this category: *early postoperative* and *spontaneous* (Brooke et al 1977, Hawker et al 1993). Early postoperative fistulas are not always due to failure at the anastomosis, but can be due to exacerbation of the disease elsewhere. *Early postoperative fistulas* from diseased bowel may be very difficult to treat, they are often of high output associated with major intraabdominal sepsis and cannot be expected to close spontaneously. Their management follows the lines we have set out in Chapter 15 for postoperative fistulas in general.

Spontaneous fistulas vary greatly in their complexity. The simpler ones usually arise from a terminal ileum involved in active disease. The implicated bowel becomes attached to an area of scar on the deep surface of the abdominal wall which in turn becomes inflamed. An abscess forms and spontaneous discharge or surgically induced drainage results in an enterocutaneous fistula. Much more complex fistulas may arise in association with abscesses secondary to spontaneous penetration of the wall of the intestine. These abscesses usually present as brawny bluish swellings on the abdominal wall and may spontaneously discharge faeces, pus or mucoid material at several sites. A mistake is to assume that if only pus or mucoid material escapes, there is no deep connection with the intestine. Some claim that such fistulas may close with TPN azathioprine, 6-mercaptopurine (Kozarek et al 1989, Present et al 1980), cyclosporin (Sachar 1989) or elemental diets, but most authorities remain sceptical, and it is safe to assume that such fistulas will never close without surgical intervention. Spontaneous fistulas associated with Crohn's disease are treated as other fistulas in that the initial stages are concerned with controlling sepsis, correcting metabolic defects and nutritional support. The problem with these patients is the timing of surgery. Our studies have shown that nutritional support is valuable while sepsis is being brought under control but once that has happened there is no point in further delay. *While a Crohn's mass remains in the abdomen it seems almost impossible to have appreciable gains in total body protein in spite of aggressive nutritional support* (Hill et al 1988). The operative procedures required are discussed in Chapter 15, Section V.

SECTION V
RADIATION ENTEROPATHY

INTRODUCTION

Gastrointestinal symptoms occurring during and after radiotherapy are common but usually resolve spontaneously within a few weeks of stopping the treatment. Many patients go on to develop chronic problems but most of these result in symptoms that are minor consisting of minimal change in bowel habit and little else. Others may develop symptoms such as proctitis, diarrhoea or malabsorption which can be managed by dietary manipulation and constipating agents. Less than 5% of patients who receive radiotherapy will ultimately come to the surgeon with symptoms caused by bleeding, fistula, perforation or chronic obstruction from stricture formation. The majority of patients requiring surgical treatment have had pelvic irradiation for carcinoma of the cervix, endometrium, ovary or bladder (Hauer-Jensen 1990).

AETIOLOGY

The determining factor in radiation injury is probably the dose. Whereas tumour doses of below 4500 cGy are only rarely associated with radiation injury, it has been shown that small bowel injuries increase from a range of between 1 and 5% at the dose of 4500 cGy to 25–50% at 6500 cGy.

Previous abdominal surgery, particularly when it has involved the pelvic viscera, is an important factor in the development of radiation enteritis. It is thought that the normal mobile distal small bowel becomes trapped in pelvic adhesions where it becomes particularly vulnerable to the radiation beam. A similar problem occurs in patients who have had previous pelvic inflammatory disease. There is some evidence that chemotherapy and radiation produces more intestinal damage than either of these treatments used alone.

PRESENTATION

Radiation affects the intestine in two main ways. First there is a direct effect on the mucosa that occurs during the course of the treatment. Secondly there is an indirect effect caused by obliterative endarteritis which may cause ischaemic change in the irradiated bowel. This may produce mucosal necrosis with ulceration and bleeding or it may produce a complete infarct of a portion of the bowel with chronic perforation and the symptoms of pelvic sepsis and incomplete obstruction. The development of a stricture appears to be due to a more chronic type of ischaemia resulting in considerable fibrosis of the bowel wall. These pathological findings help in understanding the three classic clinical presentations of radiation enteropathy (Carr et al 1984).

Radiation enteropathy presenting within 1 month of radiotherapy

Many patients develop proctitis either during or soon after the course of treatment is finished. A few patients develop an acute ileitis which may cause diarrhoea or even obstructive symptoms and exceptionally this may need surgical relief. Most of the early symptoms settle with conservative treatment and the patients have no further symptoms although a small minority develop symptoms later.

Radiation enteropathy presenting between 2 months and 2 years of radiotherapy

Chronic perforation, rectal bleeding and *anal pain* and *fistula* are the problems that occur in this intermediate period. Some patients have more than one of these presenting symptoms. The usual picture is of a patient with moderate to severe PEM of the marasmic-kwashiorkor type suffering severe pain from incomplete intestinal obstruction. There is usually evidence of pelvic sepsis and chronic perforation. The perforation may be in the upper rectum or sigmoid colon or in the ileum and some develop a fistula into the vagina. Severe rectal bleeding can be the predominant symptom and anorectal ulceration can be severe; if this encroaches on the anoderm severe pain is the result.

Perforation. Patients with perforations secondary to radiation injury fall into two main groups. There are those who have a perforation alone, usually within the first year after radiotherapy and there are those who have a perforation later, sometimes 5 or 6 years after radiotherapy, in whom it is found that the perforation occurs immediately proximal to a radiation induced stricture. Both small and large bowel (usually at the rectosigmoid junction) may perforate and present as generalised peritonitis. Occasionally where local intraabdominal defences react effectively, the patient will present with an intraabdominal abscess. The usual presentation, however, is with pelvic sepsis and incomplete intestinal obstruction due to chronic perforation and these patients present with deep abdominal pain, often severe weight loss, sometimes with diarrhoea and evidence of low grade sepsis. They may be hypoalbuminaemic and present a classic picture of marasmic kwashiorkor. The diagnosis is not always thought about. Severe bowel disease after pelvic radiotherapy is relatively uncommon. It is unusual for any surgeon unless he works in a major oncological unit to encounter many patients with this disease. A high index of suspicion is the key to early diagnosis, particularly in the group with chronic perforation. The surgeon must be vigilant in order not to overlook a potentially curable situation and not dismiss the patient as suffering from incurable residual or recurrent malignancy.

Bleeding. This usually results from proctitis and on sigmoidoscopic examination local reaction varies from mild erythema suggestive of early inflammatory bowel disease to a pale thick and fibrotic mucosa with multiple telangiectasia to a markedly hyperaemic mucosa with many superficial bleeding ulcers. The upper rectum and rectosigmoid junction are usually narrowed and fixed and it is difficult to pass the sigmoidoscope beyond this area of narrowing. A chronic rectal ulcer also may develop from the anterior rectal wall just above the anal verge. This necrotic yellowish grey appearing ulcer usually 3 or 4 centimetres in diameter also appears characteristic of radiation necrosis, and not at all like a malignant ulcer of the rectum.

Fistula. Fistulas characteristically form between the vagina and rectum just proximal to the site of rectosigmoid stenosis. They may involve small bowel, uterus, bladder, and skin and the clinical presentation varies with their site. Both small and large bowel (again at the recto-sigmoid junction) may perforate and present as generalised peritonitis.

Radiation enteropathy presenting more than 2 years after radiotherapy

Although chronic perforation, bleeding and pain may present many years after radiotherapy most late presentations are secondary to incomplete intestinal obstruction due to a fibrous stricture which may involve the sigmoid colon or the ileum or both. An ileal stricture or entrapment of the ileum in a pelvis full of dense fibrous tissue is the commonest late presentation. It is usually manifested by crampy central abdominal pain, nausea, occasional vomiting and malabsorption in the patient who appears chronically ill, is undernourished and has persistent pain after meals. These patients are classically suffering from marasmic kwashiorkor of moderate to severe degree. They are hypoalbuminaemic, with over-expanded extracellular water, a small red cell volume and severe physiological impairments. Not only does malnutrition impact on the wound healing response but the local tissues damaged by the radiation heal poorly, the combined effect being a high chance of an anastomotic breakdown after excisional surgery.

It is important to understand that a number of patients with radiation enteropathy will have symptoms due to recurrent tumour and this becomes a diagnostic problem in patients who develop symptoms within 2 years of treatment. After that time it is rare for a recurrent tumour to be the cause of symptoms. Also, patients with radiation enteropathy suffer other radiation injuries sometimes involving the skin or, more commonly, the bladder where haematuria and/ or a small fibrosed bladder causing gross frequency and incontinence may be particularly troublesome.

MANAGEMENT

Early stage

Acute radiation sickness is characterised by

nausea, vomiting and/or diarrhoea. It usually subsides quickly with modification of a dose or termination of the radiation. Acute proctitis during the latter part of the course may persist for 1 or 2 weeks after completion of radiation but in the vast majority does not persist thereafter. The patient with small bowel adherent within the pelvis may develop an acute enteritis which, if severe, is associated with vomiting and diarrhoea. These symptoms usually respond to a low residue diet, loperamide, and adequate fluid and salt replacement. Gluten free and lactose free diets have been tried with success by some authors, more commonly elemental diets and medium chain triglycerides are appropriate when there is excessive diarrhoea and steatorrhoea. If malnutrition becomes severe, and this is rare in these patients with early enteritis, TPN may be indicated. Chronic recurrent bleeding sometimes occurs at this early stage and leads to iron deficiency requiring either oral iron supplements or, if bleeding is severe, blood transfusion.

Management — perforation and fistula

Diagnosis, investigation and preparation for surgery. The patient may appear unwell and cachectic and the surgeon has the problem of deciding whether this is recurrent malignancy or some complication of the radiotherapy. Recurrent malignancy usually occurs within 2 years of radiotherapy and also because these conditions can coexist makes the diagnosis quite difficult at times. Investigations will include barium studies and computer aided tomography and will also include an evaluation of the patient's metabolic and nutritional status. Whilst investigations are proceeding, repair of the metabolic and nutritional deficits should be underway. Thus vitamins, trace metal deficiencies, concentrated albumin and red cell transfusion may all be required and, if the intensity of protein energy malnutrition is sufficient to cause physiological impairments, then a short course of nutritional replenishment is advisable. A typical plan for repair of a patient such as this would include:

Day 1
Clinical examination, looking for the intensity and type of protein energy malnutrition and for any physiological impairments including hypoalbuminaemia, avitaminosis, oedema, impaired wound healing, and skeletal muscle dysfunction. These are patients whose postoperative course may be complicated by poor wound healing, intestinal obstruction and low grade sepsis. Our practice is to return all the plasma values to the normal range, provide ample vitamins and sufficient protein and energy and seek a marked improvement in physiological function. Thus red cells are given to bring the haematocrit to 35%, albumin is given to bring the level above 35 g/L and intramuscular injections of vitamin B_{12}, folate and vitamin K are given before starting TPN.

Day 2
Rest while radiological studies and other evaluations are under way. Commence TPN containing sufficient energy to provide RME × 1.5 kcal/day and protein to provide 1.5 g of protein/kg/day with appropriate electrolytes and vitamins but excluding sodium if the patient is profoundly hypoalbuminaemic. The energy should be provided as 30–50% fat. Enteral nutrition is not appropriate for these patients because of the leakage of intestinal contents into the pelvis.

Day 3, 4, 5
Continue with TPN and vigorous physiotherapy.

Day 6
If investigations have been completed, the diagnosis made and the patient is free of major physiological impairments, then surgery can be planned. Particularly so if the patient has a normal plasma albumin and is free of oedema, and has clear lung bases. It is not uncommon, however, for this preparation to take a further week until more obvious improvements can be detected clinically. Continuing TPN beyond 2 weeks is unlikely to be helpful.

Surgery for perforation or stenosis. The operation may be an extremely difficult one and the decision has to be made whether the involved intestine has to be resected or bypassed. We, like many others, favour resection where possible (Schofield et al 1986), although if the intestine is a mass of dense concrete-like fibrous adhesions in the pelvis bypass is the preferred option. The important point is to make any anastomoses in bowel that is free of oedema, friability, and any evidence of radiation change. Ideally radiation induced lesions should be widely excised while two ends of bowel free of radiation disease are used for the primary anastomosis. Unfortunately, it is usually impossible to guarantee that two ends of gut are free of radiation disease. Frozen section is unreliable in deciding at what level a resection should be made. Similarly, even gut that appears macroscopically normal may ultimately be shown to be damaged when examined by microscopy. However, it has now been demonstrated that the ascending, transverse and descending colons are usually free of radiation induced lesions. Whenever possible then these parts of bowel should be used for one end of an anastomosis. Thus terminal ileal resection is followed by an ileotransverse anastomosis and rectosigmoid resection by mobilisation of the splenic flexure to bring it down for anastomosis. The problem of performing a bypass and leaving irradiated bowel in situ is that further problems may arise in the affected bowel. Perforation in bypassed bowel has been reported. After either a Hartmann's procedure or simple colostomy for bleeding the patient may continue to bleed and may still require an abdominal perineal resection of the rectum.

Division of adhesions should be accomplished with great care since small enterotomies may be made inadvertently during this procedure and, since the irradiated bowel heals poorly, minute enterotomies may leak later. *It is for these reasons that we usually advise a 2-week period of total gut rest with TPN postoperatively. After 2 weeks a soft diet is slowly introduced and when the patient is voluntarily eating 1000 kcal/day the TPN is stopped.*

Surgery for radiation fistula. The management of fistulas deserves special mention. Small bowel fistulas to either the skin or vagina should be treated by isolation or bypass rather than resection since the latter requires a considerable dissection which in these patients is potentially hazardous. Similarly there is often no need to resect rectovaginal fistulas. Parks et al (1978) described a technique in 4 patients whereby the rectum is divided just above the fistula and a length of rectosigmoid is resected. The mucosa is then stripped from the remaining rectum and the descending colon is pulled through the muscular tube leaving the fistula in situ. Others have used this technique and have achieved satisfactory results in terms of a cure of the fistula and incontinence.

Management — late stricture

Clinical example

The management of a radiation stricture presenting many years after pelvic irradiation can best be described by considering a patient we treated recently.

> The patient was a 66-year-old woman who was admitted acutely to hospital, complaining of severe abdominal pain, bloating and constipation over the previous 3 or 4 days. Examination revealed a tender abdomen with high pitched bowel sounds. A plain radiograph showed fluid levels typical of a small bowel obstruction. Her past history revealed a radical hysterectomy for stage IIa carcinoma of the cervix some 20 years previously. The hysterectomy was followed by external beam cobalt irradiation which lasted for 2 or 3 weeks but the dosage was not obtainable. Since that time she has had intermittent diarrhoea and constipation but has been relatively well. 2 years previous to this admission, however, she was admitted acutely with small bowel obstruction and laparotomy revealed thick vascular adhesions causing obstruction to the terminal ileum. No other abnormality was noted during that laparotomy.

The past history of hysterectomy followed by radiotherapy, the intermittent periods of diarrhoea since then and particularly the observations at surgery 2 years prior to this admission all raise the possibility of radiation enteropathy. A flexible sigmoidoscopy was performed and this showed a pale rectal mucous membrane with telangiectasia and readiness to bleed. At 14 cm from the anal verge it was not possible to pass the instrument further because of an apparent stricture. Nutritional evaluation revealed a small woman who was extremely thin with very little subcutaneous fat and wasting of her temporalis muscles, supraspinatus muscles, biceps and triceps and the interossei of the hands. She was tired and exhausted even after resuscitation and said she had felt that way for some many months. Her grip strength was weak although her breathing seemed normal but she was tired and rather lacking in energy when asked to walk around the ward. Weight loss had not been a prominent feature of the past weeks, but she was more than 10 kg lighter than her ideal weight prior to her hysterectomy many years ago. Blood investigations revealed a haematocrit of 33% and a plasma albumin of 31 g/L. There was no evidence of oedema on physical examination. This was moderate to severe marasmic kwashiorkor. Her RME was not raised.

Over the next day or two the abdominal distension settled quickly and radiology showed improvement, less distension and loss of fluid levels. It is clear that full investigations were necessary and that surgery might be indicated. She was commenced on a course of central TPN while these investigations continued in the hope that some improvement in nutritional state could be obtained and repair would be well on the way if surgery was indicated. The first day was spent restoring red cell mass, vitamin status, trace metals and albumin. A 2-week course of TPN was then commenced. Over the next few days a barium study which involved both a barium enema and a small bowel enema were performed revealing a stricture about 30 cm long in the terminal ileum and another stricture at the rectosigmoid junction measuring 12 cm in length. There was also clear evidence of radiation proctitis on the double contrast barium enema. By the end of 2 weeks she was much improved. She was up and about the ward and a decision was made to see if oral intake could be recommenced. Thus a soft diet was started and before long she was consuming 1500 kcal and 40 g of protein per day orally and the TPN was stopped. The patient herself was not keen to proceed to surgery although continuing to have symptoms, she felt that they were not sufficiently bad to warrant an operation. *One can expect about 30% of patients to manage indefinitely without surgery but the rest will require surgery.*

6 months later, the patient was admitted again with an acute episode of small bowel obstruction very similar to the previous admission. Radiology revealed fluid levels again, and barium studies again demonstrated the ileal stricture and the rectosigmoid stricture although the latter now allowed the passage of a colonoscope and it was not involved in the obstruction. She was neither anaemic, nor hypoalbuminaemic at this stage. Marked functional impairment was apparent on physical examination and her chronic malnutrition state persisted.

After 1 week of intensive nutritional and metabolic preparation which included vitamins, albumin infusion and TPN she demonstrated much improvement in her physiological status and surgery was planned.

Laparotomy was done through a midline incision and after very careful dissection of the many adhesions it was possible to demonstrate the stricture of the terminal ileum which involved about 25 cm of intestine. 50 cm of ileum were resected as was the caecum and ascending colon and an end-to-end anastomosis was performed in healthy looking intestine between the ileum and the proximal ascending colon. TPN continued for 2 weeks after the surgery, at the end of which time she commenced on a soft diet which soon proceeded to a normal diet. Unfortunately she had difficulty eating dietary fat and after dietetic advice she was placed on a 40 g fat diet which resulted in freedom from the symptoms of disabling steatorrhoea. She was discharged from hospital on the eighteenth postoperative day. She remains well but has a vitamin B_{12} injection on a regular basis.

14. Alimentary tract — massive resection

INTRODUCTION

Massive resection of the small intestine may have profound effects on nutrition and metabolism. The effects depend not only on how much intestine remains after resection but what part has been removed. Jejunal resection is tolerated much better than ileal resection and concomitant removal of the ileocaecal valve may result in greater symptoms than anticipated from the small bowel resection alone. Generally speaking most adult subjects have about 6 m of small intestine (Treves 1924, Backman & Hallberg 1974). It has been shown, however, that when less than 3 m of small bowel remain a number of serious metabolic and nutritional abnormalities occur. When 2 m or less remain, most patients are unable to perform a full day's work and many patients with less than 1 m of small intestine remaining need TPN at home on an indefinite basis.

The symptom complex that develops after massive resection is called *the short gut syndrome.* Besides extensive small bowel resection it comprises *diarrhoea, steatorrhoea* and *malnutrition.*

SECTION I
WHAT IS MEANT BY 'REMAINING INTESTINE'

After the operation of massive enterectomy it is important for the surgeon to say quite specifically in his operation note how much intestine remains and what part of the intestine it is. It is not how much that has been removed that counts but how much remains. Even here there are a number of pitfalls because measurement of the length of intestine in sick people is liable to major error. Firstly, the intestine may change its length during the operative procedure. Although there is a close relationship between the patient's fat free body mass and the length of his or her intestine when first measured soon after the abdomen is opened, measurements taken throughout the duration of the operative procedure show that the length is often much shorter by the end of the operation. Secondly, there are errors in the measurement itself. Measuring tapes made of cotton may shrink and shorten on becoming wet during the measurement procedure and rigid rulers can be very difficult to manipulate within the abdominal cavity. We ourselves measure the length of the small intestine in relation to the length of our index finger. Starting at the duodenojejunal flexure, loops precisely the length of the index finger are separately lifted and counted until the ileocaecal junction or the point of resection is reached. The result is expressed in centimetres of remaining bowel measured from the ligament of Treitz. Estimates made in this way have been found to be within 6% of those made by the painstaking use of a special non-shrinking tape applied approximately 1 cm from the mesenteric border of the intestine (Hill 1986).

Having made this estimate of the remaining intestine the ultimate test is the physiological length that remains and the clinical course that is followed by the patient in the weeks and months that lie ahead.

SECTION II
INDICATIONS FOR MASSIVE ENTERECTOMY

In the past, mechanical disasters such as massive intestinal infarctions within strangulated hernias, small bowel volvulus and mesenteric thrombosis were the major causes of massive enterectomy. Recent series have shown that those patients surviving massive resection and requiring long term care usually have Crohn's disease although mesenteric thrombosis (both arterial and venous) and volvulus are still significant causes (Table 14.1).

These days, therefore, the surgeon is liable to encounter the short gut syndrome in young people with Crohn's disease and in the elderly after intestinal infarction. It is important, however, to realise that long term management problems usually belong to the group of patients who have had a resection for Crohn's disease or volvulus. Patients with mesenteric vascular occlusion are often elderly and their overall prognosis is poor; thus only a few survive to become long term management problems.

Table 14.1 Comparing the indications for massive enterectomy in two recent series compared with a 1935 series

	Haymond 1935	Bambach & Hill 1982	Stokes et al 1988
Volvulus	76	—	4
Strangulated hernia	45	—	—
Mesenteric thrombosis	34	3	10
Female pelvic disease	21	—	1
Mesenteric disease	19	—	—
Trauma	16	—	1
Tuberculosis	16	—	—
Crohn's disease	—	31	21
Radiation enteritis	—	1	1
Polyarteritis nodosa	—	—	2
Multiple fistulas	—	1	1
Miscellaneous	30	—	3
Total	257	36	44

SECTION III
INTESTINAL ADAPTATION

For a 1 to 2 year period after massive resection, the remaining small intestine dilates though it probably does not elongate (Dowling 1982). There is hyperplasia of the mucosa, with an increase in the villus surface area. This results in enhanced absorption per unit length of intestine (Bristol & Williamson 1985). Many years ago, Flint (1912) studied the effects of extensive resection of the small intestine and showed a significant increase in villus height. He calculated that the absorptive area of the remaining bowel had increased fourfold. This enhanced absorption is non specific and the absorption of all substances is increased. *The adaptation is particularly prominent in younger patients and probably does not occur at all in patients over the age of 65.*

There are three factors which affect postresection intestinal adaptation:

- *The presence of enteral nutrients*
  Throughout the small intestine the crypt cell production rate is dependent on the presence of enteral nutrients. If, following resection, patients are maintained on total gut rest and TPN, then intestinal adaptation does not occur. Enteral nutrition increases gut blood flow and provides specific nutrients for the enterocyte. It appears that chyme is required for adaptation to occur. Chyme consists of both food and intestinal secretions (Bristol & Williamson 1985).
- *The amount of intestine which has been excised*
  With massive resection the adaptive response is directly proportional to the length of bowel removed.
- *The site of resection*
  The adaptive response to ileectomy is not as strong as that after jejunectomy. This is probably because after ileal resection the jejunal luminal contents remain unchanged, whereas if the jejunum has been resected

the ileum receives more chyme than usual and responds accordingly. If the ileum is resected the jejunum does not inherit the specialised transport functions of the jejunum which include vitamin B_{12} absorption, bile salt absorption, and the ability to regulate sodium and water absorption.

SECTION IV
SURGICAL PHYSIOLOGY OF MASSIVE ENTERECTOMY

This can be better understood if it is remembered that there are differences in *motility, nutrient absorption* and *fluid and electrolyte transport* between the proximal and distal small intestine.

MOTILITY

Chyme passes through the upper half of the small intestine in less than one third of the time it takes to pass through the distal half. The ileum has a marked effect in slowing transit and the effect of the ileocaecal valve and the colon is to slow transit even further (Singleton et al 1964). The clinical effect is that proximal small bowel resection does not raise the rate of intestinal transit whereas ileal resection may have a dramatic effect. The colon has the slowest motility of the intestine so ileal resections that include the colon as well further increase the rate of intestinal transit.

WATER AND ELECTROLYTE ABSORPTION

Again the effects of resecting the proximal or distal small intestine or the colon are quite different. This is because the jejunum keeps its contents in an isotonic state whereas the contents within the last metre of ileum and in the proximal colon become progressively more concentrated. The distal ileum and colon in particular are powerful conservers of salt and water, particularly when mineralocorticoid activity is high. Thus, jejunal resection results in little malabsorption of salt and water because the ileum absorbs much of the increased fluid and electrolyte load and any excess is absorbed in the colon. In contrast, after ileal resection there are two problems with which the colon has to cope. Firstly there is an increased isotonic fluid load and secondly there is the presence in the chyme of irritating and diarrhoeal producing bile salts (Binder 1973). Bile salts are usually absorbed in the distal ileum. If more than 100 cm of ileum have been resected bile salts become depleted and as a consequence, fat is malabsorbed. Fatty acids reach the colon and like bile salts they reduce the reabsorption of water and electrolytes resulting in diarrhoea (Hofman & Poley 1972). If both the ileum and colon are resected and the patient is left with a jejunostomy the fluid that is discharged has not been concentrated and isotonic water and salt losses can be high. Salt and water depletion are common in patients with jejunostomies as are hypocalcaemia, hypomagnesaemia and zinc deficiency.

If there has been a massive enterectomy and an enterocolic anastomosis, diarrhoea may not be excessive unless the fluid load entering the colon exceeds its absorptive capacity. This appears to be (in the intact colon) about 5 L a day (Debongnie & Phillips 1978).

NUTRIENT ABSORPTION

Most nutrients are completely absorbed within the first 150 cm of the small intestine (Borgstrom et al 1957). The last metre of the ileum has the specialised function of vitamin B_{12} absorption and bile salt absorption, and it has some control over salt and water absorption as well. In patients who are salt and water depleted mineralocorticoids act on the terminal ileum as well as on the colon and cause them to conserve salt and water. Patients with less than 100 cm of ileum are not usually troubled by steatorrhoea but greater ileal resections result in steatorrhoea with accompanying malabsorption of the fat soluble vitamins. Lesser ileal resection may interfere with the absorption of vitamin B_{12}. It can be seen therefore that when the jejunum alone is removed the ileum takes over its absorptive function fairly readily and there is little problem with steatorrhoea or diarrhoea. By contrast, ileal resections of a metre or so cause steatorrhoea and markedly decreased fluid and salt absorption.

SECTION V
STAGES OF RECOVERY AFTER MASSIVE ENTERECTOMY

Pullan (1959) has described three clinical stages which are experienced by the patient after massive enterectomy.

THE POSTOPERATIVE STAGE

In the early days after massive enterectomy, management may not always be easy. Fluid and electrolyte losses from diarrhoea and nasogastric aspiration, bowel complications such as fistulas, and often intraabdominal sepsis may have to be contended with. In some patients, however, the early postoperative course is quite benign and the surgeon may be lulled into thinking that the problem is not going to be as great as he or she had at first thought. Diarrhoea may not start for several days and may even be delayed until the patient makes attempts at feeding. Although gastric hypersecretion can be a real problem after massive enterectomy, not infrequently there is very little drainage from the nasogastric tube and some patients never develop excessive gastric juice. A major concern at this stage is for the management of the stoma and protection of the skin around it from excoriation. If the patient is passing motions via the anus the problem of anal excoriation and fissures secondary to diarrhoea may become severe.

THE STAGE OF DISCOURAGEMENT

As the problems from disabling diarrhoea subside, appetite returns and abnormal bowel function settles and the output reaches a plateau providing the patient is not eating. Unfortunately, the diarrhoea and its associated electrolyte and fluid difficulties return as soon as attempts are made to return to normal eating. It is here that a discouraging battle is often fought to balance nutritional needs against a limited absorptive capacity without producing intolerable side effects from diarrhoea and bowel dysfunction. The intestinal adaptive processes mentioned above aid this recovery process with time, and an improvement results over the next several months as protein and carbohydrate absorption improve.

THE STAGE OF EMERGING NUTRITIONAL AND METABOLIC PROBLEMS

The patients who survive to reach this stage arrive at a period in which maximum weight gain is achieved, a relatively normal diet can be eaten and home care can be contemplated. The interval between the resection and this stage is quite variable. It may be only 3 months, but occasionally may be as long as 18 months to 2 years. Complex nutritional and metabolic problems are common during this stage and later. Table 14.2 shows our study of the long term nutritional effects of resection of the intestine which we found in a group of patients after enterectomy in which the average length of bowel remaining was 3 m. It can be seen that 15% of the patients were below their normal weight and there were appreciable but not great deficiencies of body fat and protein. *Deficiencies* of *iron*, *vitamin* B_{12} and *folate* were common but most of the patients were not anaemic. *Vitamin* and *trace metal* deficiencies were also common. The surprising fact was that two thirds of the patients in spite of these abnormalities were back to their normal occupation full time and said they felt reasonably well. Those who did not return to normal work had appreciably greater nutritional deficits and the length of bowel resected was much greater.

Urinary tract calculi of all types are more common after extensive enterectomy. Patients who have had an enterectomy and are left with a small bowel stoma have low urine volumes and there is reduced calcium excretion. The concentration of urinary oxalate and urate is increased and the risk of both uric acid and calcium stones is high. Patients with small bowel resection alone and an enterocolic anastomosis have hyperoxaluria and an increased risk of calcium stones despite a low urinary calcium.

Table 14.2 Nutritional and metabolic abnormalities found in 36 patients with extensive resection of the small intestine (after Bambach & Hill 1982)

	% reduction	% with low values
Body composition		
Body weight	14.8	—
Total body fat	23.8	—
Total body protein	9.3	—
Total body water	12.7	—
Plasma proteins		
Plasma albumin	—	8
Plasma prealbumin	—	14
Plasma transferrin	—	0
Haemintics		
Haemoglobin	—	17
Serum iron	—	47
Vitamin B_{12}	—	55
Folate	—	46
Vitamins		
White cell vitamin C	—	49
Vitamins B_1 and B_6	—	6
Vitamin A	—	33
25-hydroxyvitamin D	—	36
Minerals		
Serum potassium	—	20
Serum calcium	—	17
Serum magnesium	—	37
Serum zinc	—	14

In any event, our own studies (Table 14.3) and those of others show that patients after massive enterectomy have higher levels of urinary risk factors both for uric acid and calcium stone formation and that this risk of forming a urinary stone persists for the remainder of their lifetime.

Osteomalacia is frequently present in these patients but is not always recognised unless bone biopsy is performed (Compston et al 1978).

Hypomagnesaemia associated with severe neuromuscular symptoms and frequently accompanied by hypocalcaemia may be seen in patients who pass over 1.5 L/24 h from the stoma. The problem occurs in patients with high output stomas who are on the edge of metabolic equilibrium after a period of increased stoma activity.

Some patients develop hypersecretion after massive enterectomy and this may persist for years. It is more marked after jejunal resection and may improve with time. We have encountered patients after extensive resection, however, who have almost no gastric juice even after stimulation with pentagastrin.

Table 14.3 Abnormal urinary constituents in patients after intestinal resection — 24-hour excretion (adapted from Bambach C P, Robertson W G, Peacock M, Hill G L 1981 Gut 22: 257 by permission of the publishers)

	Normal controls (n = 85)	Ileostomy and enterectomy (n = 17)	Enterectomy with ileocolic anastomosis (n =17)
Volume (L)	1.7	0.72*	1.36
pH	6.1	5.4*	5.8
Calcium (mmol)	4.6	2.5*	1.5*
Oxalate (mmol)	0.29	0.31	0.60*
Uric acid (mmol)	3.6	2.9	3.1
Sodium (mmol)	172	23*	135
Potassium (mmol)	59	52	68

*$p < 0.001$ compared with normal controls

SECTION VI
PATIENT MANAGEMENT

AT THE TIME OF SURGERY

When small bowel resection is necessary it is important for the surgeon to remember that the distal intestine is more important physiologically than the proximal intestine, the ileocaecal valve if preserved can improve the quality of the patient's life immensely, and any length of ileum or colon that can be preserved is of benefit. Unfortunately one doesn't usually have the luxury that allows decisions based on these principles for the pathology usually dictates the length and site of resection. There are a few things that might help:

- Sometimes one cannot be firm about the extent of ischaemia and it is not easy to decide on the viability of the bowel. Techniques have been described such as fluorescein dye infusion which delineates the extent of the ischaemia and so reduces to a minimum the amount of bowel needing to be resected (Gorey 1980). There is, however, no substitute for dividing the bowel at a questionable site and proceeding proximally into an area where the blood supply is clearly adequate before the definitive resection is made. If doubt continues, rather than removing an excessive length of intestine, the safest course is to exteriorise the gut ends and observe the stomas for 24 hours or so. If they continue to look healthy then there is a place for a second laparotomy with reinspection of the remaining intestine and the creation of a new anastomosis if all is well.

- Patients in whom there is extensive Crohn's disease requiring resection are a special category. The surgeon needs to remember that such patients may require a number of resections over the years and strive to preserve as much intestine as possible. Only bowel that is obstructing or is fistulated or is involved in an abscess needs to be resected and it is a mistake to try and resect all the macroscopically diseased bowel. Even then, meticulous surgical technique in mobilising the intestine is vital for success and one needs to take down adhesions and matted bowel with the utmost care. These patients can ill afford to lose bowel that need not have been resected because the surgeon has handled it roughly or it has become ischaemic through an inadvertent mesenteric tear.

Conservative surgery therefore is the rule in Crohn's disease and the extent of resection may be judged by the extent of mesenteric fat creeping on to the bowel wall itself. Where the creeping ceases, generally speaking macroscopic mucosal and submucosal changes have also ceased and it is safe to do a primary anastomosis a centimetre or two beyond this into healthy intestine.

Stricturoplasty has added a new dimension to the surgery of small bowel Crohn's disease and it is possible to relieve obstruction without resection at all in some patients. Like others (Alexander-Williams & Haynes 1985) our practice is to carefully dissect out the entire small intestine in patients with extensive Crohn's disease and through a small enterotomy in healthy jejunum pass a Foley catheter with the balloon inflated to fit comfortably within the intestine at that site. The balloon is then milked distally along the length of the intestine and where it encounters a stricture this is divided longitudinally and repaired transversely. Where the stricture is longer or clearly the site of acute inflammation, then a limited resection is carried out. It is possible to perform 8 or 10 stricturoplasties on the same patient or, alternatively, perform some stricturoplasties and some small bowel resections and in these ways large losses of bowel can be avoided. If one encounters extensive sepsis at the site of disease, it is sometimes wiser to form a stoma proximal to this and return later when the sepsis has resolved to perform a limited resection and a primary anastomosis.

- Faced with acute mesenteric infarction careful consideration must be given to whether massive enterectomy should be done at all. A very old patient with massive infarction of almost the whole intestine is better left untreated. Intestinal adaptation can not be expected at this age and the quality of life is quite intolerable for an elderly patient with a high output stoma. There needs to be at least 1 m or more of healthy intestine which allows anastomosis either to the terminal ileum or to the colon before one can feel that it is right to proceed to surgery in a very elderly person.
- Because home parenteral nutrition has made it possible to live a reasonable life with almost no small intestine it is tempting to extend the indications for massive enterectomy. Some patients with extensive radiation enteritis, widespread neoplasm, or multiple fistulous disease associated with massive sepsis and multiorgan failure may occasionally fall into this category. We feel that such indications must be few and far between and our practice in most of these situations is to perform a gentle laparotomy for drainage purposes and attempt to obtain a loop of proximal jejunum to bring out as a loop stoma. High jejunostomy can be life saving in these circumstances and knowing this we have not yet been tempted to perform a near total enterectomy.
- Because in many patients requiring massive enterectomy there may be doubt over the safety of a planned anastomosis a stoma is

not uncommonly required. It is for this reason that in every patient in whom massive enterectomy may be expected we mark a stoma site on the skin prior to surgery. This is marked out in 4 sites, one in each quadrant of the abdomen, but preferring of course to use the lower quadrants, particularly that on the right if at all possible. Modern stoma care systems enable patients even with high output jejunostomies to be managed without undue difficulty (Hill & Pickford 1979).

DURING THE POSTOPERATIVE PHASE

It is important that the patient should receive nothing by mouth over the days and possibly weeks following massive resection. Increased secretion is encouraged by the osmotic stimulation of salt and water secretion that follows malabsorption of orally taken nutrients. With massive resection there may also be substantial fluid losses because of gastric hypersecretion and malabsorption of endogenous secretions from the gut. Rather than using nasogastric aspiration for a long period, gastric secretion can be dramatically reduced by intravenous ranitidine which is given as a continuous infusion. Somatostatin may have a place in particularly difficult patients (Ladefoged et al 1989).

As soon as the patient is haemodynamically stable central TPN is commenced, the goal being to maintain body fat and protein stores and to control within close limits hydration of the body. We measure the resting metabolic expenditure and calculate the energy requirement as 1.3 times this, and give 1.5 g of protein/kg/body weight together with appropriate sodium, water, potassium, magnesium and trace metal requirements. Zinc is required in increased amounts in these patients and for every litre of intestinal contents lost, an extra 15 mg of zinc is prescribed (Wolman et al 1979). These components together with the H_2 blocker are mixed together in a single container. Losses should be accurately measured and replaced accordingly. If the surgeon is finding difficulty in accurate fluid and electrolyte balance it is simpler to provide the nutrient solution through the central line via a single container than to put up a peripheral line to replace the fluid and electrolyte that is being lost through the stoma or via the stool. These losses can be replaced litre for litre with crystalloid. Most often, Ringer's lactate is used although if there is much continuing gastric hypersecretion this should be replaced litre for litre with 0.9% saline to which 15 mmol of potassium is added to each litre. At this stage, thorough attention to care of the stoma is important. When leakages occur, the entire skin must be gently washed with warm water and soap and the area dried with a hair dryer before a new skin barrier is applied. In patients who have an intact colon, similar attention to the perianal skin is required and after each bout of diarrhoea the area is gently washed with warm water and soap and dried with a hair dryer before a barrier cream is applied.

The duration of this difficult postoperative phase in which nothing by mouth and TPN are required varies from 1 month or so to 2 or 3 months. The end of this stage is marked by a plateau in the stool volume, and electrolyte losses which become predictable. Because adaptation does not begin before enteral feeding is given, this should be initiated as soon as faecal output and electrolyte losses reach a predictable plateau (Purdum & Kirby 1991).

DURING THE TIME WHEN ORAL INTAKE IS BEING ESTABLISHED

Resumption of enteral feeding, preferably by the oral route must be gradual and it is best accomplished with only a fraction of the intake that the patient desires. In those who have more than a metre of small bowel remaining the surgeon should attempt progressive introduction of refeeding with a view to achieving as normal a diet as possible. For those with less than a metre of intestine remaining the initial target should be a small intake of isotonic fluids containing carbohydrate and electrolyte. For patients with intermediate lengths, progressive feeding should begin with isotonic carbohydrate electrolyte feeds with an aim of ultimately achieving a normal or modified normal diet. We use a glucose polymer, Caloreen (Roussel) (34 g/L) to which is added 85 mmol/L of sodium, 12 mmol/L of potassium,

9 mmol/L of bicarbonate and 109 mmol/L of chloride. Isotonic carbohydrate electrolyte feeds such as these are usually well absorbed by patients even after extensive enterectomy (Griffen et al 1982).

Next it must be decided when to commence normal foods or whether a balanced enteral diet should be used first. We use the metre rule again; for those patients with more than a metre of small intestine an ordinary diet of natural ingredients is tried. Dry solids are taken first, followed an hour or two later by isotonic fluids. It is an important principle to separate the dry components of food from the liquid ones because of the faster rate of gastric emptying following massive resection. How much fat should be included in the diet is controversial (Woolf et al 1983). We recommend a low fat diet since after ileal resection fat is poorly absorbed and increases diarrhoea dramatically. Furthermore, a high fat diet impedes the absorption of divalent cations and for this reason they need to be given in increased quantities. In any event patients who have had an ileal resection, should always receive a low fat diet. They will not tolerate animal fat and dramatic effects can be obtained by giving a 40 g/day low fat diet.

Patients who fail to tolerate oral intake such as this are given a constant infusion of a defined formula diet. We start with half strength Osmolite at 25 ml/h gradually increasing to full strength and then to 100–125 ml/h.

Synthetic opioids such as loperamide can improve the patient's quality of life and reduce diarrhoea considerably. We use up to 4 mg of loperamide hydrochloride 3 times a day and even in these dosages side effects are extraordinarily rare. Somatostatin (SMS 201–995) is often effective in patients with very high stool outputs but it is our impression that the effect wears off and the net result is disappointing (Stokes & Hill 1990b).

It should be remembered that this second stage of transition to oral feeding can be a disheartening business. There is a battle being fought to balance nutritional needs against grossly restricted absorptive capacity and trying to do this without causing intolerable side effects particularly with uncontrollable bowel function. If oral diet used in the ways mentioned here causes severe and massive fluid and electrolyte losses, one has to back off and continue with TPN, waiting for the situation to plateau again before attempting oral intake once more. In most patients intrinsic adaptive processes aid recovery and improvement often leads to independence of external therapy over the next 3 to 6 months.

In patients in whom there is less than 1 m of remaining bowel the process is more difficult. Once the patient has reached a plateau on small amounts of carbohydrate feeds a tentative attempt at an oral feeding schedule such as that described above is tried. TPN can be gradually reduced as oral intake increases. Sometimes these patients need additional water and electrolytes only, others need TPN intermittently (say 3 times per week) whilst others remain on home TPN indefinitely.

LONG TERM NUTRITIONAL AND METABOLIC SUPPORT

The aim of management is to progress through the stages as the patient adapts firstly to TPN with some oral intake, then through an oral diet with additional fluid and electrolyte parenterally and then through to an oral diet supplemented by a defined formula diet and finally as an outpatient to a fairly normal diet.

From Table 14.2 it can be seen that there are deficits in fat stores, showing the difficulty in providing adequate energy intake for these patients, and total body protein is usually well below normal levels. This stresses the importance of good dietetic help encouraging high energy intake, good quality protein and especially added vitamins. We frequently give 1-α-hydroxylated vitamin D metabolites and magnesium hydroxide to prevent hypomagnesaemia and osteomalacia.

Those with less than a metre of ileum resected are helped often by cholestyramine. If more ileum than this has been resected and steatorrhoea is troublesome a fat restricted diet is useful. Cholestyramine is also useful in patients with hyperoxaluria. Trace element provision can sometimes be forgotten about. It is helpful from time to time to measure the volume of stool and add an extra 15 mg of zinc to the diet for each litre of stool being lost.

SECTION VII
HOME ENTERAL AND HOME PARENTERAL NUTRITION

Some patients who do not progress to oral diet can be managed by nasogastric tube feeding at home. A fine bore tube is passed through the nose into the stomach each night and while the patient is asleep a balanced enteral diet can supply the needed energy, protein, fluid, and electrolyte requirements (McIntyre et al 1983). Unfortunately such feeding is not always tolerated by the patient and home parenteral nutrition (HPN) is required (Scott et al 1991).

HPN was developed in North America in the early 1970s by Scribner and Jeejeebhoy. The procedure is now well established throughout the world and many publications have shown that the life style for patients on HPN can be good and the inconvenience of the treatment is less than might be expected (Jeejeebhoy 1983, Stokes & Irving 1989, Dudrick et al 1984).

HPN may improve the patient's quality of life enormously. A patient may eat 12 meals a day and have 20 bowel movements a day as a consequence and yet remain free of HPN. Such a life, however, would allow little time to pursue a career, let alone work, and little time for normal social intercourse. HPN will revolutionise the outlook for such a patient. Others will need HPN only for a time and then may come off it whilst others may need it for decreasing amounts of time and end up requiring to receive their infusions only 3 or 4 times a week. Jeejeebhoy (1983) has pointed out how management on HPN should proceed. 'The infusion rate and energy intake are gradually reduced as the patient can maintain his weight on an oral diet. The decision to reduce intravenous feeding is made on the observation that weight gain is occurring beyond desirable limits and that reduced infu sion does not result in electrolyte and fluid imbalance.'

Life style is good on HPN as shown by Mughal and Irving (1986). Patients are required to be connected to their pump and their nutrient solution for 12 hours a day most days of the week. In spite of this many successfully run their homes and businesses, have babies and pass exams. The treatment is extraordinarily expensive though, up to $US100 000 per year in some institutions. There are complications and deaths that can be attributed to HPN but most deaths occurring in these patients are due to their underlying disease. Septicaemia, superior vena cava thrombosis, and hepatic failure have been reported in patients on TPN (Stokes & Irving, 1989).

The central venous catheter is different to that described in Chapter 10. It is a cuffed silastic catheter which is inserted by a cut down on either the cephalic or external jugular vein. The catheter is then tunnelled to appear on the chest wall at a site which the patient can easily see and handle so that they may perform their own dressings and connections. The principles of catheter care, as discussed in Chapter 10, are not different, however.

SECTION VIII
THE PLACE OF FURTHER SURGERY

RECONSTRUCTIVE SURGERY

Mitchell et al (1984) and Thompson & Rikkers (1987) have thoroughly reviewed the large number of surgical procedures that have been employed experimentally to maximise absorption from the small bowel (Table 14.4).

At the present time in adult subjects we feel the only surgical approach that can be contemplated in the clinical setting is the reversal of segments of small intestine. We have not, though, been encouraged by our small experience of reversing 10 cm lengths of small intestine. Although often dramatic early on, in terms of reducing diarrhoea we have found later that the segment can behave quite variably. It may actually cause an obstruction or an intermittent obstruction or appear to have no effect at all. Our experience, however, does not agree with others

Table 14.4 Experimental and clinical surgical procedures for the short bowel syndrome

Controlling gastric hyperacidity
Highly selective vagotomy
Slowing intestinal transit
Antiperistaltic sequence of small intestine
Interposition of segment of colon
Construction of intestinal valves
Artificial sphincters
Baffles and strictures
Intestinal pouches
Recirculating loops of small intestine
Electrical and intestinal pacing
Increasing the area of absorption
Intestinal lengthening by longitudinal split of mesentery and intestine
Growing new mucosa
Intestinal transplantation

in the literature with whom it has been more encouraging. In a review of 29 published cases, Barros D'Sa et al (1978) found satisfactory to excellent results in 23 patients. In practice the sort of patient in whom an intestinal reversed segment can be used is hard to find. To reoperate on someone who already has a very short length of small intestine and create two new anastomoses within it is, we feel, foolhardy and particularly so if the primary disease is Crohn's disease with the consequent risk of fistula formation. The technique of Bianchi (1980) in which the two leaves of the mesentery are separated and two tubes of bowel are created by longitudinal division and subsequent end to end anastomosis is finding a place in paediatric surgery.

Retrograde electrical pacing promotes peristalsis in a reverse direction and seems to work well in dogs but not in humans (Thompson & Rikkers 1987).

Although some have suggested that a vagotomy to reduce gastric hyperacidity improves the lot of these patients we have found that the use of ranitidine probably achieves as much. It needs to be stressed that if vagotomy is used in any patient with a small bowel stoma it must be of the parietal cell type for a pyloroplasty or gastrojejunostomy in such patients may lead to uncontrollable diarrhoea.

INTESTINAL TRANSPLANTATION

Clearly, and the future may prove it to be so, intestinal transplantation would seem to be the ideal treatment for the short gut syndrome. Although the operative technique is not difficult, the function of the graft and its long term viability are proving to be almost insurmountable problems. Preservation of the donor intestine is possible but the major problem is graft versus host rejections in addition to the usual host versus graft reactions due to the presence of abundant lymphoid tissue in the donor intestine (Iwaki et al 1991). This may require radiation to the graft preoperatively, and triple combination immunosuppressive therapy (F.K. 506, azathioprine and prednisone). At the present time there are only a handful of patients who are surviving with intestinal transplants and in most cases the transplant has been done together with the liver and duodenal loop (Tzakis et al 1992).

15. Alimentary tract — enterocutaneous fistulas

INTRODUCTION

There is little in general surgery that is quite so devastating as the sight of small bowel contents coming through the wound in the early days after a difficult operation. Most enterocutaneous fistulas arise postoperatively as complications of a surgical procedure in which the surgeon has encountered extensive adhesions, inflammatory bowel disease, or radiation injury to the intestine. Before the widespread availability of safe and effective nutritional support, attempts at early surgical closure of the fistula were usual but the results were dismal. Recurrence of the fistula with fluid, electrolyte and acid base imbalance, sepsis, and marked wasting caused a high mortality rate.

The impact of total gut rest and TPN on the outcome of patients with small bowel fistulas has been dramatic. Nowadays about 50% of properly managed patients will experience spontaneous fistula closure within 4–6 weeks (Tarzi & Steiger 1988). Overall, more than 80% of these patients can be cured. There are, of course, a group of patients in whom spontaneous closure of the fistula does not occur. *When there is total discontinuity of the bowel ends, distal obstruction, persisting intraabdominal sepsis, Crohn's disease, radiation damage to the bowel and a short track to the skin spontaneous fistula closure is unlikely.* In such situations, direct surgical intervention, performed after sepsis is controlled and the patient is in a sound nutritional state, may be the only way to cure the patient. Although such definitive procedures are ideal, many patients in whom continuing sepsis is a problem will first require temporary procedures to control the fistula.

Like others, we have an established plan of management that procedes through a number of sequential but overlapping stages. These are:

- resuscitation, control of sepsis and protection of the skin
- assessment of nutritional requirements and commencement of TPN
- nutritional repletion, ambulation and anticipation of spontaneous closure of the fistula
- radiological investigations and definitive surgery when the fistula has failed to close spontaneously.

SECTION I
RESUSCITATION AND CONTROL OF SEPSIS

RESUSCITATION

Septicaemia and abdominal pain frequently herald the onset of the fistula and continue until small bowel contents discharge through the abdominal incision or drain site. Resuscitation with crystalloids, control of circulatory and pulmonary failure and the administration of antibiotics are the keystones of treatment at this time.

CONTROL OF SEPSIS

A CT scan is essential if there are signs of continuing sepsis. Many fistulas are associated with one or more intraabdominal abscesses which often drain incompletely when the fistula first discharges so that persistent sepsis is a common feature. Focal collections within the abdomen around the fistula, under the diaphragm, in the colic gutters or in the pelvis require drainage either by needle aspiration under radiological guidance or sometimes surgically through an appropriately sited incision. We are increasingly treating these abscesses by aspiration, guiding a flexible catheter into the cavity under CT or ultrasound control. A surprising finding has been that many abscesses interconnect and often the communication with the bowel is more complex than first thought. Most of the smaller connections between abscesses and bowel tend to close spontaneously and should not be a cause for undue concern. Multiple abscesses or complex abscesses associated with continuing sepsis are better managed by surgical drainage. Where the sepsis is extensive, or when the site of abscess is not certain, a full laparotomy should be undertaken with a thorough exploration of the peritoneal cavity. One thing is certain, however, and that is that the surgeon should not attempt a formal repair of the fistula at this stage. It is almost invariably associated with a recurrence which carries a high mortality rate (Hill & Bambach 1981, Reber et al 1978). It is wise to confine the procedure to the location and drainage of the sepsis using a sump drain down to the opening in the bowel in order that the discharge may be localised. Sometimes when it is clear that the output from the fistula can not be controlled this way it is better to resect or defunction the fistula and perform a proximal defunctioning stoma (Goligher 1971). These temporary procedures used to control the fistula in the presence of continuing sepsis are discussed more fully below.

PROTECTION OF THE SKIN

With the exceptions of a fistula opening near the symphysis pubis in a very emaciated patient or a fistula at the base of a large wound we seldom use suction drainage for small bowel fistulas. We prefer spontaneous drainage directly into a skin-tight adherent bag. The aim is to provide a leakproof stomal adhesive seal which is manufactured by the stomal therapist for each individual patient.

SECTION II
NUTRITIONAL REPAIR

The impact of the sepsis can be catastrophic and on occasion it can be difficult to control. Here lies the mortality in these patients – 15–20% of them die at this early stage from uncontrolled sepsis. Many of those who survive present with profound protein malnutrition. Table 15.1 shows body composition changes in 3 patients with continuing intraabdominal sepsis who had high output enterocutaneous fistulas. It can be seen that, as a group, they were protein depleted (mean protein index 0.62) and metabolically stressed (mean stress index 1.4). Over the 14 day study period, during which time sepsis was not controlled there was a profound fall of body protein (1.4 ± s.e. 0.4 kg) which is equivalent to 24% of total body protein or nearly 2% of total body protein per day. This protein loss occurred in spite of a gain in fat (or glycogen) of 1.9 ± 1.2 kg. These findings are similar to those we have found in seriously septic intensive care patients and occurred in spite of aggressive nutritional support (Chs 19 & 22).

We learn from this that until sepsis is under control TPN can be expected only to limit protein loss but not prevent it. Once the sepsis has been controlled, however, the nutritional metabolic goal changes and is directed at gaining both protein and fat, improving physiological function, restoring body hydration to normal and ensuring that the wound healing response is restored so that the fistula has the maximal opportunity to heal spontaneously. Although some authorities treat these patients almost exclusively by the enteral route, we feel enteral nutrition is appropriate only for low output fistulas in the distal small bowel or colon and that it is much more satisfactory and easier to control the situation if TPN is used. Before commencing TPN we return plasma albumin to the normal range, ensure loading doses of vitamins have been

Table 15.1 Body composition changes during 14 days of TPN in 3 patients with incompletely drained intraabdominal sepsis who had high output external small bowel fistulas. Day 1 measurements were made soon after resuscitation. Over the 14 day study period the patients received an average of 35 ± 7 kcal/kg/day and 1.5 ± 0.2 g protein/kg/day.

						Components of body composition (kg)							
						Weight		*Water*		*Protein*		*Fat*	
Sex	Age	Fistula site	Fistula output	Protein index*	Stress index†	Day 1	Day 14	Day 1	Day 14	Day 1	Day 14	Day 1	Day 14
M	60	Duodenal stump (gastric carcinoma)	900 ml	0.83	1.4	73.7	69.8	39.7	35.8	9.5	7.8	20.4	22.2
F	23	Lateral duodenum (Crohn's disease)	1,500 ml	0.48	1.2	39.3	40.4	23.3	21.1	3.7	3.1	9.7	13.6
F	47	Proximal jejunum (Crohn's disease)	700 ml	0.55	1.6	38.8	29.1	24.9	17.2	4.4	2.4	7.0	7.0

* Measured protein/predicted protein † Measured RME/predicted RME

given, trace metal deficiencies have been repaired and red cells have been given where required. Then energy requirements are measured with the indirect calorimeter and RME × 1.5 kcal/day are given. Once free of sepsis these patients behave like growing children and 1.5 g protein/kg/day are more than adequate to ensure maximal increases in total body protein. If fistula outputs are high the losses are collected and measured and their equivalent amounts of water and electrolytes are added to the calculated nutrient requirement. Of special note is the need for additional zinc and we add 15 mg of elemental zinc for each litre of fistula output.

SECTION III
NUTRITIONAL REPLETION AND AMBULATION

Now sepsis is under control, the fistula output is being collected into a skintight adhesive appliance and TPN is underway the patient is encouraged to look positively into the future. He or she has a 50% chance of spontaneous closure and if that does not occur and surgery is required it will almost always be successful. Most of the deaths are septic deaths which occur in the early stages after the fistula has first developed. To aid mobility, sutures, drains and tubes are removed as soon as practicable and the patient is encouraged to walk whenever this is feasible. It is hard to overestimate the benefit of these simple measures. It is worth trying to reduce the fistula output by physical and pharmacological means. In the past we insisted on a nasogastric tube until the fistula drainage was less than 500 ml per day. Now with H_2 blockers and somatostatin (octreotide) we sometimes see quite dramatic reductions in fistula output and can dispense with the nasogastric tube. Thus we add an H_2 blocker to the nutrient solution and give somatostatin to every patient. Octreotide (Sandostatin), with a 113 minute half life after subcutaneous administration, inhibits secretion of pancreatic polypeptide, gastrin, secretin and motilin (Lancet 1990a) but our results with it have not been as dramatic as some have reported (Nubiola et al 1989). There is no question, however, that fistula output is lessened and stomal management is much easier when somatostatin is used but fistulas that will ultimately require surgery still require surgery whether somatostatin is given or not.

A trial of conservative therapy is now started in the hope that spontaneous fistula closure will occur. By 3 weeks or so it should be obvious that the fistula is closing; the output will be considerably less and the opening will have granulated and have become much smaller. On average, spontaneous fistula closure occurs 4–6 weeks after all signs of sepsis have been eliminated. The use of somatostatin has changed this clear guideline. In the past, we saw an orderly reduction in fistula drainage in patients in whom spontaneous closure was occurring. Once drainage stopped and there was no obvious collection developing, the fistula opening crusted over and within 7 days or so the patient could safely begin oral intake. It was almost unknown, except in patients with Crohn's disease, for the fistula to reopen again. Now, with dramatic and rapid reductions in fistula output occurring in response to somatostatin, the result can be more indefinite. The wound may crust over but when the patient begins eating or somatostatin is stopped the fistula recurs. This can be an 'on and off affair' and may serve to delay the decision to proceed to surgery. For this reason we stop the somatostatin when the fistula output is less than 50 ml per day and if there is no increase, or the increase is small, then we are confident that spontaneous closure will occur. If the output increases markedly, we do not resume somatostatin preferring to see the natural progression. In this way, we have shortened the period of uncertainty that has surrounded the treatment of fistulas with somatostatin and yet have obtained the enormous benefit of this new therapy.

An encouraging feature of this period of waiting for spontaneous closure is the dramatic effect of TPN on body composition and physiological function. Table 15.2 shows the changes in body stores of protein and fat that occurred in 16 patients who received TPN over the 3-week period prior to successful fistula closure which occurred either spontaneously (4 patients) or after definitive surgery (12 patients). It can be seen that these patients, now free of sepsis, gained protein avidly. Their physiological function and hydration status (although not shown in the table) had improved similarly.

Table 15.2 Effect of TPN on body stores of protein and fat during the period of nutritional repletion, ambulation and anticipation of spontaneous closure. Shown are the changes that occurred over a 3-week period in 16 patients prior to fistula closure

Spontaneous closure	4
Energy intake	40 ±3 kcal/kg/day
Protein intake	1.8 ± 0.1 g/protein/kg/day
Change in total body protein	0.9 ± 0.1* kg
Change in plasma transferrin	40 ± 13 mg/dl
Change in plasma prealbumin	10 ± 1* mg/dl
Change in total body fat	0.3 ± 0.4 kg

* $p < 0.01$

SECTION IV
DEFINITIVE TREATMENT

RADIOLOGICAL INVESTIGATIONS

If after 3 weeks or so, all signs of sepsis have been eliminated and there is no appreciable diminution in fistula output, it is unlikely that the fistula will close spontaneously and full investigation is necessary to determine the reason for its persistence. Radiological investigations are required to outline the anatomic site and nature of the fistula and the cause of failure of closure.

Fistulography through the mouth of the discharging fistula is the best means of demonstrating the fistula and the cause of its persistence. Thin barium is injected through a soft balloon catheter which is introduced down the track. If there are several orifices, then each is cannulated, the flow of barium examined under the fluoroscope and films are taken in two directions at right angles to each other. The radiologist will note the origin of the fistula, the route of the track, the presence or absence of granulomatous disease or tumour in the underlying bowel at the site of anastomosis, and whether there is distal obstruction. It is unlikely that all this information will arise from the fistulogram, and it is always necessary to demonstrate by further barium studies along the length of both the small and large bowel. The small bowel is demonstrated best by intubation of the duodenum or upper jejunum and infusion of dilute barium (small bowel enema). Sometimes, in a very difficult case, the best result is obtained by a fistulogram performed by injecting a water-soluble contrast medium through the external opening at the same time as a small bowel enema is given.

In our experience the usual causes for failure of spontaneous closure are disease at the base of the track, e.g. Crohn's disease, irradiated bowel, or tumour invasion. Distal obstruction is also a frequent cause and discontinuity of bowel ends, mucocutaneous continuity, and abscess formation around the point of opening of the fistula all occur. When such are present, it is clear that the fistula is unlikely to close and a definitive procedure is required to cure the patient.

TIMING OF SURGERY

Following many major procedures, and especially when the bowel has fistulated, there is a dense peritoneal reaction that is maximal from 10–21 days and lasts about 6–8 weeks before resolution. If the abdomen is opened during this period, a form of obliterative peritonitis may be encountered that renders dissection almost impossible. For this reason formal elective closure of the fistula is postponed until about 6–8 weeks after all clinical signs of intraabdominal sepsis have disappeared. Unfortunately, there are times when, because of poor localisation of the fistula within the abdominal cavity and spreading or continuing sepsis, surgery must be undertaken before this. In these circumstances a definitive procedure with excision of the fistula and end-to-end anastomosis is doomed to failure, and minimal dissection with some form of defunctionalising should be done.

Before surgery it is important to ensure that there is no evidence of protein, vitamin, or trace metal deficiency, and bacteriological cultures are carried out in order that the best antibiotic regimen to cover the operation is selected.

SURGERY FOR FISTULAS OF THE JEJUNUM AND ILEUM

The definitive procedure required to close a fistula of the small bowel is a radical one, for lesser procedures frequently result in recurrence. The entire small bowel is dissected free of adhesions, the involved segment of bowel is excised, and an end-to-end anastomosis is carefully performed in bowel free from disease, oedema, and friability.

The first step in this radical procedure prepares the abdominal wall and gains access to the peritoneal cavity. The adherent drainage collection apparatus is removed from the skin, and the abdomen and the fistula opening are thoroughly sterilised. A small gauze swab is wedged into the mouth of the fistula and the whole abdominal wall, including the swab, is covered with the largest transparent adhesive drape (Opsite) (Fig. 15.1).

The abdomen is first entered through an extension (about 5 cm long if possible) of the original incision into an area of abdominal wall free of scars (Fig. 15.1). This allows safer entry to the peritoneal cavity before the old scar is reopened, although very special care is still required to avoid damaging the underlying bowel, which is invariably adherent to the deep surface of the old abdominal wall scar.

As soon as the abdominal cavity has been entered, firm traction is exerted on the wound

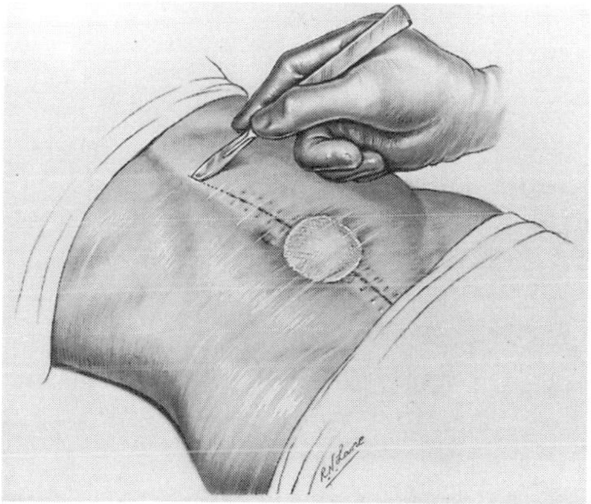

Fig. 15.1 Skin preparation and abdominal incision. A gauze swab is wedged into the fistulous opening and the entire abdominal wall has been covered by a transparent adhesive drape. Note that the skin incision has been made as an upward extension of the old incision into an unscarred area of the abdominal wall. (From Hill G L, Bambach C P 1981 A technique for the operative closure of persistent small bowel fistulas. Aust NZ J Surg 51: 477, with permission from Aust NZ J Surg, Royal Australasian College of Surgeons, publishers.)

edges and the parietal peritoneum is dissected from the underlying mass of adherent coils of intestine (Fig. 15.2). Dissection is carried under the abdominal scar, which is progressively opened, and far out into both flanks, separating the peritoneum widely up to the area where the bowel is densely adherent around the site at which the fistula passes to its opening on the surface. During the course of this dissection, an identifiable loop of small bowel is sought, although frequently in difficult cases it may only be found far on in the course of the dissection and located well laterally in one of the colic gutters.

Once a coil of intestine has been identified, the painstaking task of dissecting the entire length of small intestine, both proximal and distal to the fistula, can proceed. We have found that the application of 5-inch straight Mayo dissecting scissors frontally to an adhesion (Fig. 15.3) is the safest and surest way to perform this dissection. The bowel near the fistula itself will often be surrounded by particularly dense adhesions, but with sharp dissection and separation of the tissues by compression between finger and thumb nearly all fistulas can be mobilised. It cannot be emphasised too strongly that further damage to the bowel wall must be avoided at all costs, and with these techniques and considerable patience it is quite difficult to perforate the bowel.

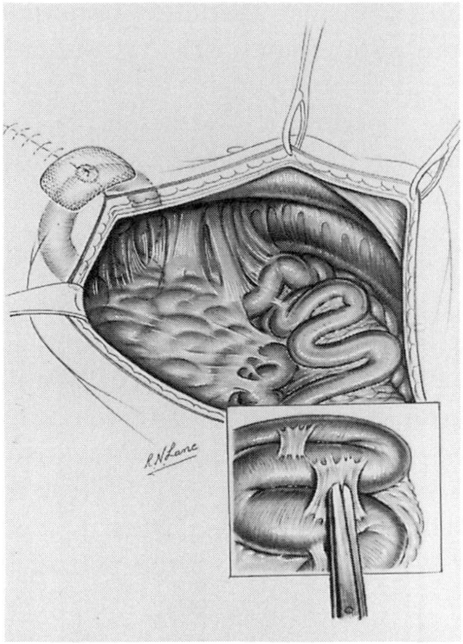

Fig. 15.3 Dissection of intestine. Once a loop of small bowel has been located in the flank, the entire length of the small bowel is dissected free of adhesions. The straight Mayo scissors are applied frontally (inset) to avoid further damage to the bowel. (From Hill G L, Bambach C P 1981 A technique for the operative closure of persistent small bowel fistulas. Aust NZ J Surg 51: 477, with permission from Aust NZ J Surg, Royal Australasian College of Surgeons, publishers.)

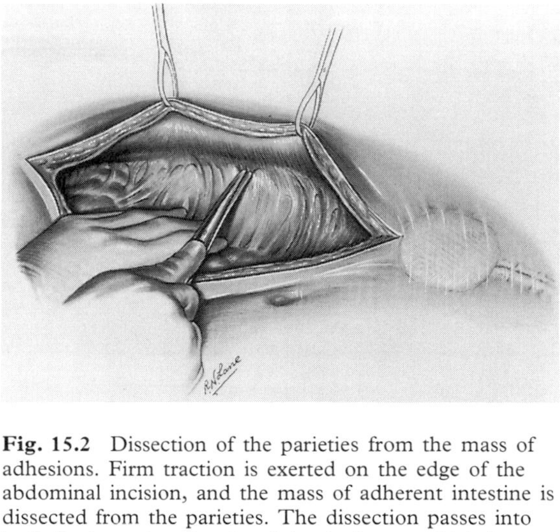

Fig. 15.2 Dissection of the parieties from the mass of adhesions. Firm traction is exerted on the edge of the abdominal incision, and the mass of adherent intestine is dissected from the parieties. The dissection passes into both flanks and under the abdominal scar, which is progressively opened as the dissection proceeds. (From Hill G L, Bambach C P 1981 A technique for the operative closure of persistent small bowel fistulas. Aust NZ J Surg 51: 477, with permission from Aust NZ J Surg, Royal Australasian College of Surgeons, publishers.)

Once the entire length of small intestine has been dissected, there remains the loop (or loops) of intestine that is densely adherent to the area of abdominal wall that contains the fistula itself. The skin immediately adjacent to the fistula is circumcised (Fig. 15.4) and the incision deepened through all layers of the abdominal wall so that the entire segment of bowel containing the fistula can be completely mobilised and excised (Fig. 15.5).

A standard 2-layer anastomosis with an inner continous layer of a 3–0 absorbable suture and an outer layer of 3–0 serum-proof silk completes the operation. We try to avoid using occluding bowel clamps and the silk sutures are lubricated to prevent drag on the delicate tissues. After closure of the mesentery and a thorough washout of the abdominal cavity (with warm saline), the

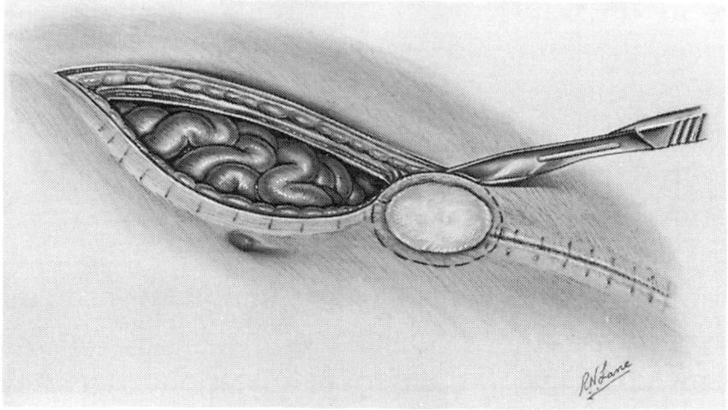

Fig. 15.4 Circumcision of the fistula. The entire length of small bowel both proximal and distal to the fistula has been dissected and the normal anatomy restored. The fistulous opening is circumcised and the remaining length of the old incision is opened. (From Hill G L, Bambach C P 1981 A technique for the operative closure of persistent small bowel fistulas. Aust NZ J Surg 51 477, with permission from Aust NZ J Surg, Royal Australasian College of Surgeons, publishers.)

abdomen is closed with interrupted synthetic absorbable sutures. Drains are not used.

Antibiotic administration is continued for the first 5 postoperative days. We have found that after such an extensive dissection the return of coordinated bowel activity is frequently delayed, and for this reason it is our practice to continue TPN for at least 2 weeks (during which time the patient takes nothing by mouth) and until he or she is able to eat voluntarily about 1,000 kcal per day.

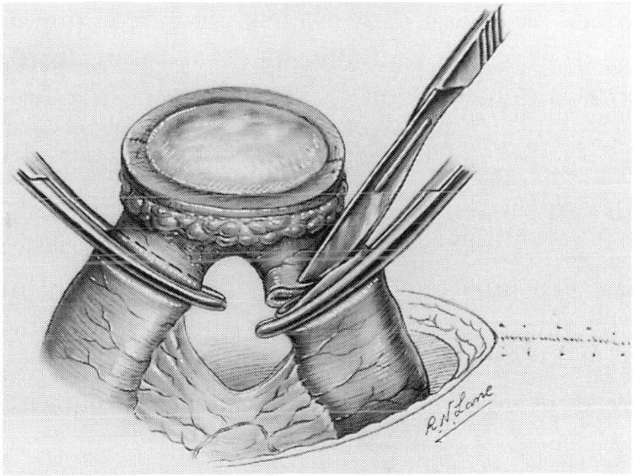

Fig. 15.5 Fistulous bowel is resected. After the fistula-containing segment of bowel has been detached from the abdominal wall, a generous segment is excised so as to reach above and below into bowel free from oedema and friability. (From Hill G L, Bambach C P 1981 A technique for the operative closure of persistent small bowel fistulas. Aust NZ J Surg 51: 477, with permission from Aust NZ J Surg, Royal Australasian College of Surgeons, publishers.)

SURGERY FOR FISTULAS OF THE SECOND PART OF THE DUODENUM

Clearly, excision of the diseased bowel and end-to-end anastomosis is not possible for fistulas of the second part of the duodenum. These are best dealt with by the serosal patch technique (Wolfman et al 1964). The duodenum is mobilised by the Kocher manoeuvre and a closed Roux-en-Y jejunal limb is brought up behind the transverse colon to lie alongside the fistula opening. An outer seromuscular layer of silk sutures is placed between the lateral jejunal wall and the posterior aspect of the duodenal defect. After these sutures are tied, an absorbable continuous suture is inserted between the edge of the fistula opening and the seromuscular layer of the jejunum until the entire circumference of the opening is sutured to the wall of the jejunum. The anterior layer of the anastomosis is completed with a row of interrupted seromuscular silk sutures.

SURGERY FOR FISTULAS OF THE THIRD AND FOURTH PARTS OF THE DUODENUM

A fistula arising in the third part of the duodenum adjacent to the superior mesenteric vessels can be a formidable surgical proposition. Nevertheless, it is possible to completely mobilise the third and fourth parts of the duodenum, resect the diseased segment, and perform an end-to-end anastomosis which comes to lie in front of the superior mesenteric artery and vein. Sometimes the base of the fistula is firmly attached to the superior mesenteric vessels, and in these circumstances it is safer to leave it in place and excise the bowel wall around the margins of the adherent area.

BYPASS PROCEDURES

In some situations it is not possible to dissect safely the distal small intestine because particularly dense adhesions are present. This is often the rule when the fistula has arisen from the terminal ileum after abdominal irradiation where the bowel is densely adherent within a frozen pelvis. In these circumstances, resection of the fistula with end-to-end anastomosis is not possible, and it is safest to locate the most distal loop of small intestine that is free of the pelvic obliterative process and to anastomose it directly to the transverse colon. This usually results in the drying up of the fistula over the next few weeks.

TEMPORARY PROCEDURES USED TO CONTROL THE FISTULA IN THE PRESENCE OF CONTINUING SEPSIS

It has already been pointed out that sometimes the drainage from the fistula cannot be localised within the abdominal cavity to a single track, and until this occurs it is difficult or impossible to deal with the consequent sepsis. Formal dissection of the bowel and end-to-end anastomosis in these circumstances is associated with almost certain recurrence and a high mortality rate (Reber et al 1978). It is much safer to resect the fistulated segment of bowel, perform a proximal jejunostomy or ileostomy, and exteriorise the distal segment (Goligher 1971). Even this requires mature judgment, and sometimes it is safer to refrain from dissecting the bowel and resecting the fistula and to leave it undisturbed, defunctionalising it by means of a loop jejunostomy or ileostomy. Later, when all sepsis has settled and the patient is in a sound nutritional state, a definitive procedure as described above can be performed.

SURGERY FOR CROHN'S FISTULAS WHICH HAVE ARISEN SPONTANEOUSLY

We saw in Chapter 13 that enterocutaneous fistulas associated with Crohn's disease may occur either postoperatively or spontaneously from an area of active Crohn's disease. Although the management of postoperative Crohn's fistulas differs in no way from that of other small bowel fistulas the surgical treatment of spontaneous fistulas requires special mention. As pointed out in Chapter 13, spontaneous fistulas arising from a Crohn's mass always need surgery to obtain closure and there is little point in trying to restore nutritional state before doing this. Whilst a Crohn's mass remains in the abdomen protein accretion cannot occur and the best that can be achieved is the correction of metabolic deficits, normalisation of body hydration and an improvement in physiological function. Thus after sepsis is under control we proceed to surgery after a week or so of TPN providing these goals have been achieved. The operation is not the sort of procedure that is easily conducted by the surgeon unaccustomed to dealing with patients suffering from Crohn's disease. Our approach involves reentering the abdomen through the previous laparotomy scar and opening the peritoneum at a point above or below the previous incision. We then take down the mass of intestine from the parieties and locate a loop of bowel in the flank. Once this is located, the tedious task of dissecting the entire small intestine is undertaken using sharp scissor dissection to separate loops of bowel and the bowel itself from the abdominal wall. Great care is taken to avoid damage to the intestine and adjacent structures. Eventually the fistulated segment of bowel is isolated on a pedicle of mesentry and after its detachment from the abdominal wall and from the site of the fistulous opening it is resected. If there is no sepsis and the intestine is not oedematous or friable, a careful end-to-end anastomosis is performed. When necessary, particularly if considerable residual sepsis is encountered, the alternative of bringing the two bowel ends out through the abdominal wall as separate stomas may be preferred. A few months later, when the patient is free of sepsis, fully mobile and restored to a good state of general health, intestinal continuity is restored by relaparotomy and end-to-end anastomosis.

Under proper conditions the results of this sort of surgery can be quite gratifying. In most patients successful closure is possible and the mortality rate should be less than 10% (Irving 1983).

SECTION V
RESULTS

Overall, the mortality rate for high output small bowel fistulas is about 20% (Ryan et al 1986). Nearly all of these patients die early on in the course of their illness from uncontrolled sepsis. Figure 15.6 shows the overall results of our own series of 86 patients with external small bowel fistulas. There were 35 males with a mean age of 49.6 ± 17.3 years and 51 females with a mean age of 47.1 ± 17.4 years. 26 fistulas arose from the jejunum, 44 from the ileum, 10 from a duodenal stump and 6 from the lateral aspect of the second part of the duodenum. 24 of the jejunal fistulas, 11 of the ileal, 2 of those from a duodenal stump and 5 of the lateral duodenal fistulas were classified as high output fistulas – that is with an output greater than 500 ml/24 h.

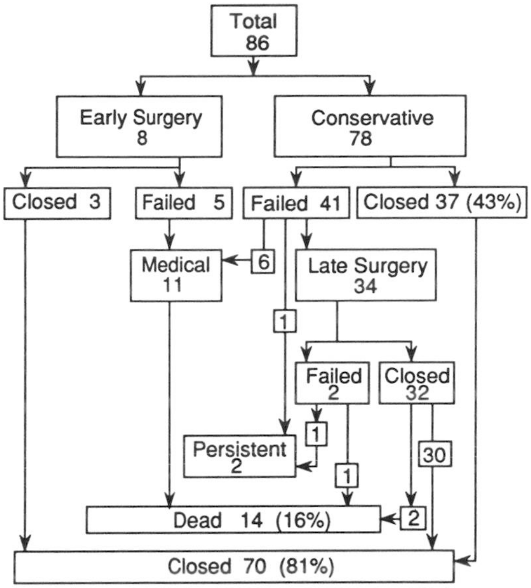

Fig. 15.6 Results of management of a personal series of 86 patients with external small bowel fistulas.

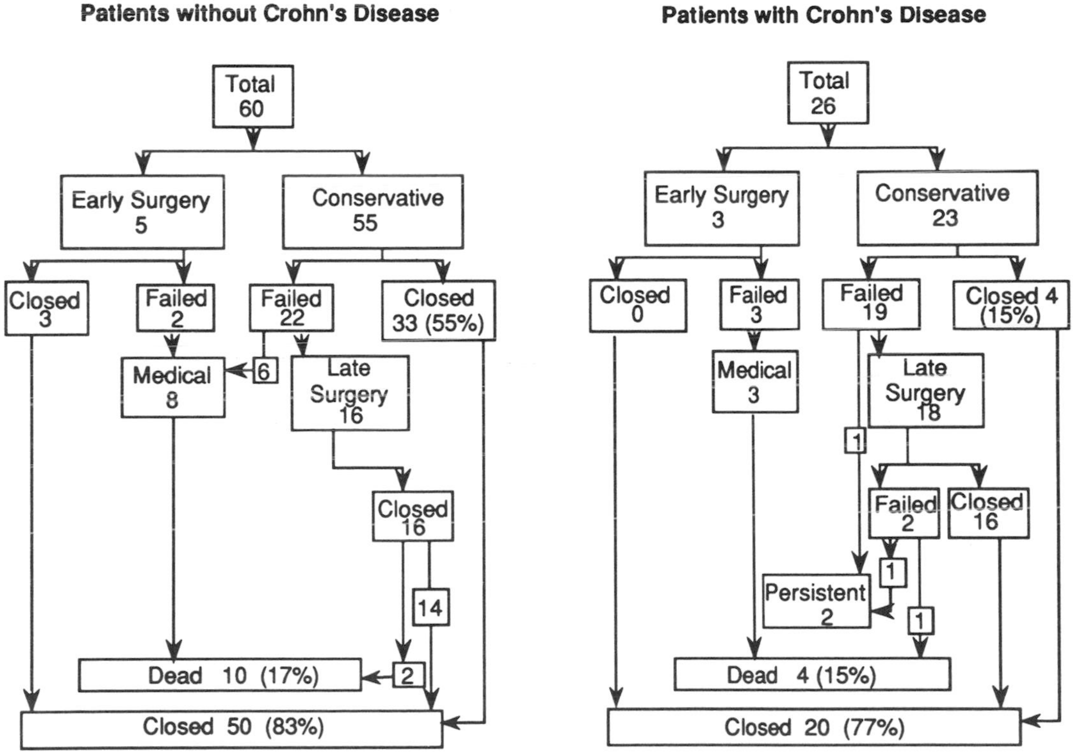

Fig. 15.7 The results shown separately for patients with (n = 26) and without Crohn's fistulas (n = 60).

20 patients had multiple fistulas and 8 had a major defect of the abdominal wall. Figure 15.6 shows that 43% experienced spontaneous closure, and most of the remainder required some form of operative control and resection of the fistula. Overall the mortality was 16%, and 81% of the patients finally had their fistula successfully closed.

Figure 15.7 shows that in patients with Crohn's fistulas spontaneous closure is much less common (15% versus 55%) but the ultimate closure rate is the same as in those patients without Crohn's fistulas (77% versus 83%).

It can be seen that a surgeon with experience in this type of work who performs a definitive procedure at the right time in a patient who is free of sepsis and in a sound nutritional state should almost always be successful.

Acknowledgements

We are indebted to the World Journal of Surgery for permission to reproduce much of the material which was contained in our two papers in the World Journal of Surgery 1983 7: 495–501 and 1988 12: 191–197.

16. Alimentary tract — massive bleeding

INTRODUCTION — CAUSES AND PRIORITIES

Peptic ulcer, portal hypertension, gastritis, diverticular disease and *angiodysplasia* are the usual causes of haemorrhage from the alimentary tract. Because massive haemorrhage occurs in a small proportion of patients who present to hospital acutely, with alimentary bleeding, all of them should be managed as though exsanguination is imminent. Haemorrhage from the alimentary tract is a clinical situation in which the surgeon should have a clear set of priorities in mind. These priorities fall into three broad areas and in order of importance they are:

- correction of hypovolaemia
- location of the source of bleeding
- identification of those patients in whom early aggressive surgery is needed.

SECTION I
HAEMORRHAGIC SHOCK

Many patients are admitted to hospital with bleeding from the alimentary tract which is not severe, causing only mild shock which responds rapidly to a bolus of crystalloid. If their risk of rebleeding is low they can be discharged early and investigation and treatment continued as an outpatient. On the other hand there are, exceptionally, patients whose bleeding may be such that intravascular volume cannot be maintained and surgery must be proceeded with, almost immediately, to avoid exsanguination.

Of particular interest here, however, are those in whom moderate to severe shock develops and blood replacement is required to stabilise the patient before endoscopy and possible surgery is proceeded with. It is of importance that the surgeon rapidly assesses the extent and rate of alimentary blood loss and replaces it as necessary. To do this, the clinical signs relating to the severity of the haemorrhage, the pathophysiology of the hypovolaemic state and how volume replacement can be monitored need to be understood.

CLINICAL SIGNS OF HAEMORRHAGIC SHOCK

Table 16.1 shows the clinical signs of shock which reflect the underlying shock pathophysiology.

Hypovolaemic shock produced by alimentary tract bleeding usually follows the orderly progression of the physical signs shown in Table 16.1 through cutaneous pallor and clamminess, oliguria, tachycardia and hypotension to cerebral and myocardial signs. These findings make it possible not only to recognise the shock state but also to gauge its severity.

SEVERITY OF HAEMORRHAGIC SHOCK

Table 16.2 describes the clinical classification of the severity of the shock state. Its severity may be either *mild, moderate* or *severe.*

Table 16.1 Physical signs of haemorrhagic shock

Physical sign	Detailed examination shows	Mechanism
Pale and clammy skin	Pale, cold, clammy, moist extremities progressing to involve the trunk	Adrenergic discharge constricting the vasculature of the skin and adipose tissue and affecting the sweat glands
Blanch test	Pressure over the plantar or volar aspects of phalanges or over the nail beds produces blanching that persists for several seconds if not indefinitely	Adrenergic discharge constricting the vasculature of the skin and subcutaneous tissue
Collapsed subcutaneous veins	Percutaneous insertion of venous catheter difficult if not impossible	Adrenergic discharge
Oliguria	Urine output <0.5 ml/kg/h	Renal vasoconstriction and tubular response to aldosterone and vasopressin
Tachycardia	Rapid, thready pulse	Discharge of adrenergic nerves to heart
Hypotension	In very young patients pressure may be normal until marked depletion in blood volume. In older patients progressive drop in blood pressure usually parallels volume lost	Inadequate stroke volume
Cerebral symptoms	Restlessness, agitation, confusion, lethargy	Inadequate blood flow to brain
Cardiac symptoms	Angina, ECG signs of myocardial ischaemia	Inadequate blood flow to heart

It can be seen from Table 16.2 that *mild shock* which indicates a loss of somewhere between 15 and 30% of the circulating blood volume is manifested by poor perfusion of the skin. The patient appears pale and the skin is cool and moist, changes starting first in the extremities and progressing to involve the trunk. The patient usually complains of feeling cold and is often thirsty. Tachycardia may or may not be present.

Table 16.2 Severity of shock – clinical characteristics

Classification	Mild shock	Moderate shock	Severe shock
Loss of blood volume	15–30%	30–40%	>40%
Skin perfusion	Pale, cold	Pale +	Pale ++, blood drained
Urine output	Low	Low	Low +
Pulse rate	Normal or high	High	High +
Blood pressure	Normal	Normal or low	Low +
Mental status	Normal or thirsty	Thirsty, anxious	Restless, agitated
Cardiac output	Low	Low	Low +, pain, ECG changes

A low urine volume and increased specific gravity are present. Loss of 30–40% of the blood volume is *moderate shock* and virtually always results in the classic signs of hypoperfusion, that is rapid pulse rate, rapid breathing, changes in mental status, hypotension and oliguria. Most of these patients will require blood transfusion. *Severe shock* occurs when more than 40% of the blood volume has been lost. Table 16.2 shows that clinically severe shock means inadequate perfusion of the heart and brain. The cardinal cerebral symptoms are restlessness and agitation which progress to stupor and coma. Cardiac manifestations may include pain from ischaemia or evidence of myocardial ischaemia on ECG.

ATYPICAL PRESENTATIONS OF SHOCK

There are exceptions to the orderly progression of the signs that have been mentioned in Table 16.1. They include *inebriated* and *cirrhotic* patients whose skin perfusion may be maintained despite poor cardiac output. Clinically, however, hypovolaemia is easy to recognise for although patients have lost the ability to constrict their peripheral vasculature in response to the shock insult their blood pressures fall and their pulse rates rise early. Of particular importance in alimentary tract haemorrhage are the *elderly* and especially those with coronary artery stenosis or widespread arteriosclerotic disease. They may manifest signs of myocardial ischaemia before changes in vital signs. Furthermore elderly patients with widespread arteriosclerosis or a low cardiac output may not be able to vasoconstrict or to redistribute blood flow when they become hypovolaemic and as little as 10–20% loss of blood volume may cause symptoms of moderate or even severe shock (Aviolio et al 1983). It is *young patients*, however, who can pose the biggest problem in the recognition of hypovolaemia. They sometimes constrict their vasculature to a remarkable extent and maintain normal blood pressure even when their cardiac output is very low. They do not always respond to hypovolaemia with obvious tachycardia, and vasoconstriction in the skin may be enough to preserve their blood pressure without normal compensatory increases in heart rate. Some young patients maintain a normal blood pressure and heart rate up to the point of cardiovascular collapse and even arrest.

SECTION II
ALIMENTARY TRACT BLEEDING — PATHOPHYSIOLOGY

The principal result of massive haemorrhage is insufficient flow in the microcirculation. The first compensatory response to this is constriction of large precapillary arterioles resulting in reversal of the filtration pressure in the capillaries (Rothe 1983, Flint et al 1984). As oncotic pressure remains the same, interstitial fluid moves back into the capillary bed, compensating for the loss of volume (Drucker et al 1981). If this compensation is not sufficient to restore vascular volume, arteriovenous shunts open which serve to divert arterial flow directly into the venous system but in the process isolating cells previously supplied with blood which as a consequence become starved of oxygen (O'Rourke 1982). These cells metabolise anaerobically and lactic acid is produced. Histamine is also released, causing constriction of the postcapillary sphincters resulting in slowing of capillary flow and agglutination of red cells within the capillaries. Accumulation of peptide regulatory factors associated with further cellular anoxia results in the large arterioles losing their ability to constrict while the postcapillary sphincters retain their spasm. The result is engorgement of the capillaries and extravasation of fluid from the vascular space to the interstitium (Sturm et al 1986). Prolonged vasoconstriction of the capillary bed also leads to endothelial cell damage and there is increased capillary permeability, and fluid and protein are lost into the interstitial space while the capillaries distend with agglutinated red cells (sludge). Cellular anoxia leads to energy deficits within cells and impairment of membrane transport (Shires et al 1972, Cunningham et al 1971). There is cellular swelling with increased water and increased concentration of intracellular sodium and chloride. Swollen cells reduce the size of the interstitial space and further impair tissue perfusion. Arteriovenous communications remain open so that peripheral flow is diverted directly back into the venous system to provide oxygen to vital areas such as the brain and heart.

If treatment is adequate and blood volume is restored many of these processes and impaired cellular functions are capable of recovery. Over 2 or 3 days the cells become less swollen and membrane transport is restored to normal. Capillary integrity may be regained as the sludge is washed into the venules where red blood cell masses break up and return to the circulation. Some of these aggregates may be filtered out by the lungs. Platelet and white cell aggregates which have formed inside venules are also washed into the systemic circulation, sometimes causing serious morbidity. Table 16.3 summarises these compensatory and decompensatory mechanisms in response to hypovolaemia and identifies some of the mediators that cause them.

SECTION III
MANAGEMENT OF MASSIVE BLEEDING FROM THE ALIMENTARY TRACT

It used to be thought that massive bleeding from the alimentary tract should be treated by precise

Table 16.3 Some of the mediators of the shock state and their actions

Action	Mediator	Compensatory mechanism	Decompensatory mechanism
Constriction of arterioles, venules and small veins in the skin	Adrenergic discharge	Blood shunted from periphery to heart, recovery of fluid from interstitium	Capillary distension, forcing fluid from vascular space into interstitium
Constriction of arterioles in skeletal muscle, gut and kidneys	Adrenergic discharge, vasopressin, angiotensin	Blood flow diverted to brain and myocardium	—
Increased heart rate	Adrenergic discharge	Increased heart rate and myocardial contractility	Tachycardia
Low urine output	Aldosterone, vasopressin	Stimulation of recovery of salt and water from glomerular filtrate	—
Hyperglycaemia	Epinephrine, cortisol and glucagon	Increased extracellular glucose	—
Dilatation of venules and arterioles	Endorphins	—	Pooling of blood in capillary bed
Endothelial damage	Tumour necrosis factor and other cytokines	Not known	Endothelial damage resulting in passage of protein and fluid into the interstitium
Membrane dysfunction	Cytokines	Not known	Damage to cell membrane, with increase in intracellular water and concentration of sodium chloride

replacement of known blood losses with an equivalent amount of blood. In fact, resuscitation of the patient should always begin with crystalloid solution even if crossmatched blood is available (Virgilio et al 1979, Canizaro et al 1983). Administration to the shocked patient of cold, stored blood which is frequently low in pH and high in potassium can prove fatal. We begin with a bolus of lactated Ringer's solution and follow with red cells as dictated by the clinical response and by the patient's haematocrit. The procedure is as follows:

- After a history and a physical examination have been performed and it is confirmed that a shock state exists (Table 16.1), a 16 gauge catheter is inserted into an arm vein and blood is taken for crossmatch, haematocrit, creatinine, liver function tests, prothrombin time and platelets.
- A bolus of Ringer's lactate solution sufficient to provide 30 ml/kg/body weight is given. A urinary catheter and a nasogastric tube are passed and residual urine and urine output are measured and the stomach is aspirated.
- If after infusion of the fluid bolus the shock state resolves, as evidenced by the return of skin perfusion and increased urine output, slowing of pulse, increased blood pressure and normal cerebral and cardiac signs, then no further support of the cardiovascular system is necessary.
- If on the other hand, the patient remains unstable, 2 units of red blood cells with Ringer's lactate are infused. After 2–4 units of blood cells the vast majority of patients with bleeding from the alimentary tract become stable.
- With the patient stable, the surgeon should then, through a large nasogastric tube, endeavour to wash the stomach free of clots and perform endoscopy in order to find the site of bleeding. In a very small number of patients, ongoing losses exceed 100 ml/min and the patient continues to be unstable after rapid resuscitation with Ringer's lactate and red cells. Such patients must be

immediately sent for haemostatic surgery.

- If bleeding persists, however, restoration of intravascular volume and the provision of red cells will not be sufficient and a coagulopathy that will make the situation worse is likely to develop. Therefore, if the patient remains haemodynamically unstable, at least 2 units of fresh frozen plasma should be transfused as soon as it is available. The platelet count should be monitored closely and platelets given when the platelet count is 100 000/mm^3 or less and haemodynamic instability persists after administration of crystalloid, packed red cells and two units of plasma. Platelets are supplied in packs of 10 units of platelet concentrate. One unit of platelet concentrate raises the platelet count by about 10 000/mm^3.
- Monitoring of the response to volume replacement should include *examination of the peripheral circulation and measurement of the blood pressure and pulse, urine output, venous pressure, arterial blood gases, and repeated assessment of haematocrit.* In very ill patients or those with coexisting cardiac or respiratory disease, admission to the intensive care unit is necessary. Here measurements of cardiac output, pulmonary artery wedge pressure and left atrial filling pressure are performed allowing a much more accurate management of the circulatory state.

SECTION IV
LOCATION OF THE SITE OF BLEEDING

It is not usual for a patient to bleed so much that operation is required during the first 24 hours. Most patients become stable after initial resuscitation and there is time to endoscope the patient in an endeavour to find the cause of bleeding. As soon as the patient is stable, therefore, and this usually is within the first 6 hours of admission to hospital, the stomach is washed out and endoscopy is performed. In 70–80% of patients endoscopy will uncover the cause of bleeding. In some units the endoscopist may attempt to control the bleeding, using laser, electrocoagulation or some type of tissue glue. If fresh bleeding, adherent clot in an ulcer or a visible vessel are seen, or if the patient is bleeding from a gastric ulcer it is less likely to stop and the scales more firmly weigh in terms of surgery. Colonoscopy may be possible in colorectal bleeding but if bleeding is brisk (more than about 2 ml/min) then arteriography should be done and it may reveal the site and cause of the bleeding. Furthermore, the arteriographer may be able to embolise the bleeding vessel if a discrete location is found.

SECTION V
WHEN TO OPERATE

Colorectal bleeding is usually managed conservatively and the first line of the treatment of *oesophageal varices* is sclerotherapy. Bleeding from peptic ulceration, once the diagnosis has been confirmed by endoscopy, is usually managed by restoration of the blood volume, bed rest and H_2 blockers. The mortality is very low in younger patients, but in patients over the age of 60 years bleeding from a gastric or duodenal ulcer, 1 in 10 die. Adverse risk factors for rebleeding include shock on admission, concomitant medical illness, endoscopic stigmata, and a large ulcer (>1 cm diameter) (Branicki et at 1990). At particular risk are those who rebleed whilst in hospital. Putting these risk factors together, a number of units have devised guidelines which are of considerable help to the practising surgeon in deciding when surgery is required. The Birmingham group in England (Morris et al 1984) have developed the following protocol:

- *In patients over 60 years of age, surgery is performed if a bleeding vessel is identified at endoscopy. If more than 4 units of red cells or plasma are needed in the first 12 hours, or, if the patient rebleeds whilst in hospital.*
- *In patients younger than 60 years of age, the indications for surgery are a visible bleeding*

vessel at endoscopy, a requirement of greater than 8 units of blood in the first 12 hours or 2 rebleeds whilst in hospital.

A randomised prospective study comparing this set of guidelines with a much less aggressive set of guidelines showed that although twice as many operations were done by adopting it the mortality fell from 15% to 4% (Morris et al 1984).

Most surgeons would also operate early in an elderly patient who has had a previous duodenal ulcer which bled in the past or a gastric ulcer which was bleeding at present. A younger patient who has had many admissions for bleeding is a good candidate for surgery too. Of special note are those patients who have had previous aortic surgery. Massive haemorrhage in such patients is from an aortoduodenal fistula until proved otherwise.

SECTION VI
THE GUIDELINES OF NYHUS

Nyhus (1990) has modified his earlier guidelines which many surgeons found particularly helpful. These modified guidelines are set out in Table 16.4 and can be highly recommended.

Table 16.4 Guidelines to know when to operate on patients with massive upper gastrointestinal haemorrhage (Nyhus 1990)

I. Conservative medical management at outset:
- A. Keystone to this phase is adequate and rapid replacement of deficient blood volume
- B. Early endoscopy, diagnostic and possible therapeutic, must be performed

II. Operative intervention is indicated when:
- A. There is need, after initial stabilisation, for over 1500 cc of whole blood transfusion in any 24-hour period
- B. Bleeding continues for more than 24 hours from onset (in patients over 60 years of age, if bleeding continues over 12 hours from onset)
- C. After cessation of bleeding, in the presence of well-known risk factors, e.g. history of shock, increased age, concomitant disease, size and type of ulcer, perform an elective operation within 36 hours
- D. Bleeding recurs after initial cessation
- E. There is coincident perforation and haemorrhage

III. Operative approach must be seriously considered when:
- A. The patient is over 60 years of age,
- B. There is gastric ulcer
- C. There is a history of haematemesis during the current episode
- D. There is a history of chronic ulcer disease or of previous haemorrhages
- E. There is a history of severe pain preceding the haemorrhage or pain persists during the haemorrhage

SECTION VII
CASE MANAGEMENT STUDY

The practical application of the principles outlined in this chapter are seen in the management of an elderly patient who was admitted to our hospital for treatment of a bleeding duodenal ulcer.

The patient was a 64-year-old retired shop manager who had had a duodenal ulcer diagnosed endoscopically 12 years earlier. He had been taking H_2 blockers intermittently but none recently and after a flu-like illness and being generally run down recently he developed increasing epigastric pain. On the morning of admission he felt faint, went to the bathroom, felt violently ill and vomited a large amount of bright red blood. He also passed a fair quantity of melaena stool soon after. An ambulance was called and he was brought to the emergency room.

On examination he was pale and his extremities were cold and clammy, his pulse was around 120 per minute and his blood pressure was 80/60. A 16 gauge catheter was inserted into an arm vein and blood was taken for cross match, haematocrit, creatinine, liver function tests, and platelets. A urinary catheter was passed and showed only a small volume of concentrated urine. A large bore nasogastric tube was passed and the stomach was aspirated. He was given 2 L of Ringer's lactate rapidly. Over the next 30 minutes he passed only 10 ml of urine.

Physical examination showed that the heart size was within normal limits and there was no evidence of liver disease. A rectal examination showed melaena on the tip of the finger.
The haematology and blood chemistry showed haematocrit 22%, white blood count 16 000 per mm^3, plasma sodium 130 mmols per L, plasma potassium 5.2 mmols per L, and a mild metabolic acidosis. Prothrombin time and platelet count were normal.

It is very likely that this patient who showed no evidence of liver disease and had melaena and bright red vomiting of blood had some form of peptic ulceration. His past history of duodenal ulcer made it almost certain that this was the cause of his bleeding. His signs: peripheral shut-down, poor urine output, high pulse rate, hypotension, and tachypnoea suggested that there had been at least 30% loss of blood volume and blood replacement was likely to be required. This depended on the response to the initial infusion of Ringer's lactate.

He continued to be haemodynamically unstable and a further litre of Ringer's lactate was run in at the same rate. After the infusion of a total of 3 L of Ringer's lactate peripheral perfusion remained poor, pulse rate remained high and his blood pressure was not restored. Urine output was less than 0.5 ml per kg per hour. Thus, red cells were infused. 2 units of red cells with Ringer's lactate were infused immediately and although there was some increase in blood pressure and urine volume (0.5 ml/kg/hour) he remained peripherally shut down and a further 2 units of red cells were infused. 3 hours after admission to the emergency room the patient was haemodynamically stable with blood pressure 130/90, a pulse 100 per minute and he was warm peripherally. The nasogastric tube was irrigated with iced saline and clots were removed. The patient was then taken to the endoscopy suite. Just before endoscopy he continued to be haemodynamically stable, his central venous pressure was 4 cm of water, and his urine output was 1 ml/kg per hour. Endoscopy showed a stomach with a residual clot which after removal revealed oozing blood at the base of a chronic duodenal ulcer. Immediate surgery was advised.

The decision for aggressive surgery was based on the age of the patient, his requirement for 4 units of blood over an 8-hour period and the demonstration that a chronic duodenal ulcer was bleeding from a large vessel in its base. He was sent from the endoscopy suite to the operating room.

Before induction of anaesthesia the stomach was aspirated and he was given prophylactic antibiotics. Through a midline incision the abdomen was opened. There was blood clot in the stomach and much clot throughout the upper small intestine. There was a heavily scarred duodenal cap. An incision was made longitudinally through the pylorus and the ulcer identified together with the bleeding vessel. This was underrun to effect haemostasis. The duodenum was closed by fashioning a pyloroplasty. A truncal vagotomy was performed. During the procedure, because of oozing and further blood loss 2 units of plasma, 5 units of platelets and a further 2 units of red cells together with Ringer's lactate were given. On return to the ward, the patient was well perfused, and required 1 L of Ringer's lactate and 2 L of dextrose in saline over the next 12 hours to maintain a urine output of 1 ml/kg bodyweight/h. He remained haemodynamically stable throughout the postoperative course, and no further blood was required. By the second postoperative day the nasogastric tube, the urinary catheter and the CVP line were removed. The patient commenced on liquids soon thereafter. By the fifth postoperative day he was taking a soft diet and on the eighth postoperative day he was discharged home.

SECTION VIII
SHOCK STATES AND THEIR IDENTIFICATION

In this chapter we have emphasised haemorrhagic shock. Except for high output septic shock (see Table 19.2) and neurogenic shock all forms of shock produce the same clinical findings in their advanced stages. There will always be signs of adrenergic discharge to the skin as the first manifestation of shock (except in inebriated patients) and the surgeon should assume that vasoconstricted patients are in shock, until proved otherwise. A urinary catheter should be passed and if urine output is less than 0.5 ml/kg/h the diagnosis is almost certainly correct. He should not wait until more advanced signs are present before making the diagnosis. The next step is to assess the neck veins. If they are distended the problem is cardiogenic or cardiac compressive shock. If they are flat the problem, besides hypovolaemia may be traumatic shock, neurogenic shock or low or high output septic shock (Rutherford et al 1976). Here and in Chapter 21 we have looked at haemorrhagic shock in particular; in Chapters 19 and 22 we will look at septic shock in some detail.

17. Surgically created metabolic and nutritional problems

SECTION I
GASTRIC RESECTION

Although the performance of total or subtotal gastrectomy with radical lymphadenectomy for gastric cancer is more common nowadays, the overall number of gastric resections being performed is much less. This is because there are now far more effective ways of treating peptic ulcer disease than gastric resection. Nevertheless the general surgeon still encounters many patients who have had a total or subtotal gastric resection and he or she is not uncommonly asked to advise on the treatment of nutritional disorders that have developed as a consequence. The main nutritional problems encountered after gastric resection are *protein energy malnutrition*, *anaemia*, and *bone disease.*

PROTEIN ENERGY MALNUTRITION

Weight loss has been reported in nearly half of the patients subjected to subtotal gastrectomy and it is probably present in all patients who have had a total gastrectomy. Some patients after Billroth I gastrectomy have weight loss but it is a more common problem after Billroth II gastrectomy (French & Crane 1963). Many patients are comfortable at their lower body weight and do not consider it to be a problem. In a few patients serious protein energy malnutrition of the marasmic type complicates gastrectomy and it is these who need to be evaluated.

Pathogenesis

The major causes of serious PEM after gastrectomy are:

- failure to eat
- poor appetite
- small gastric reservoir
- malabsorption.

The most important of these is the *failure to eat.* This is usually due to the patient being frightened to eat certain foods for fear of provoking dumping or pain (Johnston et al 1958). The pain is usually caused by bile reflux oesophagitis and is brought on by eating almost any sort of food. Liquids can usually be taken without difficulty and some patients fall into the trap of solving their problem by consuming large quantities of alcoholic beverages. Alcoholism may therefore become a problem with its associated protein and vitamin deficiencies. *Poor appetite* is also a factor in postgastrectomy malnutrition and may be caused by bile reflux and gastric atrophy. As deficiencies of iron, folate and vitamin B_{12} occur, appetite is lost and with the detection and treatment of these deficiencies, appetite may return. It is unusual for a *small gastric reservoir* to be the cause of malnutrition and hence surgery to increase gastric capacity is almost never required. The afferent limb is usually hypertrophied after subtotal or total gastrectomy and food enters it soon after a meal is eaten, such that it acts as a reservoir with a capacity similar to a normal stomach. Patients with total gastrectomy can often take meals of normal size. *Malabsorption* of carbohydrates and protein is exceptional after gastrectomy but steatorrhoea is a constant finding, although this is usually mild and of no clinical importance. Where severe steatorrhoea and fat soluble vitamin deficiencies occur there is usually an additional abnormality such as gluten sensitive enteropathy, pancreatic deficiency or bacterial overgrowth in the afferent limb that is causing the problem.

In Table 17.1 our study of 6 patients who were followed up after curative total gastrectomy for a period of between 2 and 5 years is shown. Dietetic evaluation of these patients showed that their total energy intake (38.5 ± 6.6 kcal/kg/day) and protein intake (1.5 ± 0.3 g protein/kg/day) matched their calculated energy and protein requirements. It can be seen that the patients had failed to regain preoperative tissue loss in spite of being in energy and protein balance and this was probably related to the severe steatorrhoea that was measured (21 g fat per day). Since the haematologic values were within the normal range it suggests that pancreatic deficiency was the prime cause of the fat malabsorption and the patients would have benefited from receiving pancreatic enzyme supplementation. These patients, however, were not disturbed by the steatorrhoea and none were unduly concerned over the failure to regain body weight. Each was receiving ferrous sulphate and vitamin B_{12} but no other medications.

Investigation and treatment

When the PEM is of sufficient intensity to interfere with the lifestyle of the patient then investigation and treatment are called for. A careful history is taken and a dietetic evaluation of protein and energy intake is obtained. Where there is negative energy and protein balance, therapy is directed at removing the symptoms of dumping or pain which the patient is seeking to avoid. *Dumping* is rarely a serious problem and the treatment is principally dietary. Patients know that drinks containing carbohydrates cause the symptoms and they learn to avoid them. They also avoid drinking with their meals and should be encouraged to take dry meals separate from liquids and where possible to lie down after large meals. Most patients will respond to these measures and surgical procedures for dumping are rarely required. Pain from *bile reflux oesophagitis* which may be a most distressing problem can occasionally be helped by the administration of bile adsorbing agents such as hydrotalcite (Hoare et al 1977) but severe bile reflux can be corrected only by some form of bile diversion operation. For example, a Billroth II can be converted to a Billroth I reconstruction, or a Roux-en-Y conversion with at least 50 cm between the gastric remnant and the Y junction can be created. Even these procedures have a disappointing success rate (Alexander-Williams 1984).

Although *malabsorption* is an uncommon cause of postgastrectomy malnutrition, pancreatic function tests, jejunal biopsy and quantitative bacterial cultures are required if severe steatorrhoea is prominent. Gluten free diet for enteropathy, pancreatic enzyme substitution for pancreatic deficiency and antibiotics for bacterial overgrowth are given when abnormalities are found.

Very serious malnutrition is exceptional but, when it occurs, enteral or parenteral nutrition may be required to reverse a downward spiral. *Home enteral nutrition* through a fine nasogastric tube by continous infusion using a pump can sometimes be used to restore a patient to nutritional health. These patients generally have difficulty handling a liquid osmotic load so that enteral feeding is not always well tolerated and causes severe diarrhoea. *Home parenteral nutrition* is sometimes required for patients who have had both a gastric resection and a small bowel resection or who have a gastric resection together with severe pancreatic insufficiency. A few patients with severe malnutrition may need home parenteral nutrition indefinitely.

ANAEMIA

Iron deficiency anaemia occurs in up to 20% of patients after gastrectomy. Some suggest that the cause is iron malabsorption. It is argued that iron extraction from its organic form in the diet does not properly occur and there is insufficient time for it to be absorbed in the upper jejunum. However, the cause of iron deficiency anaemia after gastric surgery is most commonly due to bleeding

Table 17.1 Body composition, haematology, and faecal chemistry of 6 patients (median age 63 years) who had undergone curative total gastrectomy 2–5 years prior to this evaluation. Values are mean ± s.e.m. (Adapted from Curran F T, Hill G L 1990 Br J Surg 77: 1015, by permission of the publishers)

	Value when well	Value before gastrectomy	Value 2–5 years after gastrectomy
Body composition			
Body weight (kg)	66.5 ± 3.3	59.0 ± 3.7	57.7 ± 1.6
Total body protein (kg)	9.7 ± 0.7	8.2 ± 0.7	8.5 ± 0.4
Total body fat (kg)	15.9 ± 1.2	9.3 ± 2.5	10.1 ± 1.3
Haematology			
Serum iron (µmol/L)	20	—	12 ± 2.9
Serum iron binding capacity (µmol/L)	50	—	66 ± 2.9
Serum vitamin B_{12} (pmol/L)	250	—	197 ± 32
Serum folate (nmol/L)	12	—	20 ± 4
Serum 25 hydroxy-calciferol (µg/L)	40	——	30 ± 4
Faecal output			
Fat (g)	3	—	21 ± 7
Nitrogen (% intake)	7	—	6.4 ± 1.2

from damaged or friable gastric mucosa usually around the stoma. In any event, it is a relatively simple condition to treat with organic iron preparations. It is usual to try simple oral iron supplements and to resort to parenteral iron administration only in the rare event of failure to respond. Macrocytosis in patients with a normal vitamin B_{12} is caused by *folate deficiency*. This is principally the result of poor dietary intake. The dietary deficiency is due again to the fear of provoking pain by eating fresh vegetables. It is not usual to go to the trouble of investigating folate deficiency further for it is simpler to give low dose folic acid replacement therapy (5 mg of folic acid each day) which repairs the deficit and prevents its occurring again. *Vitamin B_{12} deficiency* is invariable after total gastrectomy unless supplementation is given and it occurs in a subclinical form in many patients after subtotal gastrectomy. In these circumstances it is due either to intrinsic factor deficiency caused by complete gastric mucosal atrophy or sometimes, and much more rarely, to the intestinal blind loop syndrome which causes colonisation in the upper gastrointestinal tract, particularly in the afferent limb. Bile reflux is common after a Billroth II anastomosis and gastric atrophy is an inevitable consequence. By the time gastric atrophy is established, patients are usually vitamin B_{12} deficient with macrocytosis and low serum vitamin B_{12} levels are found. The treatment is to replace the poorly absorbed vitamin B_{12} by giving 250 µg hydroxocobalamin (i.m.) every 2 months.

BONE DISEASE

Two types of bone disease may occur after gastrectomy. *Osteoporosis*, which is the loss of normal bone tissue — the remaining bone is normally calcified, and *osteomalacia* which is much rarer, occurring perhaps in only 1 or 2% of patients long after gastrectomy. Osteomalacia is a loss of calcium from bone and is due to vitamin D deficiency.

Osteoporosis is a process that occurs normally as patients become older, but after gastric resection the process occurs 10 or 20 years earlier. The clinical effect is to increase the likelihood of fractures, particularly of the femoral neck. One group observed a greater than threefold increase in the incidence of fractures in patients who had had a gastrectomy compared with matched controls. (Louyot et al 1961). The cause of increased osteoporosis after gastrectomy is unclear but is probably due to poor dietary intake and inactivity. Unfortunately, at present, there are no certain measures for either the prevention or treatment of osteoporosis following gastrectomy. A recent trial of calcium supplementation with microcrystalline hydroxyapatite produced no significant advantage for the treatment group (Tovey et al 1991). Therapy is therefore non-specific and involves general measures to improve overall good eating habits and the encouragement of increased physical activity.

Osteomalacia due to vitamin D malabsorption is associated with generalised malabsorption of fat. Serum calcium in these patients is often below normal and the serum alkaline phosphatase is elevated. Serum levels of 25-hydroxycalciferol are low. The problem is so rare after gastrectomy that no treatment is usually required. After total gastrectomy or near total gastrectomy where long term survival is anticipated vitamin D and calcium should be given for prophylaxis. It is sufficient to give a small dose of vitamin D analogue and 1–2 g of calcium orally per day. It is worth noting that vitamin D overdose can occur with excessive administration. Hypercalcaemia as a result of vitamin D overdose may be a much more serious matter than osteomalacia. The need for continuing vitamin D can be determined by measuring the levels of 25 OH vitamin D.

SECTION II
PANCREATIC RESECTION

Although the prognosis for patients with adenocarcinoma of the pancreas is appalling, patients with ampullary cancer and islet cell tumours may be cured after pancreatoduodenectomy (Whipple operation). After this procedure patients suffer from varying degrees of pancreatic insufficiency but frequently this is of nuisance value only and they are often able to live relatively normal lives. Some are troubled by severe steatorrhoea and malabsorption and require replacement therapy and nutritional guidance.

STEATORRHOEA AND ENERGY MALNUTRITION

DiMagno et al (1973) showed that significant steatorrhoea occurs only when enzyme output falls to less than 10% of normal. When enzyme output from the residual gland is between 2 and 10% of normal steatorrhoea can usually be controlled by dietary means alone, but when there is less than 2% of normal output steatorrhoea is severe and clinically disabling.

We studied 4 long term survivors after a curative Whipple's procedure and Table 17.1 shows their dietary intake and faecal chemistry. It can be seen that each consumed sufficient energy to reach energy balance and each was consuming normal quantities of fat in their diet. However, steatorrhoea was present to a greater or lesser extent in the 4 patients although in none of them was faecal protein output excessive. It is interesting that none of them was troubled by their diarrhoea and they all resumed work and lived a relatively normal life. Only patient 3 took pancreatic replacement therapy although all of them had voluntarily restricted the fat content of their diets.

Pancreatic insufficiency affects fat absorption more than that of protein or carbohydrate. Protein digestion is aided by gastric pepsin and carbohydrate by salivary and intestinal amylase. Patients with severe steatorrhoea may also suffer from malabsorption of fat soluble vitamins (Dutta et al 1982). Trace element deficiency may also occur, particularly of calcium, magnesium and zinc (Aggett et al 1979).

In summary, though, these deficiencies are rarely a clinical problem and the issue that concerns the surgeon is fat malabsorption and accompanying energy malnutrition. In Table 17.3 we show the results of our studies of the body composition of the 4 long term survivors shown in Table 17.2.

Values for when the patients were well were predicted from standard equations, and measurements were made just before pancreatoduodenectomy and at intervals from 20 to 64 months later.

It can be seen that none of the patients returned to their well weight, although further deterioration after surgery was small and the main compositional defect was that of total body fat depletion. We concluded from these data that the energy loss from faecal fat loss is not being met sufficiently by dietary means making it difficult for these patients to achieve positive energy balance and return to normal body weight.

Table 17.2 Dietary intake and faecal excretion in 4 patients after curative Whipple's resection. (From Curran F T, Strokes M A, Hill G L 1991 J R Col Surg Edin 36: 32, by permission of Butterworth Heinemann.)

	Patient number			
	1	2	3*	4
Total energy (kcal/day)				
Required†	2780	2900	3120	1440
Actual	2661	3459	2932	1709
Carbohydrate (g)	370	376	372	233
Fat (g)	96	180	114	62
Protein (g/day)				
Required‡	104	109	117	54
Actual	94	85	105	56
Daily faecal excretion				
Faecal fat (g per day)	23	13	59	16
Dietary intake (%)	24	7	52	26
Faecal protein (g per day)	3.8	3.9	4.7	5.2
Dietary intake (%)	4	5	4	9

* Patient underwent panproctocolectomy 12 years previously
† 40 kcal per kg body weight
‡ 1.5 g per kg body weight

Table 17.3 Serial measurements in body composition in 4 patients after curative Whipple's resection (From Curran F T, Stokes M A, Hill G L 1991 J R Col Surg Edin 36: 32, by permission of Butterworth Heinemann.)

	Patient number			
	1	2	3*	4
Current age (years), sex	38, M	58, M	36, M	71, F
Time since surgery (mths)	64	54	20	20
Weight (kg)				
Well	78.0	76.4	85.0	47.5
Before Surgery	70.4	68.8	78.3	38.5
Current	69.5	72.5	78.0	36.0
Total body protein (kg)				
Well (predicted)	11.7	11.6	13.2	7.2
Before surgery	11.5	10.5	10.5	5.7
Current	10.3	10.7	10.6	5.2
Total body fat (kg)				
Well (predicted)	17.3	17.0	18.9	13.4
Before surgery	15.5	14.7	24.2	5.9
Current	12.8	14.2	22.5	3.9

* Patient underwent panproctocolectomy 12 years previously

TREATMENT

After pancreatoduodenectomy the dietitian aims to give the patient 40–45 kcal/kg/day. Exact requirements are obtained by performing indirect calorimetry and multiplying the resting metabolic expenditure by 1.5. This is the energy requirement until the patient has returned to desired weight. In practice, such refinement is rarely used and a simple figure of 45 kcal/kg/day adjusted according to the patient's response is all that is required. Carbohydrate (at least 400 g per day) and protein (at least 100 g per day) should be aimed for. Dietary restriction of fat is important only in those patients who are troubled by steatorrhoea. Restriction to a 50 g per day fat diet often solves the problem of symptomatic steatorrhoea and the amount of fat then can slowly be increased until diarrhoea reappears.

Where steatorrhoea is troublesome, pancreatic enzyme replacement is used. Dosage remains unclear but 2 capsules of granular pancreatin taken immediately before or just after the commencement of a meal is a good starting point. The dose can be increased or reduced as necessary according to response.

If pancreatic replacement enzymes do not improve steatorrhoea, H_2 receptor blockers (cimetidine or ranitidine) are used. It is thought that the lipase in the pancreatin is destroyed by gastric acid.

Where energy imbalance is a major problem, medium-chained triglycerides are used. These fatty acids are more readily absorbed than long-chained triglycerides which make up 90% of the normal diet. Some patients find the ingestion of medium-chain triglycerides intolerable. They are troubled by vomiting, abdominal cramps and diarrhoea and refuse to take it.

SECTION III
INTESTINAL RESECTION AND UROLITHIASIS

It has been known for a long time that urinary stone formation is a complication of diarrhoeal disease and ileostomy. More recent information shows that there is an increased prevalence of urinary stones not only after ileostomy and ileostomy with enterectomy but also when patients have had an enterectomy and enterocolic anastomosis (Bambach et al 1981). The prevalence of urinary stones after intestinal resection is between 7% and 15% compared with 2% to 4% in the general population. Uric acid stones usually comprise less than 10% of all stones, but make up 60% of stones found in patients with an ileostomy. Table 17.4 shows the concentration of urinary constituents that we measured in 3 groups of patients who had had intestinal resections.

Compared to normal control subject's ileostomy patients had significantly lower pH and volume and higher concentrations of calcium, oxalate and uric acid. Saturation indices for both uric acid and calcium oxalate showed that these patients had an increased risk of forming uric acid and calcium stones.

A small bowel resection combined with an ileostomy increased the ileostomy output, lowered urinary volume further and reduced urinary calcium excretion. The concentration of urinary oxalate increased and the risk of both uric acid and calcium stones was high.

Patients with small bowel resection and an enterocolic anastomosis had hyperoxaluria and an increased risk of calcium stones despite a low urinary calcium. There was no increased risk of uric acid stones in this group.

This study demonstrates the marked effect of intestinal resection on the composition of urine. The high levels of urinary risk levels for both uric acid and calcium stone formation found in these patients suggest that the majority have a high risk of forming a urinary stone during the remainder of their life time. After resection patients with small bowel stomas should have measurements of ileostomy output and urinary volume and constituents. High output is suggested when patients empty their ileostomy bag more than 6 times in 24 hours and the [Na]/[K] in the urine is less than 1. If ileostomy diarrhoea and water and salt depletion is a chronic problem and there is no traceable cause for it (see under ileostomy) then loperamide should be prescribed to reduce ileostomy volume. In addition, all patients with small bowel stomas should be advised to drink sufficient water and take sufficient salt to bring urinary volume above 1500 ml per day and the [Na]/[K] ratio above 1. Such treatment will prevent stone formation. Patients with small bowel resection and an enterocolic anastomosis should be prescribed a diet low in oxalate and fat (Andersson et al 1978).

SECTION IV
ILEAL RESECTION AND CHOLELITHIASIS

Loss of functioning ileum due to disease or surgical excision is known to have an adverse effect on the enterohepatic circulation of bile acids with

Table 17.4 24-hour urinary constituents in patients after differing intestinal resections. Values are mean ± s.e.m. (Adapted from Bambach C P, Robertson W G, Peacock M, Hill G L 1981 Gut 22: 257, by permission of the publishers)

	Normal controls n = 85	Ileostomy only n = 27	Ileostomy with small bowel resection n = 17	Small bowel resection with enterocolic anastomosis n = 17
Volume (L)	1.70 ± 0.07	0.99 ± 0.07*	0.72 ± 0.11*	1.36 ± 0.14
pH	6.12 ± 0.05	5.24 ± 0.05*	5.42 ± 0.07*	5.75 ± 0.10
Sodium (mmol)	172 ± 8	79 ± 8*	23 ± 9*	135 ± 11
Potassium (mmol)	59 ± 3	62 ± 5	52 ± 7	68 ± 7
Calcium (mmol/L)	2.92 ± 0.16	4.59 ± 0.41*	3.38 ± 0.83	1.11 ± 0.25*
Oxalate (mmol/L)	0.183 ± 0.007	0.311 ± 0.098*	0.533 ± 0.069*	0.470 ± 0.062*
Uric acid (mmol/L)	2.39 ± 0.10	3.73 ± 0.23*	4.59 ± 0.37*	2.45 ± 0.29

* $p < 0.001$ compared with normal controls, using Student's t test

a consequent predisposition to the development of gallstones. We studied the frequency of cholelithiasis in a large group of patients with small bowel stomas, including some who had had no ileal resection and others with large ileal resections. The 105 patients studied were divided into two groups according to whether more or less than 10 cm of ileum had been excised. The 10 cm cut off was chosen because in a standard proctocolectomy less ileum than this is removed and the greater resection is undertaken when there is disease involved in the ileum or for some technical reason. Each of the two subgroups was again subdivided according to whether the primary disease was ulcerative colitis or Crohn's disease. In the group with resection of more than 10 cm the amount of ileum excised varied from 12 cm to 200 cm with an average of 56 cm ± 10 cm.

Table 17.5 shows the observed incidence of gallstones according to the disease and the length of ileal resection. It can be seen that in the group that had had an ileal resection there was little difference in the incidence of gallstones between those patients whose original lesion was ulcerative colitis and those with Crohn's disease. However, in those patients who had less than 10 cm of ileum removed there was a very marked difference in the frequency of gallstones depending on the nature of the primary condition, for gallstones were found in only 8 of the 54 patients who had had colitis but in 5 of the 11 who had had Crohn's disease. The increased incidence of gallstones over what might have been expected in a comparable series of the ordinary population is statistically significant in each group, other than in those patients who had undergone minimal ileal resection during standard proctocolectomy and ileostomy for ulcerative colitis.

It should be pointed out that in this group of patients only 5 had symptoms and eventually all of these underwent cholecystectomy. The management of the other 21 was expectant and in the long run it would be expected that very few of them would require cholecystectomy (Ritchie 1972). We feel therefore that asymptomatic cholelithiasis which appears in patients who have had intestinal resection should be treated expectantly. Conservative measures such as oral bile salt therapy causes troublesome diarrhoea in these patients and we feel it is meddlesome to offer surgery to patients whose abdominal cavity is the seat of multiple adhesions when the condition may never give rise to symptoms or complications.

It is not yet known if patients after ileoanal pouch surgery share this increased risk of gallstones.

SECTION V
ILEOSTOMY

A properly constructed normally functioning end ileostomy produces very few long term complications. Although a number of metabolic changes occur secondary to the increased losses from the ileostomy there are no clinically significant consequences apart from a higher incidence of urolithiasis. The life expectancy of patients with ileostomies is no different from normal. Metabolic problems that occasionally occur are the result of the differences between ileostomy fluid and

Table 17.5 Observed incidence of gallstones according to disease and length of ileal resection. (Reprinted from Hill G L, Mair W S J, Goligher J C 1975 Gut 16: 932, by permission of the publishers)

Amount of ileum resected, and original disease	Patients surveyed (no.)	Incidence observed (%)	Incidence expected (%)	Ratio observed to expected incidence
> 10 cm				
Ulcerative colitis	18	33	10	3.2:1
Crohn's	22	32	5	6.8:1
< 10 cm				
Ulcerative colitis	54	15	9	1.6:1
Crohn's	11	45	9	4.9:1

normal faeces and a breakdown in the normal compensatory mechanisms that occur in these patients (Hill 1976).

ILEOSTOMY CHEMISTRY

Table 17.6 shows the chemistry of ileostomy fluid of patients with well functioning ileostomies. It is the marked increase in the excretion of water and sodium and the low pH of the ileostomy fluid that are the factors which give rise to potential metabolic complications.

Ileostomy output is normally around 400–500 g per day but this amount is related to the size of the patient. It has been shown that a so-called normal 70 kg patient has an average daily ileostomy output around 550 g per day, the 95% confidence limits of the estimation is 100 g (Hill et al 1979b). The concentration of sodium in the ileostomy fluid is a little less than in plasma and the concentration of potassium a little more. These concentrations, however, are related to some extent to the overall sodium balance of the body. With body salt depletion, the concentration of sodium in the ileostomy fluid falls and the concentration of potassium rises. Sodium concentrations as low as 60 mmol/L of ileostomy fluid have been measured in subjects who have experienced excessive sodium losses due to diarrhoea or sweating. When an ileostomy patient becomes salt depleted the concentration of potassium rises and the ratio of sodium to potassium of around 12 may fall as low as 2. The pH of ileal excreta is weakly acidic. In the jejunum chloride and bicarbonate can be absorbed together but in the ileum chloride is absorbed and bicarbonate is excreted. There is a complex coupling of chloride and bicarbonate in the ileum which is also related to sodium and hydrogen ion transport. As the intestinal contents pass distally chloride concentration decreases and the concentration of bicarbonate and the pH rise. The concentration of chloride in the ileal excreta is around 45 mmol/L and the concentration of bicarbonate approximately 150 mmol/L. The net result of this is that the urinary pH (Table 17.4) is significantly lower in patients who have ileostomies than in normal subjects. We saw above (p. 226) that uric acid stones tend to form in the presence of elevated concentrations of uric acid

Table 17.6 Normal ileostomy chemistry (adapted from Hill G L, Bambach C P 1983 in: Williams J A, Binder H J (eds) Large intestine. Gastroenterology. Butterworths, London, p. 125, by permission of the publishers)

	Daily excretion	Range	Concentration	Range
Wet weight	500 g	200–600 g	—	—
Dry weight	38 g	28–48 g	—	—
Water content	—	—	92%	88–94%
pH	—	—	6.3	6.1–6.5
Sodium	55 mmol	30–80 mmol	115 mmol/L	100–130 mmol/L
Potassium	4 mmol	3–6 mmol	8 mmol/L	5–11 mmol/L
Chloride	20 mmol	15–30 mmol	45 mmol/L	15–140 mmol/L
Bicarbonate	70	—	150 mmol/L	—
Calcium	9 mmol	7.5–20 mmol	12.5 mmol/L	5–32 mmol/L
Magnesium	4 mmol	3.5–4.5 mmol	7.5 mmol/L	5–14 mmol/L
Phosphate*	—	4–12 mmol	—	—
Nitrogen	1 g	0.6–2.4 g	—	—
Fat	2.2 g	1.5–3.8 g	—	—
Zinc	0.13 mmol	0.07–0.24 mmol	—	—
Copper	0.02 mmol	0.006–0.038 mmol	—	—

* Very few data available

and when the urine is acidic because the pK of uric acid is 5.42. Although the output of magnesium, zinc and copper are very similar to losses in normal faeces, patients with ileostomy diarrhoea may develop deficiencies of these elements.

METABOLIC EFFECTS OF AN ILEOSTOMY

Sodium and water depletion

The normally functioning ileostomy excretes about 500 g water and 60 mmol sodium per day and these amounts are two or three times the amounts which are found in normal faeces. Urinary compensation results in decreased volume and decreased excretion of sodium. Although it was thought in the past that ileostomy patients, even those with well functioning ileostomies, were chronically depleted of body water and sodium more recent studies have shown that the body composition of ileostomy patients is no different from that of closely matched controls (Christie et al 1990).

If, however, a patient with an ileostomy develops gastroenteritis or the ileostomy output becomes excessive for any reason, these compensatory mechanisms may break down for there is little physiological reserve. Body salt and water depletion may develop rapidly since renal conservation mechanisms are already operating maximally. Patients with severe ileostomy diarrhoea often require urgent intravenous fluid therapy. A standard '70 kg patient' who is admitted for treatment of ileostomy dehydration requires around 4 L or more of Ringer's lactate in the first few hours to restore body hydration to normal.

Potassium depletion

Hypokalaemia is rarely seen in patients with excessive ileostomy output unless the water and salt deficit is profound. Then, because of increased sodium retention at the renal tubule which is accompanied by increased urinary potassium loss, total body potassium depletion may occur. The treatment is to rehydrate the patient and once renal function is adequate supply potassium according to the protocol set out in Chapter 4.

Magnesium depletion

Although the daily excretion of magnesium from well functioning ileostomies is about the same as in normal faeces, and magnesium depletion does not occur, patients with chronic high output ileostomies not uncommonly present with symptoms of magnesium depletion. Such patients present with pins and needles in the fingertips, tightness around the mouth, muscular weakness, twitching and occasionally tetany. Hypocalcaemia is usually present as well.

The acute syndrome of magnesium deficiency responds quickly to an intravenous infusion of magnesium sulphate (see Ch. 4), although patients with chronic deficiency are more difficult to manage because oral magnesium supplements are poorly absorbed. The key is to control the excessive ileostomy output (see below). Vitamin D increases magnesium absorption from the gut and we have found that patients with hypocalcaemic osteomalacia and hypomagnesaemia have their symptoms controlled by the administration of oral vitamin D supplements.

Urolithiasis and cholelithiasis

We have seen above (p. 226) that there is an increased incidence of urinary stones particularly of uric acid stones in ileostomy patients. Uric acid stones normally comprise less than 10% of stones in intact patients but make up to 60% of stones found in those with an ileostomy. In fact, as we have shown above, all types of urinary calculi occur with increased frequency in patients after ileostomy. Cholelithiasis may also be a problem, though perhaps not a clinical one, in patients who have had an ileal resection as well as an ileostomy.

Vitamin B_{12} depletion

Reduced vitamin B_{12} absorption has been reported following colectomy and ileostomy. During the first year following operation most patients show slightly abnormal vitamin B_{12}

absorption but only 25% of those who have had their ileostomy longer than a year have impaired absorption. In fact there is no evidence at all to suggest that patients with uncomplicated ileostomies require long term vitamin B_{12} supplementation.

ILEOSTOMY DYSFUNCTION — CLINICAL MANAGEMENT

After the establishment of an ileostomy the patient should be able to eat a normal diet and not require any medication. Over the months after surgery he or she will regain normal body composition, and return to work feeling entirely healthy. Ileostomy output reduces slightly over the first 6 months but from then on stays fairly constant for life. Difficulties may be encountered, however, in those in whom ileostomy output is greater than it should be (after correction for their body size). Abnormal output is suggested when the patients complain of increased leakages or of emptying their bag more than 5 or 6 times per day. Such patients should be investigated. The ileostomy appliance is removed, the peristomal skin is examined and the surgeon's little finger is passed into the stoma and through the abdominal wall looking for a stenosis. A paediatric sigmoidoscope is used to examine the mucosa of the distal 15 cm or so of terminal ileum looking for Crohn's disease. Suspicious areas are biopsied. Laboratory investigations are initially simple. A spot sample of ileostomy fluid and urine are sent to the laboratory. The concentrations of sodium and potassium are measured in both ileostomy fluid and urine and when the [Na]/[K] ratio in either is low, salt depletion is suspected. It is always present when the urinary [NA]/[K] ratio is less than 1. If there is no stenosis or recurrent ileal disease loperamide hydrochloride 4 mg b.d. is given together with effervescent salt tablets (10 g NaCl contain 170 mmol of Na^+ and 170 mmol of Cl^-). After 4 weeks, ileostomy and urinary chemistry is remeasured. If the treatment has been successful, frequency of bag emptying will be less than 5 per day, the urinary [Na]/[K] ratio will be greater than 1, the patient will be feeling less tired, be free of cramps and putting on weight. It is only patients in whom these simple investigations and treatment are not successful who need further investigation (Hill et al 1975). A small bowel enema, and a barium examination of the distal ileum through a Foley catheter and a small bowel biopsy are required. Strictures or adhesions causing partial obstruction are treated surgically, recurrent Crohn's disease is treated initially with steroids. Malabsorption and pancreatic deficiency are treated as appropriate.

SECTION VI
ILEOANAL POUCH SURGERY

An acceptable alternative to end ileostomy for inflammatory bowel disease and familial adenomatous polyposis is an ileal reservoir and a reservoir anal anastomosis. Experience with these procedures is limited and very long term follow up not yet available. We know, however, that body composition in such patients is restored to normal somewhere between 6 and 12 months after the surgery (see Table 13.6, Chapter 13).

Table 17.7 Ileostomy versus Ileoanal J Pouch anastomoses — 24-hour faecal and urinary analysis (mean ± s.e.m.). (From Christie P M, Knight G S, Hill G L 1990 Br J Surg 77: 149, by permission of the publishers)

	24-h stool analysis			**24-h urine analysis**	
	Weight (g)	Na (mmol)	K (mmol)	Volume (ml)	Na : K
Ileostomy (n = 14)	548 (40)	74 (10)	14 (5)	1171 (130)	0.96 (0.15)
J pouch (n = 20)	507 (9)	58 (10)	8 (1)	1139 (95)	1.17 (0.13)
p	NS	NS	NS	NS	NS

Preliminary chemical studies of ileal pouch effluent (Table 17.7) suggest that as far as water and salt are concerned chemical composition is very similar to ileostomy fluid.

It seems therefore that the metabolic problems accompanying ileoanal pouch surgery will in the long run be found to be very similar to those of patients with ileostomies. Urolithiasis will therefore be likely to be a problem but it is not clear if the incidence of cholelithiasis will prove to be higher.

18. Perioperative nutrition

INTRODUCTION

Patients presenting for major surgery usually have lost weight, the surgical procedure leads to further loss and the net result is that most develop protein energy malnutrition to a greater or lesser extent. After uncomplicated surgery in a well nourished patient the intensity of the malnutrition is mild, is taken as an accepted part of the surgical illness and little is done about it. Proper nutritional support can prevent postoperative loss of body tissue altogether but it has not been shown that this confers any clinical benefit on the patient.

On the other hand, surveys of surgical patients have shown that moderate to severe protein energy malnutrition occurs not infrequently in surgical patients and is often unrecognised and untreated. In this chapter we will look at the indications for perioperative nutritional support: we will look at the available evidence for its efficacy and make some attempt to evaluate its cost effectiveness.

SECTION I
NUTRITIONAL THERAPY PRIOR TO MAJOR SURGERY

In 1936 Hiram Studley, a surgeon from Cleveland Ohio looked carefully at a number of factors which he thought might contribute to the high mortality after subtotal gastrectomy for duodenal ulcer. Controlling for the age of the patient, the operating surgeon and the length of the operation, he found a correlation between the magnitude of preoperative weight loss and postoperative mortality. Most of the deaths that occurred in these patients were due to respiratory infection which was frequently complicated by wound dehiscence. Although this study is frequently quoted as proof of the relationship between malnutrition and surgical outcome it is clear that there are many factors in modern surgery which now make this relationship much less clear. Modern surgery with minimal access, prophylactic antibiotics, better anaesthetic and fluid therapy, improved suture materials, better treatments for postoperative pain and better physiotherapy has inbuilt safeguards to minimise the types of complications that occurred in Studley's patients. It is not surprising therefore that many modern studies of the relationship between weight loss and postoperative mortality are inconclusive. Nevertheless a number of recent prospective studies have shown that severely malnourished patients are still at increased risk of developing complications after major surgery. What is now clear, however, is that weight loss of itself is not a risk factor, it only becomes so when the weight loss is accompanied by clinically obvious impairments of physiological function (Windsor & Hill 1988d). Studley titled his 1936 paper *Percentage weight loss — a basic indicator of surgical risk.* We titled our 1988 paper *Weight loss with physiologic impairment — a basic indicator of surgical risk* (Windsor & Hill 1988d).

BIOLOGY OF MALNOURISHED SURGICAL PATIENTS

In Chapter 5 we looked at the metabolic, compositional and physiological abnormalities that accompany protein energy malnutrition. We saw that moderate to severe protein energy malnutrition affects fat and protein turnover with an enhanced reliance on fat as an energy substrate. In some patients there is a marked increase in whole body protein breakdown whilst in others protein is conserved. These metabolic alterations result in fat depletion, an erosion of body protein stores and often an expansion of extracellular water. Cellular function is altered with deficits in membrane potential, alterations in cellular hydration, reductions in key enzymes of glucose oxidation and deficits in high energy phosphates. These effects result in a range of functional impairments which include psychological impairments, skeletal muscle dysfunction, a range of defects in respiratory function, immune dysfunction and impairment of the wound healing response. It is not difficult therefore to appreciate that some patients with deficiencies of body protein are at increased risk of postoperative complications.

Table 18.1 illustrates this point well. It shows the results of a study of 101 patients who presented for major gastrointestinal surgery. The table compares outcome after surgery in those patients who were protein depleted (a deficit of total body protein >20%) and those in whom protein depletion was not present.

Table 18.1 Demographic data, protein nutrition and postoperative course of 101 patients undergoing a major gastrointestinal resection. Group I patients (n = 53) were not significantly depleted of protein, Group II patients (n = 48) were all significantly depleted of protein, i.e. measured body protein was less than 77% of predicted total body protein. (Adapted from Windsor J A, Hill G L 1988b Aust NZ J Surg 58: 711, with permission from the Royal Australasian College of Surgeons, publishers)

	Group I non-protein depleted patients (n = 53)	Group II protein depleted patients (n = 48)	*p*
Sex M : F	30 : 23	21 : 27	NS
Age (yr)	58.5 (1.3)*	63.4 (2.5)	NS
Weight loss (%)	7.8 (1.2)	13.1 (1.1)	<0.05
Transferrin (mg %)	264 (8)	219 (10)	<0.05
Prealbumin (mg %)	22.8 (1.1)	14.8 (0.9)	<0.01
Deficit of total body protein (%)	4 (.01)	39 (2)	<0.01
Complications Postop.			
Major complications	12	24	<0.01
Pneumonia	4	11	<0.05
Wound infection	5	9	NS
Postop. hospital stay (d)	14.6 (1.1)	19.2 (2.0)	<0.025

* Mean (s.e.m.)

EFFECTS OF SHORT TERM NUTRITIONAL REPLETION

The time available for preoperative nutritional therapy is necessarily limited and it is usually not practical or possible to consider a period of longer than 7–14 days. The accretion of body protein that can be expected over this time period is small and dependent on nutritional and metabolic factors. Patients with moderate to severe marasmus would be expected to increase their body protein stores by 5% with 2 weeks of parenteral or enteral nutrition but if resting metabolic expenditure is raised (from sepsis, trauma or other metabolic stress) the gain in body protein would be less than 1% or none at all (Hill et al 1991). In spite of this disappointing short term effect on body composition, we saw in Chapter 6 that within a few days of commencing nutritional therapy there are substantial improvements (10–20%) in many physiological functions. These improvements, which are probably clinically significant, occur maximally around 4 days after commencement of feeding and do not continue thereafter until there are demonstrable increases in total body protein. There may, however, be other effects of short term nutritional support such as hepatic glycogen repletion, repletion of the labile protein pool, enzyme induction and hormonal responses which may also be beneficial. None of these factors has yet been associated with a reduction in postoperative risk.

IDENTIFICATION OF SUBJECTS AT RISK

Some use indices of nutritional state to identify subsets of patients at high risk of postoperative complications and feel that these indices are useful tools for the selection of candidates for preoperative nutritional support. Profound weight loss, some anthropometric indices, tests of muscle function, and measurements of plasma protein levels, including albumin, transferrin and prealbumin, have been used as indicators of risk of postoperative nutrition associated complications. Others use combinations of these, the most popular being the Prognostic Nutritional Index (PNI) from Philadelphia which uses anthropometry, delayed hypersensitivity skin tests and plasma proteins to devise a prognostic nutritional index (Buzby et al 1980). These various indices of nutritional state are said by those who use them to indicate the need for nutritional repletion prior to surgery. Table 18.2 shows the results of a study in which we formally compared a number of indicators of risk in a prospective study of a large number of patients undergoing major gastrointestinal surgery. It can be seen that weight loss and a variety of anthropometric indices are not clear indicators of risk, whereas measurements of grip strength, and low levels of plasma proteins are to some extent indicators of risk of postoperative complications. Three prognostic indices, including the one from Philadelphia (PNI) have little more to offer than low levels of plasma proteins. Others have argued that a thorough clinical evaluation is just as effective as these indices of surgical risk. It can also be seen in Table 18.2 that thorough clinical examination which assessed nutritional status as well as major organ function proved to be as effective as any other indicator in identifying subjects at risk.

This idea of clinical examination being the best way of identifying patients at risk of nutrition associated complications has been validated by Detsky and his colleagues (1987b). We have developed it further by testing the hypothesis that *weight loss with clinically obvious organ dysfunction is the best indicator of surgical risk* (Windsor & Hill 1988d). On the day before surgery 102 patients underwent a clinical assessment and a series of objective tests to detect the presence

Table 18.2 Retrospective comparison of indicators of surgical risk when indicator selected 17–20% of patients as being at high risk. (Adapted from Pettigrew R A, Hill G L 1986 Br J Surg 73: 47 by permission of the publishers)

	Indicator	Cut off selecting 17–20% of population	Sensitivity (%)	Specificity (%)	Positive predictive value (%)	Negative predictive value (%)	Overall predictive value (%)	Statistical data* x^2	p
Age	Age	>73 years	30	83	29	84	74	3.5	NS
Body measurements	WL	>16%	31	84	30	85	75	4.4	<0.05
	BMI	< third percentile	30	75	22	83	67	0.5	NS
	TSF	< third percentile	21	80	19	84	70	0	NS
	MAMC	< third percentile	26	83	25	87	73	1.1	NS
Muscle function	GS-males	<64 k Pa	40	87	38	88	79	4.3	<0.05
	GS-females	<47 k Pa	30	83	21	89	76	0.3	NS
Plasma proteins	Albumin	<35 g/L	33	82	29	85	73	4.2	<0.05
	Transferrin	<174 mg/dl	41	86	40	87	78	14.2	<0.001
	Prealbumin	<12 mg/dl	43	87	43	87	79	18.9	<0.001
Prognostic indices	Philadelphia	>45	35	83	32	85	75	6.5	<0.05
	Boston	>–0.7	30	84	30	84	74	3.8	>0.05
	Leeds	<–1.0	46	85	40	87	78	18.0	<0.001
Clinical judgement	Thorough clinical examination	>6 points	41	85	32	89	78	6.3	<0.025

* Complication rate in high risk group versus complication rate in low risk group. Key: WL = weight loss; BMI = body mass index; TSF = triceps skin fold; MAMC = mid arm muscle circumference; GS = grip strength; NS = not significant

of nutritional depletion and physiological dysfunction. Clinical assessment of weight loss and physiological function was evaluated by history and physical examination as described in Chapter 7. The patients were then categorised into 3 groups — group I (n = 43) weight loss <10% with normal function, group II (n = 17) weight loss 10% with normal function and group III, weight loss >10% with physiological dysfunction present clinically in at least 2 systems (i.e. overall activity level, psychological function, respiratory function, skeletal muscle function, wound healing and plasma albumin). After surgery, which included a major gastric or intestinal resection the patients were watched for complications and length of hospital stay. The results are shown in Tables 18.3, 18.4 and 18.5.

From Tables 18.3, 18.4 and 18.5 it can be seen that the group who were particularly at risk were those with moderate to severe protein energy malnutrition, i.e. malnutrition with physiological impairments. This means that patients with more than 20% weight loss (who virtually always have clinically obvious organ dysfunction) are at risk and those with lesser degrees of weight loss who have clinically obvious organ dysfunction are also at risk. Such patients have 3–5 times the complication rate and an increased hospital stay of 4–6 days.

Table 18.3 Objective validation of the nutritional status of 3 clinical patient groups. Values are given as mean ± s.e.m. Key: TBF = total body fat; Fat index = measured total body fat: predicted total body fat; MAMC = mid arm muscle circumference; TBP = Total body protein; Protein index = measured total body protein: predicted total body protein (From Windsor J A, Hill G L 1988d Ann Surg 207: 290, with permission of the publishers J B Lippincot Company)

Clinical categories	Group I weight loss <10% normal function	I vs II	Group II weight loss >10% normal function	II vs III	Group III weight loss >10% abnormal function	I vs III	Statistical data
Weight loss	3.9 ± 0.7	‡	13.4 ± 2.4	NS	14.8 ± 1.1	‡	$F = 25.73$ ($p<0.0001$)
Body fat stores							
Anthropometric (kg)	18.3 ± 1.1	*	13.3 ± 1.3	NS	13.7 ± 0.9	‡	$F = 6.09$ ($p<0.005$)
Measured TBF (kg)	17.3 ± 1.2	NS	14.9 ± 1.9	NS	13.1 ± 1.2	NS	$F = 2.89$ (NS)
Predicted TBF (kg)	14.7 ± 0.6	NS	14.3 ± 1.0	NS	15.6 ± 0.5	NS	$F = 1.24$ (NS)
Fat index (%)	117 ± 11	NS	102 ± 26	NS	84 ± 16	‡	$F = 3.65$ ($p<0.05$)
Body protein stores							
MAMC (cm)	264.7 ± 6.1	*	236 ± 6.2	NS	223.0 ± 4.9	‡	$F = 15.66$ ($p<0.0001$)
Measured TBP (kg)	8.8 ± 0.4	NS	7.9 ± 0.9	*	6.4 ± 0.3	‡	$F = 8.30$ ($p<0.005$)
Predicted TBP (kg)	9.9 ± 0.4	NS	9.9 ± 0.5	NS	9.3 ± 0.3	NS	$F = 1.12$ (NS)
Protein index (%)	88 ± 3	NS	78 ± 6	NS	63 ± 3	‡	$F = 9.67$ ($p<0.005$)
Fat free mass (kg)	51.4 ± 1.9	NS	47.8 ± 2.9	NS	41.3 ± 1.5	‡	$F = 8.42$ ($p<0.005$)

* $p<0.05$ ‡ $p<0.01$

Table 18.4 Objective validation of the nutritional status of the 3 clinical patient categories. Values are given as mean ± s.e.m. Key: FEV_1 = forced expiratory volume in 1 second; PEFR = peak expiratory flow rate; POMS = profile of mode score (From Windsor J A, Hill G L 1988d) Ann Surg 207: 290; with permission of the publishers J B Lippincot Company)

Clinical categories	Group I weight loss <10% normal function	Group I vs II	Group II weight loss >10% normal function	Group II vs III	Group III weight loss 10% abnormal function	Group I vs III	Statistical data
Liver function							
Transferrin (mg/dl)	263 ± 10	NS	247 ± 11	NS	216 ± 12	*	$F = 5.24$ ($p<0.01$)
Prealbumin (mg/dl)	23.7 ± 1.3.	NS	18.9 ± 1.5	*	13.8 ± 1.2		$F = 15.95$ ($p<0.0001$)
Skeletal muscle function							
Grip strength (kg)	32.8 ± 1.8	NS	34.2 ± 1.9	*	22.9 ± 1.8	*	$F = 10.46$ ($p<0.005$)
Grip strength/FFM (%)	65 ± 3.9	NS	70 ± 3	‡	53 ± 3.3	*	$F = -5.56$ ($p<0.01$)
Relaxation time (m/sec)	104.5 ± 2.6	NS	100.4 ± 2.8	*	116.4 ± 2.8	*	$F = 7.71$ ($p<0.005$)
Respiratory function							
Respiratory muscle strength index (%)	106.9 ± 7.0	NS	98.1 ± 7.6	*	72.2 ± 8.6	*	$F = 3.67$ ($p<0.05$)
FEV_1 (% predicted)	97.8 ± 3.3	NS	98.0 ± 5.7	NS	88.8 ± 5.3	NS	$F = 1.33$ (NS)
Vital capacity (% predicted)	108.8 ± 2.6	NS	108.7 ± 5.6	*	82.6 ± 3.6	‡	$F = 6.35$ ($p<0.005$)
FEV_1/VC(%)	75.9 ± 1.8	NS	78.3 ± 2.8	NS	78.8 ± 2.1	NS	$F = 0.81$ (NS)
PEFR (% predicted)	90.9 ± 2.5	NS	89.0 ± 4.9	*	75.2 ± 3.4	‡	$F = 7.21$ ($p<0.005$)
Maximum voluntary ventilation (% predicted)	81.1 ± 3.8	NS	84.4 ± 6.8	*	63.5 ± 4.3	‡	$F = 5.66$ ($p<0.01$)
Psychologic function							
POMS fatigue score	5.8 ± 1.5	NS	7.5 ± 1.8	NS	9.8 ± 1.4	*	$H = 6.61$ #($p<0.05$)

* $p < 0.05$ ‡ $p < 0.01$ # Kruskal–Wallis statistic

Table 18.5 The postoperative course of the 3 clinical categories of patients (from Windsor J A, Hill G L 1988d Ann Surg 207: 290, with permission of the publishers J B Lippincot Company)

Clinical Categories	Group I weight loss <10% normal function	Group II weight loss > 10% normal function	Group III weight loss > 10% abnormal function	Statistical data
Major complications	6	3	15	$\chi^2 = 5.98$ ($p<0.05$)
Septic complications	8	4	18	$\chi^2 = 6.36$ ($p<0.02$)
Pneumonia	4	1	10	$\chi^2 = 4.83$ ($p<0.05$)
Wound infection	4	1	7	$\chi^2 = 1.79$ (NS)
Death	0	1	4	NS
Hospital stay (d) (mean ± s.e.m.)	15.9 ± 1.3 .....NS...	12.7 ± 2.5 ....*......	19.2 ± 2.2	$F = 3.11$ ‡($p<0.05$)
	Group I vs Group III: NS			

* $p<0.05$ ‡ ANOVA

PREOPERATIVE TPN AND THE OUTCOME OF SURGERY

A lot has been written about the efficacy of preoperative nutrition and the situation has only recently become clear. A detailed meta-analysis of the available studies up to August 1986 was performed by Detsky et al (1987a). These workers evaluated 18 controlled trials but only 11 met the minimal criteria laid down for proper analysis. The pooled results of these 11 trials showed *trends suggesting* that TPN reduced the risk of complications from major surgery ($p = 0.21$) and fatalities ($p = 0.21$). However, the design flaws in these studies (for example admitting both well nourished and malnourished patients to the trials and employing sample sizes that were too small) made it difficult to show the effectiveness of TPN. These authors concluded that 'future studies should concentrate on selected subgroups of patients at high risk and may show that perioperative TPN is both effective and cost effective.'

When it was announced that a large multicentre randomised clinical trial of TPN in malnourished surgical patients was underway (Buzby et al 1988) surgeons realised that a definitive answer would finally be forthcoming. The study, now completed, has shown, not surprisingly, that a very small number of surgical patients (around 5% undergoing major elective surgery) benefit substantially from a week or so of preoperative TPN (Buzby et al 1991). The beneficial effect is confined to those with very severe malnutrition but in those with lesser degrees of malnutrition it may do more harm than good. Buzby's study was in fact a huge logistical exercise, never likely to be repeated, in which a study population of 3259 patients from 10 institutions were identified as being potentially eligible. 459 of these patients who were malnourished and available to enter the trial were randomly assigned to receive TPN (an average of 8 days) prior to operation and 3 days after operation, or no perioperative TPN. After surgery the patients were monitored for complications for 90 days. More infectious complications (mainly pneumonia and wound infections) occurred in the TPN group (14.1% versus 6.4%, p = 0.01) but more non infectious complications occurred in the control group (22.2% versus 16.7%, $p = 0.2$). On closer analysis it was found that the increased rate of infections was confined to patients categorised as well nourished or mildly malnourished and these patients experienced no benefit from preoperative TPN. Around 6% of the study population were classified as suffering from severe malnutrition and they experienced fewer non-infectious complications (mainly anastomotic breakdown) with TPN than without TPN (5% versus 43%, $p = 0.03$) but no increase in infectious complications.

In summary therefore, it can be said that a small number of very malnourished patients, probably about 5% of all patients coming in for major abdominal surgery, should receive a course of 7 days or so of total parenteral nutrition. They will include patients with massive weight loss, either with hypoalbuminaemia or clinically very obvious impairments of organ function or both. It can be expected that they will suffer fewer postoperative complications and have a shorter postoperative course.

GENERAL GUIDELINES FOR THE PRACTISING SURGEON

Although very sophisticated decision trees have been suggested for selecting patients for preoperative nutrition in clinical practice the process can be more straightforward (Fig. 18.1). There are three factors which must be considered when a patient is being assessed for preoperative nutritional support:

- his/her nutritional state with its associated functional impairment
- the magnitude of the projected operative procedure, particularly in terms of the known risks postoperatively and
- the anticipated response to the nutritional therapy.

The use of this schema is shown in Figure 18.1. It can be illustrated by two clinical examples.

Example 1

A male patient aged 63 years with 22% weight loss presented with clinical evidence of wasting, associated muscular weakness and breathlessness on walking at a normal pace. On physical examination he had marked wasting of subcutaneous fat stores and muscle stores of protein, and grip strength and respiratory function were obviously impaired. There was an unhealed scar on his right forearm but there was no clinical evidence of sepsis. His plasma albumin was normal. He complained of 6 weeks of dysphagia secondary to a small adenocarcinoma of the gastric cardia and required a total gastrectomy — a procedure associated with a high postoperative complication rate. It was clear that he suffered from advanced protein energy malnutrition and there was clinical evidence of functional impairment. Since the planned operative procedure was to be a large one with a significant morbidity he was considered for preoperative nutritional repletion (Fig. 18.1). He spent 7 days undergoing metabolic/nutritional repair. On the first day in hospital he was given parenteral vitamins, a fine nasogastric tube was passed endoscopically through the cancer and a course of Osmolite was commenced. After 2 days he was receiving 40 kcal/kg/day and 1.6 g protein/kg/day and towards the end of the week he was clearly much improved being up and around the ward and feeling stronger. Table 18.6 shows the changes in body composition, plasma proteins and physiological function that occurred over the 7-day period. There was a small gain in body protein (about 4%), a rise in plasma proteins and improvements (4%–10%) in various physiological functions. These objective data, his subjective improvement, and the fact that he was now up and around the ward, had clear lung bases and normal renal function suggested that the time was right for surgery.

The operation was performed on the seventh day after admission to hospital, he had a total gastrectomy and a Roux-en-Y oesophagojejunostomy performed. Postoperatively, his feeding continued as parenteral nutrition rather than enteral nutrition because technically it was not possible to safely intubate the small bowel without interfering with the Roux limb. On the 11th postoperative day a gastrografin swallow showed that the anastomosis was intact and the patient was started on oral diet. 3 days later he was consuming 1000 kcal and 40 g protein and the TPN was stopped. He was discharged on the fifteenth postoperative day without complication.

Example 2

A 30-year-old woman was admitted to hospital with partial obstruction from small bowel Crohn's disease. This, together with chronic ill health and lack of response to steroids, necessitated surgery. Her well weight was 67.6 kg; she now weighed 49.2 kg (27% weight loss). Her Crohn's disease activity index was 254 (<150 indicates inactive disease) and she was tired, listless and depressed. Examination revealed an emaciated young woman with gross depletion of fat and protein stores. She was reluctant to leave her bed and clinical evaluation of physiological function revealed very weak grip strength, poor respiratory muscle strength, unhealed scratches on her legs and a plasma albumin of 29 g/L. Reference to Figure 18.1 suggests that preoperative nutrition was indicated although her chronic septic state and high disease activity would mitigate against a substantial improvement in protein nutriture. The goal was to try to improve physiological function with a 1-week course of TPN (TPN was chosen because of the partial obstruction) before embarking on surgery to a point where she was up and about, feeling stronger and showing

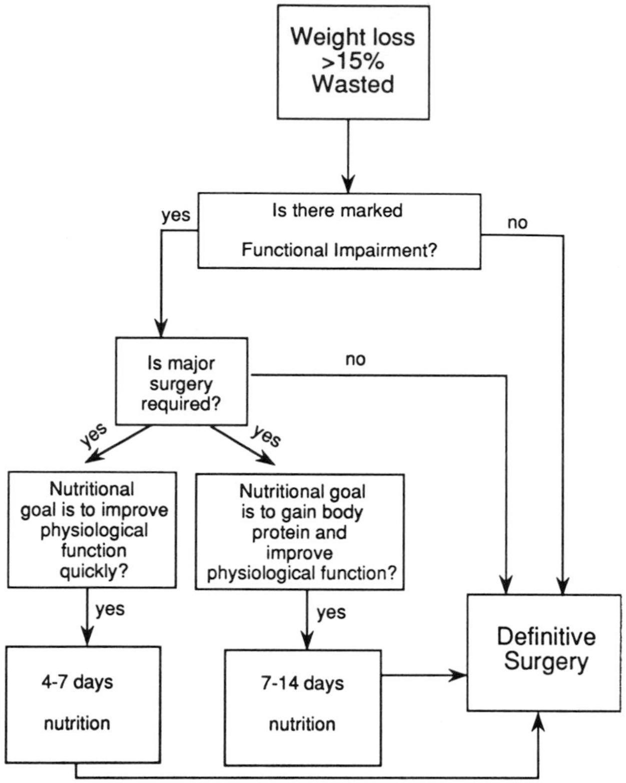

Fig. 18.1 Simplified decision tree for selecting patients for preoperative nutritional therapy.

Table 18.6 Changes in body composition, plasma proteins and physiological function that occurred over a 7-day period of preoperative enteral feeding (41 kcal/kg/day and 1.6 g protein/kg/day) in a 63-year-old man presenting with localised adenocarcinoma of the gastric cardia

	Estimated value when well	Measured value day 0 of enteral nutrition	Measured value day 7 of enteral nutrition
Body composition			
Body weight (kg)	62.4	52.2	52.4
Total body fat (kg)	14.3	10.7	10.8
Total body protein (kg)	9.5	6.3	6.5
Total body water (L)	35.1	31.4	31.2
Plasma proteins			
Transferrin (mg/dl)	263	176	219
Prealbumin (mg/dl)	24	15.7	23.4
Physiological function			
Grip strength (kg)	38	24	28
Respiratory muscle strength (cm H_2O)	95	32	36
Forced expiratory volume$_{1\ sec}$ (L)	3.8	2.3	2.8
Vital capacity (L)	4.6	2.9	3.3
Peak expiratory flow rate (L/min)	540	351	453
Maximum voluntary ventilation (L/min)	230	122	154

Table 18.7 Changes in protein nutriture with 2 weeks of TPN: 30-year-old woman with active Crohn's disease

	Day 0	Day 7	Day 14
Weight (kg)	49.2	49.4	49.1
Total body protein (kg)	7.3	7.4	7.5
Plasma transferrin (mg/dl)	215	223	253
Plasma prealbumin (mg/dl)	19.0	23.6	27.6

objective evidence of substantial improvement in skeletal muscle function and respiratory function. The results of the course of TPN are shown in Tables 18.7 and 18.8. The preoperative TPN in fact continued for a further 7-day period for the nutrition support team felt that after 7 days she had shown insufficient clinical improvement to undergo major surgery.

The results show a steady but small improvement in protein nutriture over the 2-week study period (Table 18.7). Most of the improvement in physiological function occurred during the first week rather than the second week. It is arguable therefore if TPN should have continued beyond the first week where clearly it was most effective. The study of Buzby and his colleagues (Buzby et al 1991) showed a significant reduction in postoperative risk with 7–15 days (average 8 days) of feeding and taking this together with the lack of improvement in physiological function during the second week of feeding suggests that 7 days of replenishment may have been all that was required for our patient. On the other hand, as Example 1 shows, depleted non septic patients may be expected to gain much more protein than this and if the clinical circumstances allow TPN for longer than 7 days in such patients it can be expected that further gains in physiological function will occur as a result of protein accretion. Significant protein accretion may be of vital importance to some very depleted patients but longer than 7 days of replenishment is required to achieve this.

Table 18.8 Effect of TPN on respiratory and skeletal muscle function with 2 weeks of TPN: 30-year-old woman with active Crohn's disease

	Day 0	Day 4	Day 7	Day 14
Respiratory muscle strength (cm/H_2O)	50	61	60	62
Forced expiratory volume$_{1\ sec}$ (L)	3.0	3.4	3.4	3.5
Peak expiratory flow rate (L/min)	411	447	444	442
Grip strength (kg)	26	31	32	33

SECTION II
NUTRITIONAL THERAPY AFTER MAJOR SURGERY

In Chapter 2 we saw how major surgical procedures in patients who are not malnourished result in postoperative weight loss and mild protein energy malnutrition. It was also pointed out that postoperative nutritional therapy could prevent this loss of protein, fat and weight but no clinical advantage could be shown by doing so. In Chapter 2 also we saw how postoperative fatigue develops postoperatively and some have sought to associate this with the loss of muscle protein. Unfortunately recent studies have shown that prevention of protein loss in the postoperative period has not prevented the development of postoperative fatigue (Schroeder et al 1991).

There are, however, some patients who do need nutritional support in the postoperative period and in this section we will look at the indications for this treatment and how it might be administered.

MALNUTRITION IN THE POSTOPERATIVE PERIOD

Postoperative malnutrition does exist and many studies have shown that it is more common than previously thought. In clinical practice postoperative malnutrition, that is, malnutrition of a degree sufficient to affect physiological function occurs in three broad groups of patients. In some patients *preexisting malnutrition* is untreated prior to surgery and hence persists and is made worse by it. Postoperative malnutrition may also occur in some patients directly because *oral intake is not possible for technical reasons*. The most severe form of postoperative malnutrition occurs in those patients who have developed a *complication* (particularly a septic one) as the result of the surgical procedure itself.

Preexisting malnutrition as cause of postoperative malnutrition

When malnourished patients are subjected to a major surgical procedure in which further oxidation of both fat and protein occurs, severe protein energy malnutrition may develop. Patients with severe marasmus may show surprisingly little response to surgical trauma and providing eating is resumed promptly little weight may be lost. However, there are few extra reserves in such patients and it is important to remember that after most major gastrointestinal surgery only 50% of normal intake is taken over the first 2 postoperative weeks (see Fig. 2.8).

Thus patients who present for a major procedure having already lost 15% of their body weight may lose a further 5–6% as a result of the operation before normal oral intake is restored. It may take months before this weight is regained and normal function restored.

Postoperative malnutrition occurring as the result of enforced gut rest

After a difficult anastomosis of the oesophagus, stomach, duodenum, small bowel, pancreas or biliary tract it is not uncommon for the surgeon to forbid normal food intake until all risk of anastomotic breakdown has passed, usually about the tenth or twelfth postoperative day. Since adequate voluntary food intake will not be achieved for another 2 weeks or so after that, all but those patients who are normally nourished will suffer an overall weight loss around 15% unless some form of enteral or parenteral feeding is instituted. Patients who have undergone massive bowel resection for Crohn's disease, tumour or infarction are unable to take oral food until compensatory bowel adaptation has occurred. As pointed out in Chapter 14, TPN is required until daily output of stool plateaus at something less than 1.5 L per day. Without such treatment profound or even lethal protein energy malnutrition will develop.

Postoperative complications as a cause of malnutrition

Whenever a major complication develops in the postoperative period it is certain that protein energy malnutrition will occur as a direct consequence. A protein and energy deficit develops not only because oral intake is delayed but also because energy output and whole body protein breakdown are increased. A good example of this is the patient with an intraabdominal abscess presenting during the second postoperative week. The patient is nauseated, there is paralytic ileus and no oral intake is possible. Body tissues are being consumed at an increased rate because of increased energy requirements and markedly increased protein breakdown. The lack of energy intake, together with the increased energy output result in a large energy deficit which continues until the abscess is drained and the patient resumes eating.

Even then it will be another 10 or 12 days before normal voluntary food intake is resumed adding a further substantial energy and protein deficit. Although there are some patients with huge fat and protein stores who may be able to cope with such a nutritional assault, most patients require nutritional support when such complications develop. The patient who develops a high output small bowel fistula will have a much greater problem. Not only must oral intake cease, but the accompanying sepsis results in raised energy expenditure and increased protein losses. The energy and protein deficit will continue until the fistula closes either spontaneously or is closed directly by surgery and the patient is eating again. Such a patient requires nutritional support for at least 6 weeks and the surgeon should institute TPN soon after the establishment of the fistula to avoid the otherwise inevitable development of protein energy malnutrition.

PREVENTION OF PROTEIN ENERGY MALNUTRITION AFTER SURGERY

The guidelines published by the American Society of Parenteral and Enteral Nutrition (1986) are helpful in deciding on the use of postoperative nutritional support. These guidelines suggest nutritional support following major surgery if adequate intake is not anticipated within 7–10 days. If the patient is severely catabolic or if severe preoperative malnutrition is present, the guidelines suggest support when 5–7 days of postoperative starvation is anticipated.

At the present time there are three methods being used to prevent protein energy malnutrition after surgery:

- nasogastric decompression with jejunal feeding
- fine needle catheter jejunostomy
- total parenteral nutrition.

Nasogastric decompression with jejunal feeding

Postoperative nasojejunal feeding has been used intermittently over the years and has been shown to decrease postoperative weight and protein loss and possibly to shorten hospital stay (Sagar et al 1979). Such treatment, however, is not without its risks (Smith et al 1985) and cannot be recommended for routine use. Moss has suggested a technique of simultaneous nasogastric decompression and jejunal feeding which when used for 2–3 days in the early postoperative period seems to be associated with few disadvantages and some remarkably beneficial effects. These include early discharge from hospital because of early and rapid resumption of oral intake and a theoretical improvement in the strength of bowel anastomoses (Moss et al 1980, Moss 1984).

We were taken by these remarkable results and as a consequence put the technique to the test in a randomised trial of 32 patients who were undergoing colorectal surgery (Schroeder et al 1991). 16 patients received simultaneous naso-oesophago-gastric decompression and jejunal feeding with Osmolite. Over the first 4 postoperative days they received an average of 1200 kcals per day. The control group given routine postoperative care received an average of less than 400 kcals per day. 4 out of the 16 patients who received the enteral feeding, however, were unable to tolerate the tube and were withdrawn from the study. Although the beneficial effects were not statistically significant, there was an increased caloric intake, a reduced loss of body protein and a shorter time to pass flatus in the enterally fed group. Wound healing, which was assessed by the Goretex implant technique (Ch. 6), was improved ($p < 0.2$). There were no differences in postoperative complications, the incidence or degree of postoperative fatigue or the postoperative deterioration of muscle function. We also found the technique to be quite demanding in terms of nursing time.

From our own results and those of others (Elmore et al 1989) we have concluded that this technique does have a small place in some types of gastrointestinal surgery, particularly in patients with marginal malnutrition undergoing major surgery in whom further protein loss is to be avoided (Schroeder et al 1991).

Fine needle catheter jejunostomy

Most often when it is anticipated that enteric feeding will be required in the postoperative period fine needle catheter jejunostomy is recommended. As a general rule the technique of jejunostomy feeding should be reserved for patients in whom the surgeon knows that voluntary food intake will be delayed and moderate–severe PEM will develop as a consequence. Others have shown improved nitrogen balance, reduction in septic complications and more rapid rehabilitation with this treatment (Ryan et al 1981) but others are more cautious (Smith et al 1985).

We compared the changes in body composition and plasma proteins, and the clinical outcome of 20 patients fed by fine needle catheter jejunostomy after major colorectal surgery and compared the results with those of 20 matched controls. Body weight, fat free mass and plasma prealbumin fell significantly in the control patients but not in those fed by jejunostomy (Fig. 18.2).

Surprisingly, the voluntary food intake was no different between the control patients and those fed via the jejunostomy (Fig. 18.3).

We found there was no significant difference in clinical outcome in terms of complication rate or duration of postoperative hospital stay. Nevertheless, the technique proved to be relatively safe, and we have concluded that although it cannot be recommended for routine use after surgery it can be of real value in patients in whom gut rest

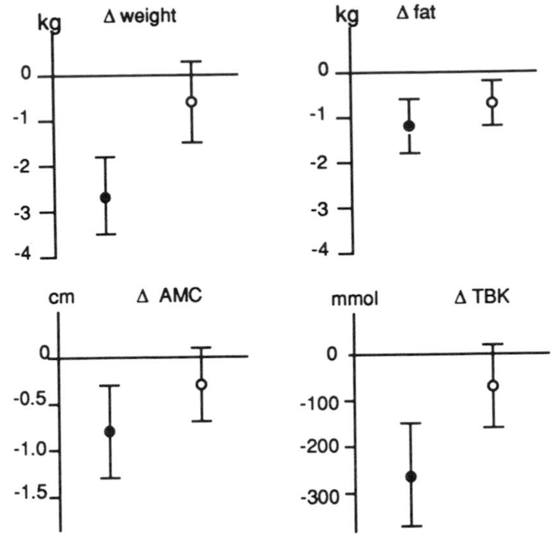

Fig. 18.2 Mean changes (with 95% confidence limits) in body weight, body fat, arm muscle circumference (AMC) and total body potassium (TBK) in the 2 groups of patients. Key: ● = controls ○ = patients fed via jejunostomy. (Redrawn from Yeung C K, Young G A, Hackett A F, Hill G L 1979 Brit J Surg 66: 727 by permission of the publishers.)

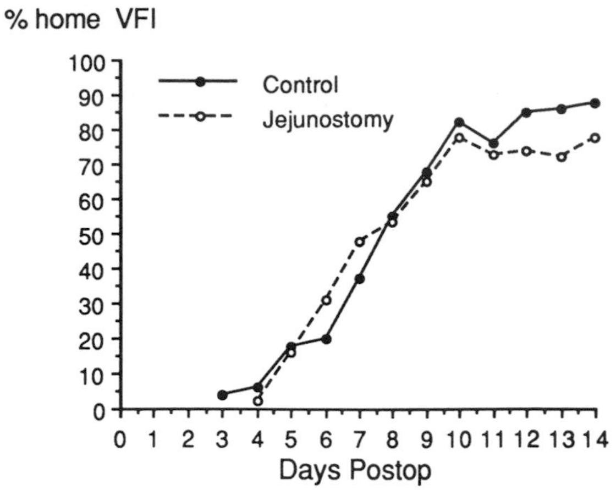

Fig. 18.3 Voluntary food intake (VFI) in the two groups of patients expressed as a percentage of the home voluntary food intake during the first 14 days after operation. Key: ● = controls ○ = patients fed via jejunostomy. (Redrawn from Yeung C K, Young G A, Hackett A F, Hill G L 1979 Brit J Surg 66: 727 by permission of the publishers.)

is required for an extended period. We now use it instead of total parenteral nutrition in selected patients after total gastrectomy or Whipple's resection (Hamaouie et al 1990).

Postoperative jejunal feeding may find new favour if the promising results of the first trial of a new organ specific enteral feed are confirmed in a larger trial. As we saw in Chapter 6, a preliminary report (Daly et al 1992) describing the use of an enteral diet enriched with arginine, RNA and N-3 polyunsaturated fatty acids appeared to show considerable advantages for such a diet. The results of a multicentre trial of this new enteral diet are awaited (Bower 1990a).

Total parenteral nutrition

A number of workers have shown that protein and fat loss can be prevented by the administration of TPN in the postoperative period. It has been much harder, however, to demonstrate any positive clinical benefit to patients in whom postoperative complications have not occurred (Yamada et al 1983). In a major study of postoperative parenteral nutrition we (Young & Hill 1980) studied the changes in body composition, plasma proteins and the clinical response obtained before and 15 days after surgery in each of three groups of patients who were receiving in addition to a restricted oral diet:

- no TPN
- parenteral amino acids without an energy source
- full TPN.

Infusion of amino acids alone spared body protein but there were no increases in plasma proteins other than those of the acute phase type. In contrast full TPN spared more body protein and fat, increased plasma proteins and the clinical outcome was more favourable (see Ch. 10, Fig. 10.3).

We have concluded from this study that TPN has a place in the prevention of further protein losses in patients who come to very major surgery already with moderate–severe PEM and in whom a large and extensive wound will be made. Clearly patients who have received TPN preoperatively should have that continued in the postoperative period until adequate oral intake is established. It is clear that full TPN prevents further tissue loss after surgery, restores plasma proteins to normal rapidly and, in some circumstances, improves clinical outcome.

Enteral nutrition versus parenteral nutrition

In studies that compared enteral with parenteral postoperative nutrition in gastrointestinal surgery no significant reduction in morbidity or mortality was achieved by either feeding route. Cost savings were, however, considerable when patients were given enteral nutrition (Bower et al 1986, Quayle et al 1984, Muggia-Sullam et al 1985).

Clearly, cost savings are a factor and we conclude that postoperative parenteral nutrition should therefore be restricted to malnourished patients whose operations are major, who cannot tolerate enteral nutrition and in whom prolonged ileus is anticipated.

SECTION III
COST EFFECTIVENESS OF PERIOPERATIVE NUTRITION

The cost of healthcare is increasing at an alarming rate. With limited resources and necessary reductions in hospital expenditure, hospital managers are asking about the cost effectiveness of perioperative nutrition. Although the average daily cost of enteral nutrition is not much more than hospital meals the cost of TPN is more than ten times higher.

Two types of analyses may be done to look at cost effectiveness. There is a *cost-benefit analysis* which relates the monetary cost of the treatment to the value of the good it produces. The problem in this sort of analysis is that it places monetary values on such things as complications and lives saved and thus becomes very difficult to do. In *cost-effectiveness analysis* the good to be achieved is selected and the costs of differing strategies to achieve it are compared.

As far as enteral nutrition is concerned the costs are so low that the major concern is to demonstrate benefit and safety. We have already discussed some of these aspects.

Table 18.9 Cost-benefit analysis of preoperative TPN: 100 severely malnourished patients presenting for major gastrointestinal surgery

Benefit	
24 major complications avoided @ $US50 000 per complication	$US1 200 000
Total benefit	$US1 200 000
Costs	
TPN (100 patients × 7 days of TPN @ $US500/day)	$US350 000
Hospital Bed (100 patients × 7 days @ $US400/day)	$US280 000
Total costs	$US630 000
Net savings = Total benefits − Total costs	
= $US1 200 000 − $US630 000	
= $US570 000	
= $US5 700 per patient	

With available data it is possible to do a cost-benefit analysis of the use of preoperative TPN (Table 18.9).

In constructing this analysis we have used the data from Twomey & Patching (1985) who estimated that an economic benefit of around $US50 000 accrues from the avoidance of a major complication such as anastomotic leak. For the benefit of TPN we have used the data from the Department of Veterans Affairs cooperative study of TPN (Buzby et al 1991). As we saw above, however, this study showed that TPN increased the rate of infections in patients categorised as well nourished or mildly malnourished and these patients experienced no demonstrable benefit from TPN. However the small number of patients (about 5–6% of all patients coming forward for major surgery) who were categorised as being severely malnourished were helped substantially by TPN. Not only were non-infectious complications not increased but there was a substantial reduction in non-infectious complications in these patients treated with TPN. From these data it can be expected that if 100 severely malnourished patients were given TPN for 7 days 24 major complications would be avoided. A calculation based on the value of these benefits and the cost of TPN (Table 18.9) yielded a net saving of $US5 700 per patient as a result of 7-days preoperative TPN even if nutritional support is the sole reason for the patient being in hospital.

PART 4

Metabolism and Nutrition in Serious Surgical Illness

Part 4 Contents

19. Metabolic and nutritional management in surgical intensive care

INTRODUCTION — THE HYPERDYNAMIC–HYPERMETABOLIC STATE

Seriously ill surgical patients frequently require a period of intensive care after major elective surgery, severe trauma, or serious sepsis. During this time they often require respiratory and inotropic support and are at high risk of other organ failures. In most of these patients the lung is usually the first organ to fail and other organs follow in a characteristic sequential pattern. Respiratory failure is followed in order by cardiac, hepatic, renal, haematologic and gastrointestinal failure. Many patients with multiple organ failure develop a hyperdynamic–hypermetabolic state with high cardiac output, low peripheral resistance, increased oxygen consumption and excessive protein catabolism. The increased blood flow (*hyperdynamic circulation*), especially to the damaged and septic tissues, supports the increased cellular metabolism and enhanced oxygen requirements within them. The total consumption of oxygen by the body is greater than normal because of the increased oxidation of carbohydrates, fats and proteins which are being used to drive the metabolic processes of the body at an accelerated pace. As a result the patient produces more heat and is said to be *hypermetabolic*. Other features of the hyperdynamic–hypermetabolic state are fever, marked expansion of the extracellular fluid (leaky capillaries) and glucose intolerance (insulin activity is antagonised by growth hormone and epinephrine).

SECTION I
SURGICAL METABOLISM

INTERORGAN SUBSTRATE EXCHANGE IN CRITICAL SURGICAL ILLNESS

There is an integrated metabolic response to critical illness which involves the wound or focus of inflammation, the liver, muscle, kidneys and intestine. The heart plays a major role by increasing output to produce the high rate of flow required to allow these interchanges to occur. This integrated metabolic response is initiated and propagated by cytokines and the nervous and endocrine systems are involved in regulation of the response. The intensity of the response is related to the wound size, or the mass of necrotic or inflammatory tissue; the larger the wound the more intense is the integrated metabolic response. Figure 19.1 shows the exchange of substrates that occurs in critical illness.

The wound or inflammatory mass is the site of intense cellular activity. Necrotic tissue is lysed and removed, bacteria are immobilised and destroyed, and collagen synthesis and wound repair are underway. These processes require a variety of substrates, particularly glucose and glutamine as respiratory fuels and amino acids for protein synthesis. Glucose is the principal fuel supplying the relatively hypoxic inflammatory mass and the cells within it (Daley et al 1990) and lactate is produced and released into the circulation for transport back to the liver for the further production of glucose (Cori cycle) (Fig. 19.1). Most of the glucose required for the inflammatory mass is produced by the liver not only

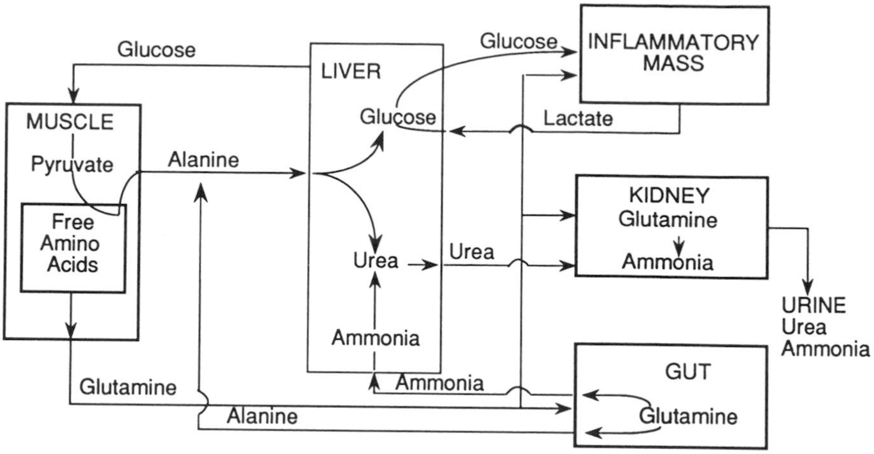

Fig. 19.1 The metabolic response to the presence of an inflammatory mass is shown. The substrate exchanges between the organs support the inflammatory cells in the septic area which have substantial requirements for glucose and glutamine for energy and amino acids for protein synthesis. These exchanges are facilitated by a hyperdynamic circulation. Most of the glucose required is produced in the liver from lactate, amino acids (mainly alanine) and glycerol from the hydrolysis of triglycerides in adipose tissue (not shown). The carbon skeletons of the amino acids are used for gluconeogenesis and the nitrogen is excreted as urea. As can be seen muscle is the major source of the amino acids. Glutamine levels fall to low levels in muscle cells of septic patients. Glutamine serves as a primary fuel for the gut where it is processed into ammonia (which buffers acid loads in the kidney) and alanine which is processed in the liver.

from lactate but also from alanine and other glucogenic amino acids. These reactions require energy which comes from the oxidation of fatty acids. It is the carbon skeleton of alanine that is the main structure for new glucose formation; the amino group is cleaved off and forms urea which is excreted in the urine. Muscle is the major source of amino acids which are used for protein synthesis both in the wound and the liver. The most abundant amino acids released from muscle are alanine and glutamine (Salleh et al 1991). Glutamine serves as a primary fuel for the gut producing ammonia and alanine which are processed by the liver. In addition, glutamine may help buffer filtered acid loads in the kidneys by the formation of ammonia. Glutamine is also a primary fuel for macrophages and lymphocytes (Newsholme et al 1988). It is a nonessential amino acid which accounts for only about 5% of protein but it is the most abundant intracellular free amino acid, accounting for about 60% of the total intracellular free amino acid pool. The intracellular concentration of glutamine falls under many catabolic conditions including starvation, inactivity, elective operation, trauma and sepsis. This decrease occurs early in the course of the condition, persists until late convalescence and appears to be related to the severity of the critical illness. Figure 19.2 shows how the increased rates of protein breakdown in muscle provide branched-chain amino acids within muscle which then donate their nitrogen for the synthesis of alanine and glutamine. From Figure 19.2 it can be seen that glutamine is formed from α-ketoglutarate and the amino group from branched-chain amino acids. Because it is much easier to provide parenteral α-ketoglutarate than glutamine (as ornithine α-ketoglutarate) some have suggested that it might be a practical proposition to prevent or reduce muscle proteolysis by its use (Wernerman et al 1990).

ENDOTOXIN AND THE ROLE OF THE GUT IN CRITICAL ILLNESS

A low continuous dose of endotoxin administered to animals produces a hypermetabolic state that exhibits all of the features of the response to

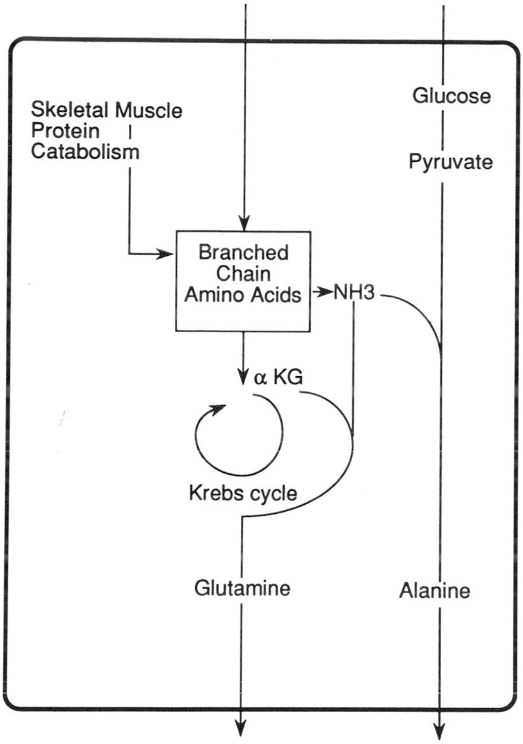

Fig. 19.2 Alanine and glutamine production in muscle from branched-chain amino acids. Branched-chain amino acids donate their amino groups for the synthesis of alanine and glutamine. The rate of glutamine release is influenced by a number of hormones and metabolites. α KG = α-ketoglutarate.

critical illness (Bessey 1989). The critically ill patient can become exposed to endotoxin from the wound, intravascular cannulae, lungs and urine. In addition, endotoxin can be absorbed from the gut directly or it can be released as a consequence of the lymphatic trapping of bacteria that have translocated from the gut lumen (Berg 1983, Alexander 1990). Formerly it was thought that the gut was a passive bystander during critical illness, especially when ileus developed or when the gut was rested by fasting. It has now been shown that gut mucosal permeability is increased in critically ill patients due to reduction in splanchnic blood flow, release of mediators from other sites of injury or sepsis which have been shown to increase permeability, e.g. endotoxin itself (O'Dwyer et al 1988) or oxygen free radicals (Deitch et al 1987), and from the lack of intraluminal nutrition, particularly glutamine (Windmueller 1982). Thus, in critically ill patients, there appears to be an adverse role played by the gut in perpetuating and augmenting the metabolic response to critical illness (Fong et al 1989a, Bounous 1990). It is for this reason that it is widely recommended that attempts should be made to prevent translocation of bacteria or endotoxin from the gut of critically ill patients. There is growing evidence that proper nutritional support of the gut may be a valuable strategy for minimising the adverse effects associated with endotoxin translocation (Mochizuki et al 1984, Border et al 1987).

SYSTEMIC MEDIATORS

The neuroendocrine changes discussed in Chapter 4 explain much of what happens in serious surgical illness but there is not enough stimulus from them to accelerate net skeletal muscle proteolysis to the degree that is seen in the hypermetabolic state (Bessey et al 1984). It is because of this that workers have looked for other mediators which must participate in the protein catabolic response to critical illness. In Chapters 1 and 4 we discussed the role of cytokines in initiating and propagating the metabolic response (Fig. 4.5). In serious surgical illness we saw how when added to the circulation they add a new dimension to the severity of the metabolic response (Gough 1991). It is now clear that the stress hormones appear to be necessary but not completely responsible for the catabolic response to critical illness.

Michie and his colleagues (Michie et al 1988b, Michie et al 1988c) administered human TNF to patients. 30 to 60 minutes after the start of the infusion, symptoms of headache, myalgia and chills developed. In addition, the patients experienced fever, tachycardia and an increase in the ACTH level indicating that the adrenal–pituitary axis was activated. These findings were compared with those of normal subjects who received endotoxin. The symptoms produced by endotoxin infusion were similar to those observed following TNF infusion but their onset was delayed. However, following endotoxin there was a sharp rise in TNF concentration which was of the same order of magnitude as that observed with TNF infusion and it preceded clinical symptoms. The clinical responses persisted for several hours until TNF was no longer detectable. When the cyclooxygenase inhibitor Ibuprofen was given to subjects before endotoxin the rise in the TNF concentration and the subsequent leucocytosis were still observed but the systemic symptoms and endocrine responses were attenuated (Revhaug et al 1988). These workers concluded that the systemic responses associated with endotoxin are due to a pulse of TNF and are mediated by the cyclooxygenase pathway.

The actions of TNF are the object of intensive research activity. In high dose it causes haemorrhagic necrosis of most organs of the body. One of its first effects is on endothelial cells causing vascular leak and shock. Although its concentration in the blood of critically ill subjects fluctuates widely, in general the higher the serum concentration the poorer the outcome.

ENERGY METABOLISM

Because of the hypermetabolic state, resting energy expenditure rises by 5–50% after major trauma and serious sepsis (Carlsson et al 1984, Clifton et al 1984, Bartlett et al 1982). It may remain elevated for a considerable period. In contrast there is little change in resting energy expenditure after major uncomplicated elective surgery (Ch. 2). We have seen how in sepsis and after trauma these increased energy needs are met predominantly by the oxidation of fat (Nanni et al 1984) and also from glucose derived by increased gluconeogenesis from body protein (Shaw et al 1985). Total body glycogen stores are small (approximately 500 g protein) and are unlikely to provide a significant contribution to energy supply after the first day or two.

PROTEIN METABOLISM

Critically ill patients in surgical intensive care all have high urinary urea/nitrogen loss — often 15–20 g of urea/nitrogen per day being found in the absence of nutritional support (Streat et al 1987). Other sources of nitrogen such as creatinine and ammonia also contribute such that urea accounts for about 75% of total urinary nitrogen. Unlike the situation seen in simple partial starvation (and perhaps in patients within a few days of major elective surgery) the starving patient with sepsis or after trauma does not have an adaptive reduction in urinary nitrogen loss and instead rapidly becomes severely depleted of body protein. In addition, the efficient almost complete suppression of gluconeogenesis from protein seen after glucose infusion and non-septic starvation is not seen in septic patients and larger amounts of glucose are required to suppress glucose production even partially (Shaw et al 1985). Much research endeavour (see Alexander & Fischer 1990 for review) is directed at ways to reduce or eliminate the huge loss of muscle protein that occurs in injured or septic patients. Endotoxin blockade (Wolff 1991), cytokine blockade (Cohen & Glauser 1991, Glauser et al 1991) and hormonal manipulation (Shaw & Wolfe 1988a) are under investigation and specific fuels such as branched-chain amino acids, α-ketoglutarate and glutamine enriched solutions have been and are being tried. Needless to say, nothing has yet improved (or is even likely to improve) on the profoundly beneficial effect of surgical drainage and elimination of the septic focus. *It is good to know that in these days of peptide regulatory factors and the like that the time honoured use of the scalpel and the surgeon's finger is still the cornerstone of the treatment of patients with serious sepsis.*

SALT AND WATER METABOLISM

In addition to changes in the energy and protein metabolism, there are in septic and injured patients profound changes in the metabolism of salt and water and in the volume and composition of body fluid compartments (Streat et al 1987). The presence of sepsis, profound shock and tissue damage leads to impaired capillary permeability with the resultant obligatory expansion of the interstitial fluid space during shock (Petrakos et al 1981). As we have seen, one of the first and most important effects of TNF is to cause vascular leak and shock.

Clinically then, the surgical patient in intensive care has rapid wasting of muscle and, to a lesser extent, fat which is initially not seen because of an expanding layer of extracellular water.

INTENSIVE CARE TREATMENT

If the patient needs ventilatory support he or she also necessarily gets bed rest, opiates, sedatives and often muscle relaxants. The resultant immobility and perhaps even curarisation itself may further increase the loss of body protein. Other intensive care treatments such as inotropic agents, particularly epinephrine (Bessey et al 1983), haemodialysis (Ward et al 1979) and steroids (Long et al 1981) may all also contribute to the catabolic process.

FUNCTIONAL EFFECTS OF PROTEIN CATABOLISM

We have shown in Chapters 5 and 6 that there is impairment of skeletal muscle strength and endurance, reduced respiratory muscle strength, low levels of plasma proteins and impaired wound healing and immune responses when more than 20% of body protein is lost. Clearly, the functional aspects are of crucial importance in the recovery from critical surgical illness.

SECTION II
CHANGES IN BODY COMPOSITION THAT OCCUR IN SURGICAL PATIENTS RECEIVING OPTIMAL INTENSIVE CARE

Surgical patients in intensive care fall into three main groups: *postoperative major elective surgery*, *major trauma* and *serious sepsis*.

MAJOR ELECTIVE SURGERY

Although these patients are not always admitted to intensive care electively they are mentioned to highlight the differences between them and the patient in intensive care after major trauma or with serious sepsis. Most patients who are admitted to intensive care after major elective surgery are there for a short period of haemodynamic monitoring or respiratory therapy and after a day or two are transferred back to a surgical ward.

We conducted a longitudinal study of the changes in body composition that occur after very major surgery. The results from 8 patients are presented in Table 19.1.

The patients had body composition measurements on the day prior to operation and again 14 days postoperatively. 3 of the patients had total gastrectomies with intraabdominal oesophagojejunal anastomoses, 2 had pancreatoduodenectomies, 2 had mucosal proctectomies with ileoanal pouch formation and ileostomy and 1 had panproctocolectomy. No patient had TPN preoperatively or during the 14 day postoperative period and none developed a serious complication.

As a group, these patients were depleted of approximately 24% of total body protein immediately preoperatively. In the first 2 weeks postoperatively there was a loss of total body protein of 0.6 kg or 5% of total body protein and at this time the patients were approximately

Table 19.1 Early body composition changes in patients after major elective surgery, severe blunt trauma, and serious sepsis (from Streat S J, Hill G L 1987 World J Surg 11: 194, by permission of the publishers)

	Major surgery	Trauma	Sepsis
Number of patients	8	10	8
Protein deficit (%)	24	8	+12
Energy intake (kcal)	—*	1691 ± 141†	2750 ± 150†
Protein intake (g)	—*	88 ± 13†	127 ± 16†
Study interval (d)	14	10	10
Changes in body composition†			
Weight (kg)	−5.3 ± 0.9	−4.2 ± 1.2	−6.2 ± 2.9
Water (kg)	−3.8 ± 1.3	−3.3 ± 1.4	−6.8 ± 2.6
Protein (kg)	−0.6 ± 0.35	−1.1 ± 0.2	−1.5 ± 0.3
Fat (kg)	−0.7 ± 1.2	+0.2 ± 0.6	+2.2 ± 0.8

* Elective surgery patients received no specific postoperative nutritional support but were allowed oral feeding as soon as clinically appropriate.
† All values are mean ± s.e.m.

29% depleted of total body protein. There was a loss of 0.7 kg of fat in keeping with a postoperative caloric deficit met by oxidation of fat as well as protein. Weight losses were moderate, the average being 5.3 kg and were predominantly due to losses of body water. Thus, this small study of patients undergoing very major surgery would suggest that these sorts of patient are frequently moderately depleted of body protein preoperatively but even without nutritional support lose only approximately another 5% or 43 g/day of body protein in the first 2 weeks following surgery (see Ch. 2).

MAJOR TRAUMA

Most trauma patients are young, seriously injured and were previously, prior to injury, in excellent health. The patients who require TPN after trauma usually require prolonged intensive care.

We performed a study of the changes in body composition seen in these very severely injured patients and the results are shown in Table 19.1. These 10 patients were chosen for study on the basis that they were likely to require intensive care for more than 10 days after reaching haemodynamic stability. They were young (median age 23) and all had severe blunt injury (injury severity scores (Baker & O'Neill 1974) range 16–57, median 34). All were ventilator dependent throughout most of the 10-day study period and all survived to leave hospital. The first body composition study was made on post-injury day 6 and the second 10 days latter. TPN was given to 7 patients, 4 of whom received small amounts of additional enteral feeding via a nasogastric tube. The other 3 patients had enteral feeding alone. Mean daily nutritional intakes for the group were 1691 ± 141 non-protein kcal, and 88 ± 13 g protein. i.e. 29 non-protein kcal/kg/day and 1.4 g protein per kg per day.

As can be seen from Table 19.l, the patients were probably slightly protein depleted at the time of the first body composition study (about 8%) and lost a mean of 1.1 ± 0.2 kg of protein (or 11% of total body protein) to end up approximately 19% protein depleted by the time of the second assessment 10 days later. There was a small insignificant gain of fat for the group of patients. An estimate of the total daily energy expenditure over the 10-day period was made for each patient from the nutritional intakes and from the body composition data. The data suggest that total energy expenditure lay between 2286 and 2410 kcal, or approximately 39–41 kcal/kg/day. Table 19.1 also shows that most of the weight loss was due to loss of water (mean 3.3 ± 1.4 kg).

Thus our study suggests that patients with major trauma in intensive care are not depleted initially but despite adequate nutritional support lose a large amount of body protein (an average of 110 g/day) in the first 10 days after trauma.

SERIOUS SEPSIS

The other large group of patients in whom nutritional problems are seen are postoperative and have sepsis as a major contributing factor to their requirement for intensive care. They are usually old and some may have preexisting nutritional depletion as a result of cancer, recent major trauma, multiple operations or semistarvation. They have serious acute diseases such as faecal peritonitis, infarcted small bowel, toxic megacolon, pancreatic abscess and the like and they consume intensive care resources at a rate vastly disproportionate to their numbers.

We measured body composition in 8 postoperative patients in intensive care with serious sepsis before and after 10 days of TPN. The patients all had serious surgical sepsis complicated by both respiratory failure and the septic shock syndrome. They suffered from toxic megacolon with perforation (1), ischaemic colon with pancreatic fistula (1), perforated colon (3), small bowel ischaemia (1), pancreatic abscess (1), disruption of rectal anastomosis (1). Mean daily nutritional intakes for the patients as a group were 2750 ± 150 non-protein kcal, and 147 ± 16 g of protein (35 non-protein kcal and 1.8 g of protein/kg/per day). All patients had recovered from the septic shock syndrome but were still ventilator dependent and most were still receiving Inotrope infusions at the start of TPN. 6 patients survived and left hospital. Results are shown in

Table 19.1. These patients were as a group not depleted of total body protein at the time of their first body composition assessment, but lost a mean of 1.5 ± 0.3 kg of protein, or 12.2% of total body protein, over the 10-day period. There was a significant gain in energy stores (fat and glycogen) for the group of patients (mean gain 2.2 ± 0.8 kg). An estimate of the total daily energy expenditure over the 10-day period was made for each patient from the nutritional intakes and the body composition data and the best estimate total energy expenditure for the group was between 2027 and 3265 kcal or approximately 26–41 kcal/kg. The weight loss was predominantly due to loss of water, with several patients losing more than 10 kg of water.

Clearly, large losses of total body protein (about 150 g/day) still occurred in patients with sepsis in intensive care despite aggressive nutritional support sufficient to result in a gain in total body fat.

SECTION III
DOES NUTRITIONAL SUPPORT PRESERVE BODY PROTEIN IN SURGICAL INTENSIVE CARE PATIENTS?

In the face of the massive loss of body protein that has been demonstrated in spite of the aggressive use of TPN it might be asked if nutritional support in these patients is of any use at all. From detailed kinetic studies of the effects of TPN on critically ill patients we now know that net protein catabolism is more than halved by its use. Figure 19.3 summarises the studies of Shaw et al (1987) on the effects of TPN in severely septic patients and the studies of Shaw and Wolfe (1989) on the effects of TPN in severely traumatised patients. It can be seen that the use of TPN results in a significant increase

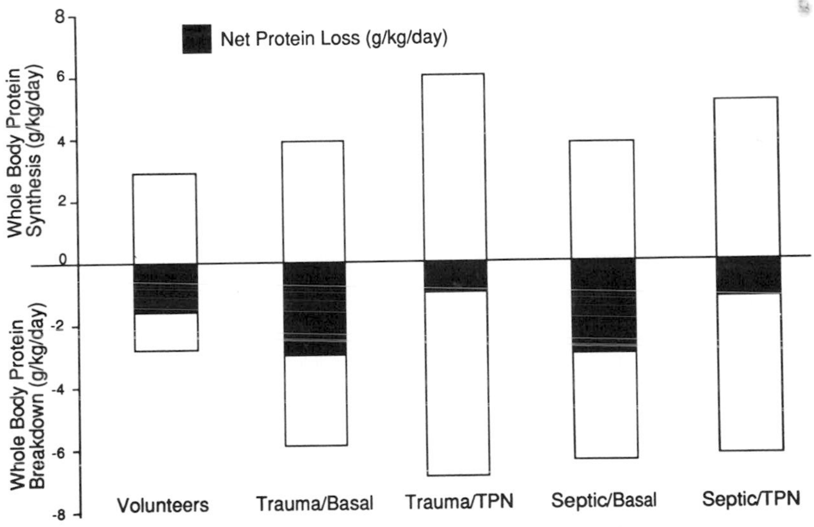

Fig. 19.3 The increase in net protein loss during trauma and sepsis results from an increase in protein breakdown not from a decrease in protein synthesis. Here the patients given TPN had an increase in synthesis of protein but there was no effect on protein catabolism. Nevertheless, the net result was a halving of the net loss of the protein from the body. A similar effect probably occurs after enteral feeding and it can be concluded that nutritional support in seriously ill surgical patients reduces protein loss from the body although it cannot be expected to eliminate the loss altogether. (Data from Shaw et al 1987, and Shaw & Wolfe 1989.)

in protein synthesis but does not affect protein catabolism. The net result is to halve the rate of net protein catabolism but not eliminate it.

SECTION IV
CLINICAL AND NUTRITIONAL MANAGEMENT OF CRITICALLY ILL SURGICAL PATIENTS

CONTROL OF SEPSIS

Drainage

The profound effect of cytokines produced from inflammatory cells within the infectious process makes it clear that the single most useful 'metabolic therapy' in patients in intensive care is the drainage of a septic focus when present. It is salutary to reflect that when sepsis develops late after trauma, with its catastrophic effect on metabolism, cardiopulmonary function and mortality, it is often as a result of early surgical failure to provide appropriate or adequate debridement, drainage or defunctioning. The majority of patients with abdominal sepsis do not develop abscesses if the initial surgery has been definitive. We have found, as have others that nosocomial pneumonia is a common cause of a persistent septic state in such patients and that in patients with persistent respiratory failure cultures obtained by fiberoptic bronchoscopy will often identify a responsible gram negative bacillus not found on conventional tracheal aspiration. Nevertheless as such organ failure is known also to be a marker of a remote septic focus (Bell et al 1983) an intraabdominal septic focus should always be suspected. Computerised tomographic scanning is of great clinical value in confirming the presence of an abscess which may be amenable to percutaneous drainage under CT or ultrasound control. Multiple or complex abscesses are better managed by surgical drainage. Failure to demonstrate a drainable collection by CT scan is usually very reassuring but occasionally can be misleading and repeat laparotomy may still be required. The disturbingly high early septic mortality from complex gastrointestinal fistulas (Ch. 15) and pancreatic abscesses (Ch. 20) may be reduced by the use of the 'open abdomen' with daily laparotomy, often in the intensive care unit until effective drainage has been established.

Immunotherapy

Apart from the early administration of appropriate antibiotics it is now apparent that another breakthrough in the management of Gram negative sepsis has become available. The successful production of a human monoclonal antibody that binds to the lipid-A domain of endotoxin has been shown to profoundly affect the outcome of critically ill patients with the sepsis syndrome (Fisher et al 1990, Khazaeli et al 1990, Ziegler et al 1991).

In more than 50% of patients the sepsis syndrome (Table 19.2) is caused by Gram negative bacteria and this is more likely to be so in critically ill septic surgical patients. It has been shown that it is highly cost effective to treat all surgical patients with the sepsis syndrome with a

Table 19.2 Definitions of sepsis syndrome and of septic shock*

Sepsis syndrome	Septic shock
Clinical evidence of infection Tachypnoea (>20 breaths per min, >10 l per min if mechanically ventilated) Tachycardia (>90 beats per min) Hyperthermia (>38.3°C) or hypothermia (<35.6°C) Evidence of inadequate organ perfusion including one or more of the following: Hypoxaemia (F_aO_2/F_IO_2 ≤280 without other pulmonary or cardiovascular disease as the cause) Elevated plasma lactate (above upper limits of normal for the testing laboratory) Oliguria (<0.5 ml/kg body weight for at least 1 h in patients with catheters)	Sepsis syndrome with hypotension (sustained decrease in systolic blood pressure <90 mm Hg, of drop >40 mm Hg, for at least 1 h, when volume replacement is adequate and the patient taking no antihypertensive medication, in the absence of other causes of shock such as hypovolaemia, myocardial function, and pulmonary embolism)

* Definition proposed by Bone 1991.

single dose of anti-endotoxin (HA-1A) as soon as possible after diagnosis (Smith, 1991).

GENERAL INTENSIVE CARE MANAGEMENT

It is obviously important that the critically ill patient receives a high standard of intensive care. All aspects of intensive care management including respiratory care, fluid and cardiovascular management, analgesia, nutritional support, microbiological surveillance and instrumentation are the combined responsibility of the surgeon and intensive care specialist. There are a number of aspects of management that have potentially relevant metabolic consequences and on which we place particular emphasis.

Respiratory management

Because of the risk of barotrauma (Kirby et al 1975) and possible unfavourable effects on salt and water metabolism (Kumar et al 1970) and intracranial pressure (Apuzzo et al 1977) we avoid high positive end expiratory pressure (PEEP) (>12–15 cm H_2O) unless indicated for severe frothing pulmonary oedema or for refractory hypoxaemia despite F_1O_2 >0.8.

Although the effects of curarisation (denervation) itself on muscle loss are unknown, we believe that they are more likely to be harmful. Therefore, we do not routinely use curarisation in the management of the ventilated patient except for patients with severe head injury in whom curarisation itself can lower intracranial pressure and ameliorate rises in intracranial pressure consequent on coughing during tracheal suctioning or against the ventilator. In all other patients, relaxants are given for facilitation of intermittent positive pressure ventilation (IPPV) only if respiratory failure is severe (e.g. $F_1O_2 > 0.6$, PEEP > 10 cm H_2O) or to facilitate cooling in hyperpyrexia.

Because of possible favourable effects on salt and water metabolism and respiratory muscle function that may result from early use of intermittent mandatory ventilation (IMV) (Downs & Douglas 1982), we predominantly use this mode of ventilation, often in association with continuous positive airway pressure (CPAP) and thoracic epidural anaesthesia.

Cardiovascular management

We believe that the prevention of renal failure is of paramount importance in the survival of the critically ill patient in surgical intensive care and we are relatively less concerned by the appearance of peripheral oedema, which can sometimes be massive, during resuscitation from shock when guided by appropriate haemodynamic monitoring. We frequently use dopamine in low doses (2–5 μg/kg/min) in such patients. When further inotropic support is required, we increase dopamine to 10 μg/kg/min before adding epinephrine. Because of the unfavourable metabolic effects of this drug, it is weaned off as soon as possible. Removal of excess salt and water after resuscitation is complete being accomplished by sodium restriction and judicious albumin infusion.

Prevention of opportunistic sepsis

Continued microbiological surveillance, especially of the respiratory tract, minimal use of invasive monitoring, and restrictions on the use of antibiotics to those for which there is a defined indication are all important in this regard.

Nutritional support and energy requirements

Energy requirements in critically ill ventilated patients are notoriously difficult to measure for technical reasons (Browning et al 1982, Ultman & Bursztein 1981). There may be wide variations in energy expenditure in an individual from day to day and at different times of the day (Carlsson et al 1984) and the relationship between measured energy expenditure and that predicted on the basis of standard predictor equations is so variable (Bartlett et al 1982) as to make such equations almost useless as a guide to the energy requirements of the individual patient. Nevertheless, although resting energy expenditure is increased in critical illness it is probably not as high as was previously thought and by virtue of the reduction in that component of total energy expenditure due to muscular work total energy expenditure in critically ill patients is not greatly increased from normal — 35 kcal/kg body weight/day is likely to be a somewhat generous allowance. Body weight is of course a rather crude index of metabolic size particularly in those patients who have large changes in body water as shown above and there will be few patients who will require more than about 2500 non-protein kcal/day.

It is difficult to meet energy needs in these patients with glucose alone (Nanni et al 1984) without pharmacologic doses of insulin and close monitoring. Although insulin promotes clearance of glucose from plasma, it does not increase glucose oxidation (Wolfe et al 1979). Hypoglycaemia, fatty liver and increased heat production are likely to result. We have found even in the most seriously ill patients that equicaloric mixtures of glucose and fat can be given simply and safely and that lipaemia and hyperglycaemia do not occur. Using this system, insulin is often not required and is not routinely given. When needed, for hyperglycaemia, moderate doses (40–60 units per day) will suffice. Although there are some who suggest that lipid infusions can result in reticuloendothelial cell and hepatocyte lipid uptake and prostaglandin mediated hypoxaemia (Cerra 1990), in clinical practice this must be very rare indeed. We give 50% of the non-protein energy as continuous fat infusion, mixed with glucose, amino acids, vitamins, trace elements, electrolytes and certain drugs, in large plastic bags. Though as a matter of principle we avoid adding drugs to the TPN solution when there is a reasonable alternative, we have added safely dopamine, dobutamine, epinephrine, cimetidine, ranitidine, pirenzepine, insulin, hydrocortisone and dexamethasone. A number of specific incompatibilities have been identified by our pharmacists as resulting either in 'cracking' of the lipid emulsion or an activation of drug additives and these are listed in Table 19.3.

Many other potential or theoretical incompatibilities can be avoided by the correct sequence of dilution and addition of the components to the TPN bag. Amino acid solutions together with some additives are added first, followed by dextrose solution, water and other additives and, finally, fat emulsion. No additives are ever added directly to fat emulsions.

Table 19.3 Specific incompatibilities in TPN mixtures containing fat, glucose, and amino acids (from Streat S J, Hill G L 1987 World J Surg 11: 194 by permission of the publishers)

PVC bags cause leaching of plasticiser and cracking of fat emulsion
Total divalent cation concentration >4 mmol/L causes cracking of fat emulsion
Total monovalent cation concentration >150 mmol/L causes cracking of fat emulsion
Low amino acid doses can cause cracking since cracking is pH dependent
Bacterial filters cannot be used since fat droplets are larger than filter pore sizes
Dopamine and albumin together cause a purple Biuret reaction
Epinephrine is converted to pink, inactive, adrenochrome by trace elements and zinc

Protein requirements

In addition to the considerations discussed above pertaining to protein loss from catabolism and starvation critically ill patients frequently lose protein from wounds, drains, and via the arterial lines. For these reasons, when giving TPN we use high protein intake at least 2 g protein/kg body weight. We have shown that critically ill ventilated patients have insensible water losses of about 1200 ml per day and relatively large volumes of free water (3–5 L per day) may be required to prevent azotaemia during TPN when such high protein intakes are given. It may be difficult to provide these protein intakes, for high intake of free water is contraindicated by brain injury or renal impairment. Although careful fluid management has resulted in our ability to give these intakes to the great majority of patients, substantial protein loss still occurs.

Enteral feeding

Because enteral feeding is much cheaper and simpler to administer in the critically ill patient than TPN it is always preferred if the gut is available for use. Enteral feeding is, however, not without the risk of pulmonary aspiration in critically ill patients unless the airways are protected by a cuffed endotracheal tube, and diarrhoea may also limit its use. Nevertheless, enteral feeding is a much underused treatment for supplying nutrition to critically ill patients. With a feeding tube placed distal to the pylorus at surgery, under fluoroscopy or by endoscopy, aspiration is rare and absorption occurs even in the presence of a mild ileus. In addition to avoiding the complications of TPN, enteral nutrition increases blood flow to the gut and this together with the provision of nutrition to the enterocyte preserves gut barrier function. Enteral nutrition, compared to parenteral nutrition reduces septic morbidity (Moore et al 1989). Patients with combined gastrointestinal losses of more than 1 L cannot be safely fed by the enteral route. Total gastrointestinal output 1 L/day is a much better indicator of the likelihood that enteral feeding could be tolerated than the passage of flatus. A balanced enteral diet which is isotonic is started at 30 ml/h by continuous infusion. If the tube is in the jejunum, half strength formula is better tolerated and full strength is only given when the full intended volume is being administered. After 24 hours, feeding tolerance and the presence or absence of aspiration is assessed. If all is well the rate of infusion is increased by 10 ml per hour every 6 hours as tolerated until the required protein and energy is being given. The details of enteral feeding are fully discussed in Chapter 9. In critically ill patients some advocate diets enriched with branched-chain amino acids (for stress) or branched-chain amino acids with decreased aromatic amino acids (hepatic failure) or renal diets with only essential amino acids. Enteral diets with an increased ratio of fat to carbohydrate may be useful in a ventilator dependent patient and may aid weaning (see Ch. 6). Tissue specific diets (see Ch. 6) enriched with arginine, branched-chain amino acids, N-3 fatty acids and RNA may prove to have a special role in intensive care patients (Peck et al 1991).

Vascular access for TPN

It is extremely difficult to care properly for a central venous line in the neck of a patient in intensive care and such sites are easily contaminated from the adjacent tracheostomy site, which is often a source of Gram negative bacteria. For this reason, an infraclavicular subclavian approach without tunnelling (in the vast majority of patients) or an internal jugular line which has been tunnelled subcutaneously to exit below the clavicle (in patients in whom there is a high risk of pneumothorax during line insertion) is preferable. In ventilated patients, a temporary increase in inspired oxygen to 100% together with removal of PEEP is used to minimise the risk of pneumothorax during line insertion. This complication should have an incidence of less than 3% but can be fatal in a ventilated patient with poor lung function. A strict protocol prohibiting the use of the central line for anything but TPN together with a careful dressing technique which prevents contamination of either the skin entry site or the junction of the line to the giving set will keep catheter sepsis to a rarity. We do not use multiple lumen central venous catheters for TPN since their relative safety over single lumen catheters in this situation is not yet established (see Ch. 10). We have demonstrated that the use of such a protocol in patients in surgical wards is associated with an incidence of catheter sepsis of 2.3 episodes per 1000 patient-days (Pettigrew et al 1985). In 20 patients in intensive care with serious sepsis who had a least 10 days of TPN there were no instances of catheter sepsis and no catheter required to be changed. We do not recommend changing these lines 'as a routine'.

SECTION V
NUTRITIONAL PHARMACOLOGY AND SURGICAL INTENSIVE CARE

Recently there have been exciting new developments in the area of feeding seriously ill patients which arise from new understandings of the interorgan exchanges in the hyperdynamic state and a realisation that enteral feeding prevents the translocation of bacteria. There is now a better understanding of energy and protein requirements in these patients and there are growing

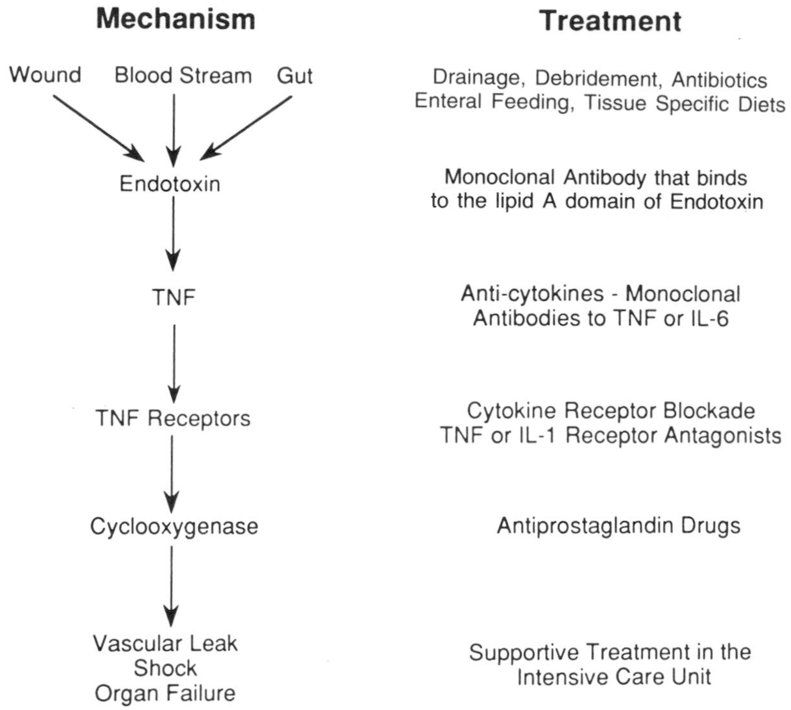

Fig. 19.4 Present and emerging strategies for the treatment of the sepsis syndrome.

insights into specific nutrients which have modulating effects on immune function (Park et al 1991), gut function (Darmaun et al 1991), respiratory function and possibly hepatic and renal function (see Ch. 6). A number of reviews of these important growth areas are available, e.g. Alexander & Fischer (1990).

SECTION VI
EMERGING STRATEGIES FOR MODIFYING THE PATIENT'S RESPONSE TO CRITICAL ILLNESS

From the discussion above it is reasonable to conclude that a sequence of events in which the inflammatory mediators of the septic response are generated may be: translocation of bacteria and endotoxin from the gut → endotoxaemia → TNF release → cyclooxygenase activation → host responses. Developments in nutritional pharmacology and immunotherapy have led to the possibility of blockade of each of these steps (Figure 19.4; see also Dunn 1988, Sagawa et al 1990, Salles et al 1989, Shimamoto et al 1988, Exley et al 1990, Ohlsson et al 1990, Hack et al 1990, Espevik et al 1990, Larrick & Bourla 1986, Wilmore 1991).

Acknowledgements

We are indebted to the World Journal of Surgery for permission to reproduce here some of the material which was contained in our paper, World Journal of Surgery (1987) 11: 194–201.

20. Pancreatitis

INTRODUCTION

Acute pancreatitis represents a wide spectrum of inflammation of the pancreas, ranging from generalised *oedema* with minimal systemic disturbance through *partial necrosis* to acute necrotising or *haemorrhagic pancreatitis* associated with multiple organ failure and a high mortality. The disease may also lead to major complications including *pseudocyst, abscess* and *fistulas* which are complex and dangerous conditions. Although the oedematous form of the disease may present as an acute and devastating illness, it usually follows a benign course with the patient out of hospital within a week or so and returning to normal life in 2 or 3 weeks. The management of such patients is conservative and designed to support the circulation during the acute illness until the patient is able to take oral fluids and food again. Patients with partial necrosis usually have a more prolonged clinical course and often require both metabolic and nutritional care for prolonged periods during which they are unable to take oral liquids or food. Patients with necrotising or haemorrhagic pancreatitis together with those who develop major septic complications, may suffer a catastrophic form of illness which requires intensive care, sometimes heroic surgery, and prolonged periods of metabolic and nutritional support.

SECTION I
PATHOPHYSIOLOGY AND SEVERITY

PATHOPHYSIOLOGY

Pancreatitis is due to enzymatic digestion of the gland and this digestion may extend into the periglandular tissues resulting in destruction not only of the gland but also of the surrounding fat planes and in very severe cases much of the retroperitoneum. In mild disease there is a swollen *oedematous* gland which may have small areas of patchy necrosis but in severe cases the whole of the gland may appear to be destroyed resulting in *haemorrhagic necrosis* not only in the region of the gland but also through the retroperitoneum; the enzyme rich haemorrhagic mass may even excavate widely as far as the upper thigh. Foul smelling infected chunks of grey necrotic pancreas and necrotic fat can be found within the haemorrhagic material. A *pseudocyst* in the plane between the pancreas and back wall of the stomach may develop in the second or third week and may grow to become quite large and threaten rupture. The cyst fluid, which may become infected, is rich in pancreatic enzymes. The necrotic material may coalesce, become infected and form an *abscess.* This is one of the most dangerous conditions in surgery which affects the patient not only from the systemic effects of sepsis, but by the propensity of the abscess to erode into major blood vessels with exsanguinating haemorrhage as a consequence.

From a metabolic point of view the most important consequences of acute severe pancreatitis are those that occur distant from the gland. The vasoactive peptides and cytokines released from the inflamed septic mass may cause profound metabolic derangements leading to multiorgan failure; principally respiratory insufficiency, myocardial depression, renal failure and gastric stress ulceration. There is loss of plasma and extracellular fluid locally around the gland as well as generally from the leaky capillary syndrome. Marked fluid and electrolyte shifts, acid base imbalance, decreased myocardial contractility, impaired liver and renal function, hypoxaemia, disseminated intravascular coagulation and alterations in calcium metabolism all occur in severe pancreatitis.

SEVERITY

Early identification of the patients who have severe disease or who are at greatest risk of developing complications allows them to be monitored and treated intensively even though, initially, they may not have seemed particularly ill. A number of grading systems have been used but the most effective are either based on the local anatomical pathology as revealed in a CT scan (Ranson et al 1985) or based on the disturbed metabolism that occurs as a consequence of the release of cytokines. The most popular scoring system for the severity of pancreatitis is Ranson's 'metabolic score' (Ranson et al 1974, Ranson & Pasternack 1977; see Table 20.1).

Table 20.1 Ranson's scoring system for the severity of pancreatitis. Morbidity and mortality rates correlate with the total number of criteria present, that is 0–2 criteria — 2% mortality rate, 3–4 criteria — 15% mortality rate, 5–6 criteria — 40% mortality rate, 7–8 criteria — 100% mortality rate.

Criteria at presentation
Age > 55 yr
White cell count > 16 000/μl
Blood glucose > 200 mg/dl (>10 mmol/L)
Serum LDH > 350 iu/L
SGOT > 250 iu/dl
Criteria developing during the first 48 hours
Haematocrit fall > 10%
Serum calcium < 8 mg/dl (<2.0 mmol/L)
Blood urea rise > 8 g/dl (>2.9 mmol/L)
Arterial oxygen < 60 mmHg
Base deficit < 4 mEq/L
Fluid sequestration > 600 ml

OVERALL CLINICAL PICTURE

The clinical picture may best be summarised by referring to the study of Sitzmann and his colleagues (1989). They found that in a prospective study of 327 patients admitted to the Johns Hopkins Hospital with a diagnosis of acute pancreatitis 73 (22%) had severe pancreatitis and required total parenteral nutrition. The characteristics of this group of 73 patients, which are described in Table 20.2, are presented to highlight the clinical features of those patients with pancreatitis who require intensive metabolic and nutritional care.

SECTION II
SUBSTRATE METABOLISM IN ACUTE PANCREATITIS

Shaw & Wolfe (1986) have described glucose, fatty acid and urea kinetics in patients with severe pancreatitis. They showed that these patients were metabolically similar to septic patients in that they proved to have markedly elevated rates of net protein breakdown which disappointingly were only minimally reduced by glucose infusion or total parenteral nutrition. When volunteers were infused with glucose, endogenous glucose production fell 94%; when the patients with severe pancreatitis were infused with glucose, endogenous glucose production fell only 45%. The effect of glucose infusion on the rate of protein breakdown was similar but considerably smaller. Shaw & Wolfe also demonstrated the reliance of the inflamed pancreatic mass on glucose as a fuel

Table 20.2 Clinical features of 73 patients with severe acute pancreatitis (data from Sitzmann et al 1989)

Age	45 ± 1.9 years (s.e.m.)
Aetiology	Alcohol 41, biliary tract 15
Ranson score	2.5 ± 0.12, >50% had a Ranson score of 3 or more
Mortality	11%
Number of days on TPN	29 days, range 7–123 days
Surgery required	cholecystectomy 6, abscess drainage 20, necrosectomy 5

for there was an enhanced rate of glucose clearance in the patients they studied. As time went on, the patients who received TPN utilised proportionately more glucose although, throughout, they relied heavily on fat as an energy source.

These kinetic data show that patients with severe pancreatitis are metabolically similar to septic patients and it can be assumed that the interorgan exchange of substrates as detailed in the previous chapter is similar as well. Roth et al (1985) have shown profound intracellular glutamine depletion in patients with acute pancreatitis and others have shown increased levels of branched-chain amino acids in muscle (Holbling et al 1982). Clinically patients with severe pancreatitis are hypermetabolic in the same way as patients with serious sepsis or major injury and they suffer from a rapid loss of body weight which is as profound as any in surgery (Blackburn et al 1976). It is now becoming clear that during the first week after the onset of severe disease endotoxaemia and high circulating levels of tumour necrosis factor and other cytokines may be detected.

SECTION III
PROTEIN ENERGY MALNUTRITION (PEM) IN ACUTE PANCREATITIS

PEM AND DISEASE SEVERITY

We have seen already the devastating effect of the disease on substrate metabolism which quantitatively and qualitatively is comparable to that seen in other critical surgical illness. In mild disease there is little metabolic upset and the inability to take food lasts only 3 or 4 days. In more severe disease where metabolism is more deranged there is also a prolonged period where the patient is unable to take food. It usually lasts 4 weeks or so but if complications develop it may last for 17 weeks or longer (see Table 20.2). Although there is little change in body composition in patients with mild disease, the catastrophic effects of severe pancreatitis lead quickly to protein energy malnutrition of the adult kwashiorkor type. There is rapid dissolution of body protein stores and an expanding extracellular fluid with profound falls in plasma albumin; up to 2% of body protein may be lost per day in patients with severe pancreatitis. Table 20.3 shows the effect on body composition and physiological function in 5 patients we measured at the end of a 5-day period after the onset of an acute attack of severe pancreatitis. These patients were previously well. From the table can be seen the expansion of body water, the erosion of body fat and the lysis of body protein that has occurred over the 5-day period in these hypermetabolic patients (RME raised 36%). They also have sustained profound falls in plasma albumin levels and in levels of

Table 20.3 Objective nutritional assessment of 5 patients with severe pancreatitis who had been quite well until 5 days before. None of these patients had received nutritional support prior to this study. The large expansion of body water associated with the resuscitation fluids can be seen (10 L) together with the loss of fat and particularly protein (700 g). Physiological function had deteriorated markedly during the short period since the onset of the illness in this group of hypermetabolic patients.

	Estimated value when well	Measured value	% change
Body composition			
Body weight (kg)	70.3	80.3	+14.3
Total body fat (kg)	29.9	28.7	–4.0
Total body protein (kg)	9.3	8.6	–7.5
Total body water (L)	29.8	39.2	+31.6
TBW/FFM	0.74	0.76	+2.7
Plasma proteins			
Albumin (g/L)	42.0	30.9	–26.4
Transferrin (mg/dl)	260	186	–28.5
Prealbumin (mg/dl)	24.0	14.2	–40.8
Physiological function			
Grip strength (kg)	37.0	31.5	–16.4
Respiratory muscle strength (cm H_2O)	114.0	48.6	–57.4
Forced expiratory volume$_1$ (L)	2.04	1.55	–23.9
Vital capacity (L)	2.85	2.30	–19.4
Peak expiratory flow rate (L/min)	520	400	–21.7
Metabolic expenditure			
Resting metabolic expenditure (kcal/24 h)	1099	1497	+36
Activity energy expenditure (kcal/24 h)	1000	50	–95
Total energy expenditure (kcal/24 h)	2099	1547	–26
Stress index	1.0	1.36	+36

plasma proteins. Marked deficits of physiological function are present.

PEM — THE EFFECTS OF NUTRITIONAL SUPPORT

Mild disease

Although protein losses similar to those seen after elective surgery occur in patients with mild pancreatitis, the early administration of TPN has no effect on outcome provided the period of starvation is not excessive (>7 days) or the patients were not previously malnourished (Sax et al 1987).

Moderate to severe disease

Although about one third of patients with severe disease develop a devastating illness complicated by serious sepsis and organ failures which require intensive care, two thirds have a more straightforward course even though there is invariably a long period where oral intake is not possible. Table 20.4 describes sequential nutritional assessments of such a patient who required 3 weeks of TPN before she settled and was able to take oral intake again. It shows how nutritional state can be preserved in patients with severe but uncomplicated pancreatitis. Over this 3-week period this woman suffered from continuing acute inflammation with hyperamylasaemia but she developed neither organ failure nor a septic complication. It can be seen that total body protein stores were preserved during the 3 weeks of TPN with a small gain of body fat and preservation of body weight. Physiological function tests showed an improvement over the first week which was maintained thereafter.

Table 20.4 Serial measurements of nutritional state on a 48-year-old female with acute pancreatitis (Ranson score 3). The first measurement was made 3 days after the onset of the disease. After 3 weeks of TPN she was able to take an oral diet without hyperamylasaemia or abdominal pain.

	Day 0	Day 7	Day 14	Day 21
Body composition				
Body weight (kg)	63.2	64.5	65.3	65.5
Total body fat (kg)	23.6	23.9	24.4	24.5
Total body protein (kg)	7.8	7.6	7.6	7.5
Total body water (L)	28.7	29.8	30.2	30.3
TBW/FFM	0.73	0.73	0.74	0.74
Physiological function				
Grip strength (kg)	17	21	17	—
Respiratory muscle strength (cm H_2O)	15.0	23.1	42.2	—
Forced expiratory volume$_1$ (L)	0.90	1.40	1.56	—
Vital capacity (L)	1.50	1.85	1.80	—
Peak expiratory flow rate (L/min)	120	320	360	—
Metabolic expenditure				
Resting metabolic expenditure (kcal/24 h)	1324	1681	1654	1585
Stress index	1.22	1.53	1.50	1.43

Severe pancreatitis

Table 20.5 shows the very different situation that developed in a patient with acute necrotising pancreatitis who eventually died. It can be seen that at the time of the first measurement, 5 days after admission, when haemodynamic stability had been reached, he already was severely protein depleted and overhydrated with an extracellular water expansion of 14.2 L. Over the next 10 days, in spite of TPN (3134 kcal of non-protein energy and 121 g protein per day), he continued to lose massive amounts of protein, even though energy intake was excessive (he gained 4 kg of fat/glycogen). This inability to preserve body protein stores in spite of high intakes of energy and protein could have been predicted from the kinetic studies described above. Patients with necrotising or haemorrhagic pancreatitis or those suffering from septic complications continue to lose 1–2% of their body protein stores each day until the inflammatory mass is brought under control.

To summarise, nutritional support has no place in mild disease; it can be expected to preserve nutritional state in uncomplicated severe disease but in complicated severe disease body protein continues to be lost at a high rate. As we saw in Chapter 6, however, the rate of protein loss is considerably less than if no nutritional support had been given at all.

Table 20.5 Changes in body composition in a 66-year-old male with haemorrhagic pancreatitis. After haemodynamic stability was reached on the 5th post-admission day he was commenced on a 10-day course of TPN. This patient later developed renal failure and died.

	Estimated value when well	5 days after admission	After 10 days TPN
Body composition			
Body weight (kg)	103.2	117.2	122.1
Total body fat (kg)	17.8	16.8	20.8
Total body protein (kg)	19.2	18.2	16.1
Total body water (L)	62.3	76.5	79.5
TBW:FFM	0.73	0.76	0.79
Metabolic expenditure			
Resting energy expenditure (kcal/24 h)	1711	—	2423
Activity energy expenditure (kcal/24 h)	1000	—	—
Total energy expenditure (kcal/24 h)	2711	—	2423
Stress index	1.0	—	1.44

SECTION IV
NUTRITIONAL SUPPORT

Nutritional support in acute pancreatitis is indicated for severe disease, for the complications of the disease, and particularly after surgery. We have seen already that there is no indication for nutritional support in mild disease (Sax et al 1987). However, in view of the rapidly developing malnutrition that occurs in patients with severe pancreatitis we advise that patients with severe disease should commence nutritional support as soon as they are haemodynamically stable. Apart from limiting protein loss and providing nutrition in a situation where it is impossible to take food orally it is generally accepted that one of the purposes of feeding these patients is to rest the pancreas by minimising the stimulation of exocrine and endocrine function. While it is clear that nutritional support cannot inhibit pancreatic secretion altogether enteral nutrition and, to a greater extent, TPN can have a beneficial effect (McMahon 1988).

ENTERAL FEEDING IN PANCREATITIS

Oral food, or oral enteral diets stimulate pancreatic secretion more than if they are given intraduodenally. Stabile et al (1984) showed that an elemental diet infused directly into the upper jejunum stimulated the gland less than a full liquid diet, particularly with respect to protein output. It is clear, however, that infusion of any nutrients into the gastrointestinal tract always induces some degree of pancreatic exocrine secretion. It is reassuring though that an elemental diet or even a balanced enteral diet infused at a neutral pH into the upper jejunum of patients with severe pancreatitis does not appear to aggravate the pancreatitis (Kudsk et al 1990).

TPN IN PANCREATITIS

There is little doubt that TPN has less stimulating effect on the pancreas than any type of enteral diet or any form of enteral feeding (Stabile et al 1984). Experimental data concerning the effects of TPN on pancreatic secretion are not always easy to interpret although 'there is sufficient agreement to conclude that TPN is the optimal nutritional technique to support patients in whom the avoidance of pancreatic secretion is considered to be important' (McMahon 1988). There is more controversy over the effect of intravenous fat in patients with pancreatitis although this is probably not clinically important, for the large clinical study of Sitzmann et al (1989) showed that lipid based TPN is a safe and effective therapy in acute pancreatitis. These workers also showed that lipid does not cause hypertriglyceridaemia nor does it aggravate the pancreatitis. The administration of lipid to these patients may actually make management easier by lowering insulin requirements and providing a more stable metabolic situation (Grant et al 1984).

ENERGY AND PROTEIN REQUIREMENTS

Our studies suggest that energy requirements are raised 30–50% in patients with severe pancreatitis. An estimated RME × 1.5 will therefore provide adequate energy which is administered in the form of glucose and lipid — 50:50. Protein requirements in patients with acute pancreatitis have not been studied directly but 1.5 g protein/kg/day is likely to be sufficient and more than this is unlikely to be utilised (Shaw et al 1987).

SECTION V
EARLY MANAGEMENT

MILD DISEASE

The goal of treatment for mild disease is to minimise pancreatic stimulation, replace sequestered fluid, correct any electrolyte abnormalities that occur, and provide adequate pain relief until spontaneous resolution occurs. To these ends, oral intake is withheld and a nasogastric tube is inserted to aspirate gastric secretion to avoid acidification of the duodenum. For the majority of patients improvement is rapid and the nasogastric tube and urethral catheter may be removed in 24 hours. Oral feeding is resumed, usually after 3 or 4 days when serum amylase levels have dropped to normal and the patient is free of pain and feeling hungry. In mild disease less than a litre of fluid is sequestered and once this is replaced with 0.9% saline maintenance fluids are all that are required. The response to fluid replacement is assessed initially in terms of peripheral perfusion, pulse rate and blood pressure, but most of all by monitoring the volume and the specific gravity of urine. Hypocalcaemia does not usually occur in mild disease and parenteral supplementation is not usually necessary.

MODERATE TO SEVERE DISEASE

When initial assessment suggests the patient is suffering from moderate or severe pancreatitis then intensive physiological support in order to prevent organ system dysfunction is required. The surgeon must focus on the following points.

The acute shock phase

Large amounts of extracellular fluid may be lost locally in the retroperitoneum, forward into the peritoneum and throughout the body from widespread leaky capillaries. In the most severely ill patients up to 8 L of 0.9% NaCl may be necessary within the first 24 hours after admission (Imrie & Shearer 1986). The response to the crystalloid is monitored in terms of the peripheral circulation, pulse, blood pressure and urine output. Urine output should be maintained above 30 ml/h. We prefer 0.9% NaCl rather than Ringer's lactate in pancreatitis because of the tendency toward alkalosis in these patients. Hypoxaemia is an important and common problem in severe pancreatitis. The degree of respiratory insufficiency is not always apparent clinically and is not necessarily related to the severity of the disease. Arterial blood gases should be measured for the first few hospital days and supplemental oxygen is administered if blood gases reveal Po_2 levels below 70 mmHg. Correction of hypoxia is particularly important and close attention to this has shown reduced mortality especially in elderly patients (Imrie & Blumgart 1975). A few patients with haemorrhagic pancreatitis require red cells. Packed red cells are infused in sufficient quantities to keep the haematocrit above 30.

These very sick patients need to be monitored carefully to determine whether the trend is towards further deterioration. Blood gases are measured every 12 hours and serum creatinine measurement, liver function tests and a full blood count (including platelets) are carried out daily. Rapid deterioration in organ function requires admission to the intensive care unit for closer monitoring and physiological support. This may include mechanical ventilation, inotropes and antibiotics.

Specific biochemical problems

Hypoalbuminaemia. There is a general extravasation of albumin from the vascular to the extravascular space because of widespread leaky capillaries. It probably is wasteful to administer albumin at this stage because of the continuing leak (see Ch. 21).

Calcium. Hypocalcaemia is quite common in acute pancreatitis and is important because of its prognostic significance. The majority of patients who are hypocalcaemic have low levels of total blood calcium because of hypoalbuminaemia (50% of circulatory calcium is bound to protein). The ionised calcium in most patients with acute pancreatitis is normal. In a few patients the ionised calcium is low and they require calcium gluconate infusions as replacement therapy (50–60 ml of isotonic calcium gluconate by slow I.V. infusion). Failure to treat low levels of ionised calcium may result in cardiac dysrhythmias and in some patients, particularly those with hypokalaemic alkalosis, tetany may occur. It has been shown that the plasma parathormone levels are high in most patients early in the course of acute pancreatitis and hence the ready tendency for ionised calcium levels to be restored spontaneously.

Magnesium. Hypomagnesaemia occurs occasionally in patients with pancreatitis. This aggravates the hypocalcaemic state and makes it more resistant to spontaneous recovery. Magnesium sulphate intravenously is given and usually both calcium and magnesium rapidly return to normal levels.

Hypokalaemic alkalosis. Acute pancreatitis accompanied by profuse vomiting of high acid gastric juice may occasionally result in hypokalaemic metabolic alkalosis. The judicious replacement of volume with 0.9% normal saline together with KCl solves this problem (see Ch. 12).

The inability to take oral nutrients

Most patients with severe pancreatitis and some with mild to moderate pancreatitis are unable to eat for a prolonged period. After haemodynamic stability has been restored and it is clear that the course will be prolonged then TPN is begun. This in practice means that on the third–fifth post admission day when it is clear that a mild uncomplicated course is not being followed TPN is started.

SECTION VI
LATER MANAGEMENT

Generally speaking the patient's illness may take one of three courses; there may be a prolonged period of ileus and obstruction, it may be complicated by a pseudocyst or an abscess, or there may be a continuing downhill course requiring admission to the critical care unit and possible urgent necrosectomy.

PROLONGED COURSE OF ILEUS AND OBSTRUCTION

Many patients with severe pancreatitis will slowly improve over several weeks following a course punctuated by setbacks and improvements before finally resolving and becoming completely free of symptoms. The swollen pancreatic mass subjected to repeated but decreasingly severe attacks of inflammation may cause mechanical obstruction of the duodenal loop and be associated with a prolonged ileus. The key to these patients is total gut rest and TPN, and after a period which may vary from 2 to 6 weeks they slowly and surely become free of pain and are able to eat again without difficulty. During this time it is possible not only to preserve nutritional status, but also to improve it somewhat (Table 20.2).

ILEUS AND OBSTRUCTION COMPLICATED BY PSEUDOCYST OR ABSCESS

A patient with severe pancreatitis may continue with epigastric pain, low grade fever and intermittent attacks of hyperamylasaemia. He/she may continue to have high gastric aspirates because of a swollen pancreas partially or completely blocking the duodenum. Extensive retroperitoneal excavation may aggravate the ileus. If a CT scan demonstrates a pseudocyst collecting in the lesser sac it should be aspirated under radiological control. The cyst may not reform after aspiration, but those that do may ultimately need surgical drainage. Open surgical drainage cannot be safely performed until the wall of the cyst has firmed sufficiently to allow it to be sutured to the back wall of the stomach. Thus, a period of 6 weeks or so during which TPN is required is embarked upon. Fortunately these patients are usually free of sepsis and are able to gain total body protein and see encouraging evidence of improvement in their overall state of fitness.

If, after 2 or 3 weeks a patient with severe pancreatitis begins to develop a fever, then a *pancreatic abscess* should be suspected. A contrast enhancing CT scan is the best technique for demonstrating an abscess, which if seen is aspirated to see if it contains bacteria (Crass et al 1985, Hiatt et al 1985). Only simple single abscesses should be dealt with by percutaneous drainage, the others need a direct surgical approach which requires exposure of the abscess, drainage and sump drainage. Throughout the illness and during the long recovery period that follows drainage the patient needs nutritional support and is often in intensive care. These patients may need frequent open drainage and packing of the abscess cavity (Hedderich et al 1986) which may be done in the critical care unit. After the packs have been removed and the sepsis has settled, leakage of pancreatic fluid from the base of the cavity often occurs. Such fistulas usually close by total gut rest, TPN and somatostatin (see Ch. 15). Patients with pancreatic abscess may prove to be among the most challenging patients to manage in the whole of general surgery. High standards of metabolic and nutritional care are required; mature judgement and courageous surgery are the components of care that are critical. Also critical is the ability to provide nutritional support with TPN; it is life saving and the key to survival of patients whose hospitalisation may run into weeks or months.

PATIENTS REQUIRING CRITICAL CARE

A small number, something less than 5% of all patients with acute pancreatitis suffer from a devastating form of necrotising or haemorrhagic pancreatitis in which multiorgan failure develops quickly. Serial monitoring of organ system function in the critical care unit is carried out to determine whether the downward trend is continuing. When it is clear that organ function is deteriorating, early surgery is required. Indications for early surgery are the need to increase FiO_2 and PEEP to keep oxygen saturation above 90%, a rising serum creatinine, deterioration of liver function tests and the need for inotropic support. If after 3 or 4 days these trends continue then laparotomy and excision of the necrotic pancreas is required (D'Egido & Schein 1991). Before that a CT scan is performed which outlines the degree of pancreatic necrosis and confirms the diagnosis. At surgery the lesser sac is opened widely and necrotic material is removed and the pancreatic bed is packed. On return to the critical care unit it is necessary to change the packs daily and debride further if that becomes necessary. These patients need the highest standards of critical care and nutritional support but even with these the mortality is above 50%.

Our own approach is to be fairly conservative at each attempt at necrostomy. Our principle is to remove all dead and devitalised tissue to eliminate the source of cytokines which are propagating the inflammatory response. It is, however, quite easy to be overeager to satisfy this fundamental principle of surgical metabolism and to find the fingers wandering on to normal pancreatic tissue which may bleed torrentially. With the highest standards of critical care and the ability to provide safe TPN one can afford to take the long view, removing only tissue which is clearly necrotic and is easily pinched from the rest of the gland. There comes a time, usually later rather than sooner, when the necrotic tissue is more clearly defined and it is then that it can be safely removed, often with dramatic and gratifying results.

THE ROLE OF PERITONEAL LAVAGE

With the knowledge that multiorgan failure occurring in association with severe pancreatitis is in large part secondary to mediators released from within the inflammatory mass it would seem reasonable to assume that benefit would be obtained by removing the peritoneal exudate by peritoneal lavage. Early uncontrolled studies of peritoneal lavage looked promising (Balldin & Ohlsson 1979, Ranson & Spencer 1978, Stone & Fabian 1980) but a more recent multicentre controlled study of 91 patients with severe pancreatitis produced no improvement in either the morbidity or mortality (Mayer et al 1985). It is a technique that should be abandoned.

THE ROLE OF IMMUNOTHERAPY WITH MONOCLONAL ANTIBODIES

The demonstration that many patients with severe pancreatitis have high levels of circulating endotoxin early on suggests that immunotherapy might have an important place in the management of these difficult patients. We suggest that patients with pancreatitis severe enough to require treatment in a critical care unit and who have the sepsis syndrome should receive a human monoclonal antibody that binds to lipid-A — the highly conserved lipid moiety that is responsible for the biological effects of endotoxin (Ziegler et al 1991). Other monoclonal antibodies that have been raised against tumour necrosis factor and other cytokines may in due course prove to be fundamental to the management of critically ill patients with pancreatitis.

21. Major trauma — metabolic and nutritional management of a patient with major trauma

Example

A previously fit 23-year-old man ran his car into a power pole. Help came quickly and he arrived in the hospital within 30 minutes of the crash. His airway was clear, respirations were shallow with a rate of 23 per minute, his face was ashen and he was white and cold peripherally with a pulse of 130 per minute and a blood pressure of 80/60. He was unconscious with a Glasgow coma score of 8. In each antecubital fossa 16 gauge i.v. catheters were inserted, blood was taken for complete blood count, amylase, electrolytes, blood group typing and cross match. 2 litres of lactated Ringer's solution were given as a bolus. After the administration of suxamethonium an endotracheal tube was passed and mechanical hyperventilation started with inspired oxygen concentration of 100%, tidal volume of 1000 ml and ventilatory rate of 12/min. On further examination he was found to have a distended abdomen and bruising over the left upper quadrant of the abdomen. The right thigh was tense from a femur fracture. A cross table lateral cervical spine X-ray and pelvic X-ray were normal as was the chest X-ray apart from fractures of the 9th, 10th and 11th ribs on the left side. After 15 minutes the patient, who was not haemodynamically stable, received a further litre of lactated Ringer's followed by 4 units of crossmatched packed red cells. During this time he underwent diagnostic peritoneal lavage which was strongly positive. He was therefore sent immediately to the operating room where emergency laparotomy was performed. The peritoneal cavity contained 4 L of blood and the spleen contained a deep laceration. Since it was amenable to salvage it was repaired. A small laceration in the left lobe of the liver was treated by compression. Finally a fine needle catheter jejunostomy feeding tube was placed in the upper jejunum. After the abdomen was closed he was sent immediately to the CT room for a brain scan which showed a haemorrhagic contusion of both frontal lobes but no surgical mass lesion. After a short period of stabilisation in the intensive care unit he returned to the operating room where the fractured femur was treated with open reduction and internal fixation. Throughout the operative procedures which took a total of 4 hours he remained haemodynamically stable. A total of 10 units of packed red cells, 1 L of fresh frozen plasma and 10 units of platelets in addition to 6 L of crystalloid had now been given.

The patient was taken to the intensive care unit and over the next 24 hours he received a further 4 L of crystalloid and 2 units of packed red cells to maintain stable blood pressure, keep urine above 0.5 ml/kg/hour, and the haematocrit around 30%. He continued to be mechanically hyperventilated with an FiO_2 of 0.5, PEEP of 5 cmH_2O, tidal volume of 1000 ml and a ventilatory rate of 10/min. He remained curarised and sedated with small doses of morphine and a benzodiazepine.

This unconscious patient was intubated to protect his airway from aspiration should it occur and to improve oxygenation. The use of mechanical ventilation with 100% oxygen ensured maximum saturation of his haemoglobin. Hyperventilation is valuable in patients such as this for it decreases arterial $P\text{CO}_2$ which in turn decreases cerebral blood flow through cerebrovascular autoregulation. By decreasing intracranial volume in this way intracranial pressure is reduced. An important point is that extracranial factors (e.g. alcohol, shock, hypoxia) are present in 50% of patients with traumatic coma although in this patient a bilateral cerebral contusion was also found.

He also illustrates the essentials of the initial treatment and fluid resuscitation of trauma (Trunkey 1991). Peripheral perfusion, heart rate and blood pressure are the keys to judging the degree of acute blood loss. The ashen grey skin of the face and the white skin of blood drained extremities implies at least loss of 30% of blood volume. When blood volume is reduced by half or more cerebral perfusion is critically impaired and unconsciousness results. For restitution of blood volume we prefer crystalloid solutions such as lactated Ringer's solution initially. This solution repletes the total extracellular compartment of the body and reduces blood viscosity by haemodilution resulting in better tissue perfusion. Of the different isotonic crystalloid solutions any solution with an electrolyte composition similar to that of plasma is suitable. Such solutions are Plasmalyte, Ringer's lactate (Hartmann's solution) and 0.9% saline (see Table 4.6).

There is a limit for the administration of crystalloid above which blood or packed red cells should be used — this limit of crystalloid infusion is around 3 L or 50 ml/kg. Uncrossmatched type specific red cells are safe for emergency volume resuscitation. Blood type can be determined in 20 minutes but crossmatch takes twice as long. If type specific blood is not available reconstituted O-negative packed red blood cells should be used. O-positive cells may be used although the patient will become sensitised to the Rh factor, but this is important only in females of childbearing age. There are red blood cell substitutes such as the perfluorocarbon fluosol-DA, stroma free haemoglobin and encapsulated haemoglobin but these are neither clinically available nor have they yet been shown to be better than Ringer's lactate solution in the clinical setting.

The response to the volume infusion is assessed initially in terms of peripheral perfusion, pulse rate and blood pressure. Soon after the initial period of resuscitation blood pressure rises above normal values. At this time the judicious administration of small amounts of intravenous morphine opens up the peripheral circulation. There is often a short period of 8–12 hours of polyuria which is caused by a combination of factors including alcohol, renal tubular dysfunction from pretreatment circulatory shock and perhaps also a degree of hypertension associated with endogenous catecholamine production. Once this initial diuresis has settled, after 12 hours or so, urine output which should be kept at greater than 0.5 ml/kg/h is used to gauge additional requirements. Serial haematocrits give guidance about red cell requirements. There is no optimal haematocrit which should always be aimed for. Young, previously fit, patients can usually be safely maintained with haematocrits around 25%–30%. If the heart is normal compensation for a low haematocrit occurs by a rise in cardiac output providing vascular volume is properly replaced. Patients with diseased coronary arteries should have red cells sufficient to bring haematocrit up to 35%.

This patient's requirement of 10 units of red cells implies replacement of the entire blood volume and clearly other blood components were required. Fresh frozen plasma to replace clotting factors and platelet infusions were used here.

The reason for abdominal surgery was to investigate the haemoperitoneum and control bleeding from the spleen. Haemodynamic stability was maintained through the time of surgery and over the subsequent 24 hours but it required a lot of fluid to do this. The fluid requirement was not just to replace the blood that was lost — say 4–5 L in the abdomen and 1–2 L in the thigh — for a total of more than 12 L of fluid were required to maintain blood pressure and urine output. This extra fluid had been lost into the interstitium and body cavities, the so-called 'third space', and the amounts lost in this way can be quite enormous — perhaps up to 10 L in patients such as this. The fluid is lost from the vascular space by virtue of increased capillary permeability locally at the sites of injury but also generally due to a body-wide tendency for capillaries to leak.

The increased capillary permeability that leads to generalised third space accumulation is caused by a large number of humoral mediators released from cells at sites of underperfusion and trauma. Histamine, serotonin, bradykinin, arachidonic acid metabolites and other cytokines are released from injured vascular endothelium, platelets and white cells at the site of injury and cause capillary permeability and loss from the circulation of massive amounts of fluid. In organs remote from the site of injury the effect of this is to cause organ failure.

Ventilatory support was continued postoperatively mainly to optimise the intracranial environment by increasing the P_{O_2} and S_{O_2} and decreasing the P_{CO_2}. Relaxation also prevents coughing and straining both of which increase intracranial pressure. It was the head injury too that suggested the high probability of a prolonged postoperative period without adequate nutrition and hence the use of the fine needle catheter jejunostomy.

By the next evening, 24 hours after injury, he was settled on the ventilator and was haemodynamically stable. Renal function was normal, urine output was 60 ml/h and plasma osmolality was 295 mosmol/L. No more red cells had been required and all resuscitation fluids had been stopped. His fluid intake was restricted to 10 ml/h of 5% dextrose in water. He was in a slightly negative ongoing water balance and the cumulative sodium balance was positive. On the morning of the third post-injury day he had direct measurements of body composition. The results were as follows:

Value	Estimated value when well	Measured
Body weight (kg)	63.0	67.1
Body fat (kg)	17.0	16.1
Fat free body mass (kg)	46.0	51.0
Total body water (L)	33.1	38.1
Total body protein (kg)	10.5	10.0
Hydration of fat free body (%)	72	75

In spite of losing 500 g of total body protein and 900 g of fat over the 3 days since injury there had been a large increase (4.1 kg) in body weight. This was due to a 5 L increase in total body water reflecting the persistence of an expanded extracellular water which had occurred as a result of the 'third space' effect described above. Clinically though, balance data showed that he was now in ongoing negative water and sodium balance and normalisation of body hydration could therefore be expected over the next week or two. These changes all indicate a decreasing stress response and a diminution of the circulatory levels of antidiuretic hormone and aldosterone — factors which show that the patient is not being subjected to further tissue destruction or continuing developing sepsis. *Diuresis of sodium is one of the best indications that the patient is on the right track towards recovery.*

The principles of fluid and electrolyte management during this period of diuresis is to provide no sodium and only sufficient water to keep plasma osmolality as near normal as possible. Here only 10 ml of 5% dextrose in water each hour was required.

On the third post-injury day, although still intubated he was now opening his eyes and responding to painful stimuli. Bowel sounds could be heard and although the abdomen was soft it was still distended. Nasogastric aspiration was 500 ml/day. Injection of a small amount of gastrografin down the jejunostomy tube showed no leak and passage of dye into and down the jejunum. Enteral feeding with an elemental diet enriched with branched-chain amino acids (Vivonex TEN) was commenced at half strength at 25 ml/hour for the first 6 hours. This caused no distention or reflux or discomfort and he was, within 36 hours, tolerating without difficulty full strength diet at 100 ml/hour. Over the next 4–5 days, abdominal distension disappeared and he was passing one loose stool each day. By this time he had been weaned from the ventilator and on day 7 he was transferred to the neurosurgical ward. By day 10 he was sitting up in a chair taking sips of fluid without difficulty. Improvement continued and on day 18 when he was eating 1000 kcal per day consistently over a 3-day period the enteral nutrition was stopped. 3 days later the jejunostomy catheter was withdrawn. After 10 days of jejunostomy feeding the body composition measurements were repeated. The results were as follows:

	Day 0 of jejunostomy feeding	Day 10 of jejunostomy feeding
Body weight (kg)	67.1	62.9
Body fat (kg)	16.1	15.9
Fat free mass (kg)	51.0	47.0
Total body water (L)	38.1	34.8
Total body protein (kg)	10.0	8.9
Hydration of fat free body (%)	75	74

Head injury patients who have had direct measurements of resting energy expenditure have been shown to have increased caloric requirements and accelerated protein breakdown (Moore et al 1989, Boop et al 1985). It is for these reasons that it made sense to provide nutritional support for the 2–3 weeks that it was estimated would elapse before a proper diet could be taken. The goal was to limit the loss of body protein and preserve gut function thereby shortening the ultimate period of rehabilitation. The nutritional/metabolic goal was to provide energy equivalent to his total energy requirements and enough protein to provide 1.5 g/kg/day; since resting energy expenditure was not measured directly his total energy requirements were calculated from the simple formula TEE = 40 kcal/kg body weight/day. Vivonex TEN containing 1 kcal/ml and 38.2 g protein per 1000 kcal was used. 2400 ml were received over the 24-hour period providing ~38 kcal/kg/day and almost 1.5 g protein/kg/day. Enteral feeding is to be preferred in these circumstances whenever possible. There was an opportunity to insert a jejunostomy at laparotomy although if there had been extensive mesenteric or retroperitoneal damage total parenteral nutrition would have been preferred because of the high possibility of prolonged ileus. Enteral feeding also ensures adequate blood flow to the gut preventing atrophy and preserving its barrier function, in this way limiting the translocation of bacteria and endotoxin across the enterocytes. A problem with jejunal feedings into a hypotonic gut may be inadequate mixing of nutrients with bile and pancreatic enzymes. Some think that this problem can be solved by the use of an elemental diet, such as Vivonex TEN. This enteral formula contains its protein in the form of free amino acids. It also is enriched, with 30% of its amino acids being branched-chain (leucine, isoleucine, valine). Although there are theoretical advantages in giving both free amino acids and also added branched-chain amino acids it has never been demonstrated that there is a clinical advantage for their use. Volume and osmolality of the nutrient solution may also prove to be a problem. Such a hypertonic diet was used here (Vivonex TEN contains 630 mosmol/kg water) and although it may be given at full strength many feel it is better tolerated if given according to the following schedule, as used here:

1. Half strength at 25 ml/hour for 6 hours
2. Increase as tolerated to $\frac{3}{4}$ strength at 25 ml/h for 6 hours
3. Increase as tolerated to full strength at 25 ml/h for 6 hours
4. Advance 10 ml/h each 6 hours as tolerated until goal of 100 ml/h is reached.

The body composition results show the hallmarks of recovering major injuries with resolving hypercatabolism.

Firstly, there had been a diuresis of 3.3 L of body water. The hydration of the fat free body had not yet normalised but improvement was noted — no doubt due to the mobilisation of 'third space fluid'.

Secondly, there was continuing protein loss with fat preservation, in spite of aggressive nutritional support. With 100 ml/h or 2400 kcal/day he was clearly in energy balance because of a small gain in total body fat. By calculating the total energy intake over the 10-day feeding period and the changes in protein and fat stores it can be calculated that his energy requirements over this period were somewhere between 36 and 38 kcal/kg/day. In spite of being in energy balance and receiving what most would accept as an adequate protein intake loss of body protein continued to occur. This continuing loss of body protein amounted to 1.1% of total stores of body protein per day. This illustrates the impossibility of preventing major losses of body protein let alone obtaining net protein anabolism in such patients. It should not be forgotten though that without nutritional support more than twice this amount of protein would have been lost.

The point when nutritional support should be stopped remains controversial. In postoperative patients an elemental diet administered through a jejunostomy does not impede the progress towards full voluntary food intake. For this reason it should be continued until at least 1000 kcal can be comfortably taken orally. In this patient after 18 days or so this amount was being consumed regularly and the jejunostomy feeding was stopped. Steady progress continued from that point until discharge from hospital.

22. Serious sepsis — metabolic and nutritional management of a patient with serious sepsis

Example

A 68-year-old man who, 6 years earlier, had had an abdomino-perineal excision of the rectum for cancer arrived at the emergency department complaining of severe abdominal pain. This had developed acutely a few minutes after he had completed his usual daily colostomy irrigation and had steadily worsened. The pain was associated with severe nausea but no vomiting. The abdomen was tender around the colostomy site where rebound could be elicited. His temperature was 38°C, the white blood cell count 20 000/mm^3 and the haematocrit 42%. An ultrasound study and plain abdominal X-ray film showed fluid outside the colon as it passed through the abdominal wall but no free air or fluid within the peritoneal cavity.

A presumptive diagnosis of a localised perforation of the distal colon near the colostomy was made. He was commenced on broad-spectrum intravenous antibiotics, intravenous maintenance fluids and n.p.o.

The next morning his status had deteriorated. His face was ashen and his extremities were pale, cold and clammy. He had a rapid pulse rate (120/min) and his blood pressure was 90/60. He was afebrile. The tissues around the colostomy were red and swollen and crepitus could be felt in the subcutaneous tissues. No urine had been passed overnight and only 100 ml appeared after catheterisation. A nasogastric tube was placed and the patient was given an initial bolus of 2 L of Ringer's lactate solution. Over the next 2 hours he received 4 L of intravenous crystalloid to maintain urine output at 30 ml/h and blood pressure at 110/80. The pulse continued to rise and now was 140/min. After a radiological study which showed contrast leaking into the subcutaneous tissues from a perforation in the colon 5 cm proximal to the colostomy, surgery was decided upon.

At surgery the abdomen was opened through the old midline incision, the colon divided just deep to its exit through the abdominal wall and a new end colostomy was constructed in the right iliac fossa in an area of abdominal wall free of the spreading infection. The abdomen was closed and the infected and partially necrotic area around the site of the old colostomy was widely excised and packed. Muscle was not involved. During surgery 4 L of crystalloid and 2 L of 5% albumin solution were used to maintain urine output at 50 ml/h.

This patient demonstrates many of the features of septic shock from invasive serious sepsis. He required substantial extracellular fluid replacement because of 'leaky capillaries' with accumulation of fluid in the interstitial tissues and peritoneal cavity. The grave nature of his condition was not recognised at the beginning but throughout there was a loss of fluid from the vascular compartment with falling blood pressure and urine output. Later when crystalloids and colloids were given in considerable quantities a total of 10 L of extracellular fluid supplementation was required to maintain peripheral perfusion, urine output and blood pressure.

A surgical approach should have been taken earlier here but the diagnosis of necrotising fasciitis was not made until the morning after admission to hospital. Necrotising fasciitis is a condition caused by invasion of a mixed bacterial flora into the abdominal wall and the infection spreads along fascial planes causing the penetrating vessels to thrombose. The skin, as a consequence, is devascularised. Proper treatment involves high dose antibiotics, radical surgical debridement and circulatory support. In spite of this the mortality is high.

As we have seen in Chapter 19 the mediators leading to the 'leaky capillary syndrome' are now becoming better understood and some of these are capable of inducing shock and the metabolic derangements that characterise septic shock. The most widely studied cytokine in this connection is tumour necrosis factor which has been shown to produce markedly increased 'third space' requirements when injected into animals. The complex network of interactions between tumour necrosis factor and other cytokines and the interrelationships between the cytokine networks and other endogenous and exogenous mediators of septic shock are not completely understood (Ch. 4). However, it is known that invading organisms and cell damage produce TNF which then affects other mediators including endocrine hormones, growth factors, cytokines themselves, acute phase proteins, reactive oxygen intermediates and eicosanoids. The magnitude of the TNF production and the response to it determine the severity of the clinical shock syndrome. Clinically the production of these cytokines is most effectively reduced by thorough surgical debridement and by maximising oxygen delivery to the surrounding tissues. This is done locally by ensuring all dead and devitalised tissue is excised, and systematically by maximising the haemoglobin concentration, degree of saturation of that haemoglobin and cardiac output. We have also seen (Ch. 19, Fig. 19.3) how new strategies are being developed for the treatment of the sepsis syndrome. This patient should have received 100 mg Centoxin i.v. as soon as the sepsis syndrome had been diagnosed (Centoxin is a human monoclonal antibody that binds specifically to the lipid-A domain of endotoxin).

At the end of the operation the patient was taken to the intensive care unit. His fluid requirement continued to be high with losses of ~250 ml/h over and above maintenance during the first 12 hours. In the intensive care unit, main arterial blood pressure was left between 90 and 110 mmHg with inotropic support (dopamine 5 μ g/kg/min). An FiO_2 of 0.6% and PEEP of 10 cm H_2O were required to maintain arterial oxygen saturation at 95%. Vigorous fluid resuscitation using crystalloid at 300 ml/h was used to maintain urine output at 100 ml/h and at this stage the patient was obviously swollen and oedematous. A total of 14 L of fluid had now been given. Central venous pressure was 14 mmHg.

The massive fluid infusions required to maintain urine output and avoid renal failure had, because of the leaky capillaries, resulted in widespread interstitial oedema. The increased lung water was manifested by the requirement for high levels of inspired oxygen (FiO_2), the necessity for PEEP (positive end expiratory pressure) to maintain oxygen saturation and the diffuse fluffy infiltrates throughout both lungs seen on chest X-ray. This is the adult respiratory distress syndrome — ARDS.

The plasma that leaks from the intravascular space fills first the perivascular tissues and, as it worsens, fluid fills the rest of the interstitial space and ultimately the alveoli themselves. First there is a diffusion defect without chest signs or X-ray evidence, later, if the patient is not on a ventilator, arterial $P\text{O}_2$ falls and arterial $P\text{CO}_2$ falls indicating pulmonary arteriovenous shunting. Now the chest X-ray film shows diffuse fluffy infiltrates throughout both lung fields.

Our patient who was curarised and sedated (morphine and a benzodiazepine) received controlled positive pressure ventilation (CPPV), an inspired oxygen concentration of 60% and positive pressure ventilation with PEEP. Intubation and mechanical ventilation helped to combat atelectasis and lung collapse. Large tidal volumes were used because the fluid filled lungs were stiff and pulmonary compliance was poor. PEEP was used to improve oxygenation although it should not be used at high pressure (>12–15 cm H_2O) for it may cause barotrauma and adversely affect intracranial pressure. High pressure PEEP is only indicated for severe frothing pulmonary oedema or for refractory hypoxaemia despite high inspired oxygen concentrations.

The damaged capillary membranes allow albumin to extravasate from the intravascular and extravascular space and the protein concentration on each side of the capillary membrane partially equilibrates. It is for this reason that some argue that it makes little sense and indeed is quite wasteful to add colloid to the resuscitation fluids at this stage. Others argue that the intravascular compartment continues to maintain an osmotic gradient in many patients and quote studies to show that patients resuscitated with colloid ultimately suffer less overhydration than those resuscitated entirely with crystalloid. The best fluid to use in hypovolaemic situations like this is the subject of much debate but it is fair to say that the answer is not known (Webb et al 1991, Vincent 1991). The debate is not whether isotonic crystalloid solutions (lactated Ringer's solution, 0.9% saline solution) should be used, for they are always necessary to a greater or lesser extent, but whether colloid solutions containing large molecules that exert an osmotic pressure (5% albumin solution, 3% solution of gelatin in saline, hydroxyethyl starch etc.) should be used at all. Accepting that microvascular permeability increases in septic shock and that much of the administered colloid passes into the interstitium, concern has to be given to the claim that colloid retention in the lung interstitium occurs and may actually attract fluid, increasing rather than decreasing lung water. Perhaps, though, the greatest argument against the use of colloid is its high cost — albumin is about 100 times the price of crystalloid solutions. It is for these reasons, and the absence of substantive evidence that real clinical benefit follows colloid usage that we recommend that most hypovolaemic surgical patients should be resuscitated with isotonic crystalloid solutions.

The patient remained curarised for 24 hours until gas exchange and haemodynamics were stable. At this stage his requirements for extra fluid had decreased. It was then possible to reduce FiO_2 to 55% and PEEP to 7 cmH_2O. Improvement continued and by the next morning the FiO_2 was further reduced to 0.5 and PEEP to 5 cmH_2O and with a ventilatory rate of 18/min an oxygen saturation at 94% was maintained. At this point the relaxants were stopped and about 12 hours later when they had been metabolised intermittent mandatory ventilation (IMV) was begun. Attempts were then made to wean him from the ventilator whilst continuing to keep arterial oxygen saturation at 95%. A day later he was extubated and able to breathe comfortably and maintain oxygen levels at around 90% saturation.

It is reasonable to initially manage a continuing defect in oxygenation with increases in FiO_2 and PEEP levels. The arterial oxygen saturation should be maintained at 95% or more if at all possible. As stated above high levels of PEEP not only risk pneumothorax but also decrease venous return and cardiac output. High levels of oxygen are undesirable. FiO_2 levels below 0.5 are not associated with lung damage but increases in FiO_2 above this may lead to inflammatory lung lesions that may, in the long run, result in chronic restrictive lung disease.

Tracheostomy was not performed on our patient at this stage. Recommendations as to when a tracheostomy should be performed vary widely but our practice is to perform tracheostomy at approximately 10 days of orotracheal or nasotracheal intubation if it is thought at that time that intubation is likely to be prolonged.

The sepsis now seemed to be under control and further extension beyond the excised area had not occurred. Volume requirements had now diminished and maintenance fluids were sufficient to maintain urine output. Total parenteral nutrition through a central venous route was now commenced. He had not had any food for 5 days now and with a very distended abdomen and no evidence of bowel sounds it was clear that the gut would remain unusable for some time yet. Just before the commencement of total parenteral nutrition a body composition study was performed. The results were as follows:

	Estimated value when well	Measured value
Body weight	74.4 kg	81.5 kg
Body fat	15.5 kg	14.0 kg
Fat free body mass	58.9 kg	67.5 kg
Total body water	41.8 L	51.0 L
Total body protein	12.7 kg	12.1 kg
Hydration of fat free body	71%	76%

In spite of losing 1.5 kg of fat and 0.6 kg of protein during the first 6 days of the illness there has been a large (7.1 kg) increase in body weight due entirely to an increase in total body water of 9.2 L–this was the net amount of 'third space' fluid that had escaped into the interstitium, the gut lumen and the body cavities. Gains in total body water of this order are common in serious sepsis and weight gain of as much as 34 kg has been reported in a survivor with faecal peritonitis treated with crystalloid resuscitation fluids only.

He received the parenteral nutrition (TPN) through an intraclavicular subclavian catheter. To minimise the risk of pneumothorax during line insertion FiO_2 was increased to 1.0 and PEEP was removed. The central line which had been on the other side of the neck had been removed 2 days before. We prohibit the use of the feeding line for anything but TPN. A careful dressing technique, which prevents contamination of either the skin entry site or the junction of the line with the giving set keeps catheter sepsis to a rarity. We do not use multiple lumen central venous catheters for TPN, feeling their safety is yet to be proven.

For total parenteral nutrition he received an average daily intake of 2 700 kcal non-protein energy or approximately 34 kcal/kg of well body weight/day. This was given as a 50:50 mixture of glucose and fat. He received 122 g of protein per day or approximately 1.6 g protein/kg well body weight/day in the form of synthetic amino acids. Appropriate electrolytes and trace elements were added to the nutrient solution. After 10 days of total parenteral nutrition body composition was again measured.

	At commencement of TPN	After 10 days of TPN
Body weight	81.5 kg	75.3 kg
Body fat/glycogen	14.0 kg	16.2 kg
Fat free body mass	67.5 kg	59.1 kg
Total body water	51.0 L	44.2 L
Total body protein	12.1 kg	10.6 kg
Hydration of fat free mass	76%	75%

It is clear that more than sufficient energy had been given parenterally for there had been a net increase in body stores of fat which more than compensated for the energy lost as protein. In spite of this and the provision of high amino acid intakes (kinetic studies show that intakes of protein greater than 1.5 g/kg/day cannot be utilised) there was a continuing massive loss of body protein amounting to 1.2% of the total stores each day. This is a fundamental metabolic problem in serious sepsis and its mechanism can be understood more clearly from the study of protein turnover that was performed on two occasions. The first study was performed just before the commencement of TPN and the second 5 days later.

	Estimated normal value (basal state)	Study 1 (basal state)	Study 2 (after 5-days TPN)
Protein synthesis*	2.8	3.9	5.2
Protein breakdown	4.0	6.3	6.2
Net loss of protein	1.8	3.0	1.3

* All values are g (protein) per kg per day.

The compositional and the kinetic studies taken together show that continuing sepsis, in spite of TPN, results in massive losses of body protein due to a marked increase in protein breakdown. In sepsis, protein synthesis is also increased but not enough to overcome the effect of continuing massive protein breakdown. The effect of TPN is to halve the loss of protein and this happens because of an increase in protein synthesis and not because of any effect on protein breakdown. Indeed, it is this continuing high catabolic rate that is the fundamental problem of serious sepsis and to date no way has yet been found to eliminate it.

The body composition study also showed the large loss of body water over the 10-day period. At 44.2 L he was still 2.4 L overhydrated and this was apparent in the hydration index of 75% compared with an estimated normal value of 71%. Nevertheless this decrease of water, mainly from the extracellular compartment shows more than anything else that sepsis was now under control and the previously high levels of antidiuretic hormone and aldosterone had fallen. *Diuresis is a vital prognostic sign which tells the surgeon in no uncertain terms that the patient is getting better.*

The patient, now extubated, less oedematous and beginning to take an interest in his surroundings continued on TPN. About this time nasogastric losses fell to low levels (< 500 ml/day), the abdomen was less distended and bowel sounds, although infrequent, could be heard. No fluid, faeces or flatus had yet passed out of his colostomy. The large, excised area of the abdominal wound was now beginning to granulate and all areas of necrosis had disappeared.

A decision was made to begin enteral nutrition. A fine bore feeding tube replaced the large nasogastric tube previously used for aspiration. He was positioned on to his right side and metoclopramide was given to encourage passage of the tube into the duodenum. A formula providing 1 kcal/ml and 37 g protein/L was used — firstly at half strength concentration at a rate of 30 ml/h. The patient tolerated this regimen, felt no nausea or distension and after 24 hours full strength formula was given. Flatus was passed via the colostomy about this stage. The next day, although abdominal distension was still present, it was less, and full strength formula was given in increasing quantities (10 ml/h each 6 hours as tolerated) until 60 ml/hr was being received. With this, abdominal distension increased and he felt nauseous but on the day after a large fluid motion was passed into his colostomy bag. The total caloric intake was now over 1200 kcal per day and TPN was discontinued. The next day the patient commenced drinking clear fluids, then took a light diet. Soon it was possible to remove the feeding tube and rely entirely on oral intake. At this point he had returned to the hospital ward. Dietetic assessment now showed that he was consuming 1500 kcals per day and 60 g protein.

A month after his admission to hospital the abdominal wound had contracted substantially but a defect of 12 cm diameter remained and this was repaired with a split skin graft. After it was ensured that this had properly healed he was discharged home. His body weight at discharge was 71 kg.

It is known that the most serious infections that occur in general surgical practice are caused by enteric organisms. Not only do regions in close proximity to the gut, such as the abdominal wall, get infected by enteric organisms but bacteraemias and pneumonia also are often caused by them. Although it is not completely clear how these distant sites become infected with gut organisms there is increasing evidence that in serious surgical illness the intestinal barrier is broken down and organisms from the lumen move out into the mesenteric lymphatic or portal venous circulations. This presumably results either in a bacteraemia or infection at a distant site or both.

The reason for this translocation of bacteria from gut to systemic circulation is due to many factors which include changes in gut flora, immune suppression due to the illness itself and diminished blood flow to the gut, but perhaps most of all to mucosal atrophy associated with deficient nutrition of the gut mucosa due to the absence of glutamine in the diet. Clearly this may occur when patients are on TPN, for glutamine, a 'non-essential' amino acid, is essential for proper nutrition of the enterocyte but is not included in standard synthetic intravenous amino acid preparations because it is unstable in solution. There is evidence that lack of glutamine in TPN formulas results in enterocyte dysfunction, increased mucosal breakdown and increased migration of bacteria out of the gut into the bloodstream. Clinical trials suggest that patients fed properly with solutions containing glutamine by the enteral route have fewer problems with invasive sepsis. Other studies have shown that most enteral diets, even those with less glutamine, have this protective effect too and it may be that there are numerous topical benefits of providing enteral nutrition including stimulation of gut flow and increasing gut hormones as well as the direct effect of glutamine.

Most importantly, this patient illustrates the basic surgical principle of the overwhelming efficacy of draining and eliminating sepsis. Above all else control and elimination of the source of the sepsis is the key to managing patients with serious sepsis. The patient is never 'too sick' to do this; without drainage deterioration is certain. Drain, excise, defunction, exteriorise, do whatever it takes to get rid of the sepsis. Once sepsis is eliminated, cytokines with their catholic effects are no longer at high levels and leaky capillaries stabilise, vascular volume can be controlled and organ failure reversed. All the steps described in this case report are temporary ones until the sepsis is under control. Once it is, with good metabolic and nutritional care and well timed and careful surgery the patient can be set on the road to recovery.

Appendices

Appendix I

SECTION I
ASSESSMENT OF NUTRITIONAL STATUS — METHODS USED

Measurement	Units	Technique 1	Technique 2	Reference
Body weight	kg	Load cell	Avery beam balance	—
Total body fat	kg	Body weight – fat free mass	DEXA	1,2
Total body protein	kg	In vivo neutron activation	In vivo neutron activation	1,3
Total body water	L	Tritium dilution	B wt – (fat + protein + glycogen + minerals)	1,4
Extracellular water	L	Bromide dilution	From total body chlorine	5,6
Fat free mass	kg	Protein + water + glycogen + minerals	Body weight – body fat	1
Albumin	g/L	Laser nephalometry	Laser nephalometry	
Transferrin	mg/dl	Laser nephalometry	Laser nephalometry	
Prealbumin	mg/dl	Laser nephalometry	Laser nephalometry	
Grip strength	kg	Vigorimeter	Vigorimeter	7
Respiratory muscle strength	cmH_2O	Pressure transducer	Pressure transducer	8
Forced expiratory volume in 1 sec	L	Spirometry	Spirometry	9,10
Vital capacity	L	Spirometry	Spirometry	10
Peak expiratory flow rate	L/min	Spirometry	Spirometry	10
Maximum voluntary ventilation	L/min	Spirometry	Spirometry	10
Resting metabolic expenditure	kcal/24 h	Indirect calorimetry	Indirect calorimetry	11
Active energy expenditure	kcal/24 h	RME × 0.3	TEE – RME	12
Total energy expenditure	kcal/24 h	RME + AEE	Energy balance	13
Stress index	—	Measured RME: predicted RME	Measured RME: predicted RME	

1 Beddoe et al 1984
2 Mazess et al 1990
3 Knight et al 1986
4 Streat et al 1985b
5 Vaisman et al 1987
6 Yasumara et al 1983
7 Windsor & Hill 1988a
8 Arora & Rochester 1982
9 Macklem 1986
10 Baldwin et al 1958
11 MacFie et al 1982
12 Durnin & Passmore 1967
13 Hackett et al 1979
14 Streat & Hill 1987

SECTION II
BODY COMPOSITION MODEL USING IN VIVO NEUTRON ACTIVATION AND TRITIATED WATER VERSUS CADAVER ANALYSIS[1,2]

	Cadaver 1		Cadaver 2	
Body weight (kg)	58.6		25.9	
Height (cm)	174		154	
	Chemical	*IVNAA*	*Chemical*	*IVNAA*
Total body fat (kg)	10.48	10.71	7.71	6.77
Total body protein (kg)	9.56	9.21	3.66	3.60
Total body water (kg)	35.00	35.00	13.27	13.27
Total body minerals (kg)	3.33	3.31	1.20	1.90

[1] Beddoe A H, Streat S J, Hill G L 1984 Evaluation of an in vivo prompt gamma neutron activation facility for body composition studies in critically ill intensive care patients: results on 41 normals. Metabolism 33: 270–280
[2] Knight G S, Beddoe A H, Streat S J, Hill G L 1986 Body composition of two human cadavers by neutron activation and chemical analysis. Am J Physiol 250: E179–E185

SECTION III
BODY COMPOSITION REGRESSIONS FOR NORMAL SUBJECTS

A = age (yr); H = height (cm);
M = total body mass (kg)

Body weight (kg)

86 women	
M = –87.665 + 0.239A + 0.852H	s.e.e. = 6.608 (10.6%)
76 men	
M = 4.060 – 0.129A + 0.441H	s.e.e. = 9.737 (12.7%)

Total body fat (kg)

86 women	
TBF = –25.284 + 0.161A + 0.223H	s.e.e. = 5.14 (29.1%)
TBF = 29.059 + 0.0134A – 0.305H + 0.620M	s.e.e. = 3.12 (17.7%)
76 men	
TBF = 20.012 + 0.0456A – 0.0159H	s.e.e. = 7.37 (47.9%)
TBF = 17.979 + 0.0091A – 0.237H + 0.501M	s.e.e = 5.56 (36.1%)

Total body protein (kg)

86 women	
TBP = –15.984 – 0.00633A + 0.150H	s.e.e. = 0.961 (11.24%)
TBP = –9.322 – 0.02449A + 0.0851H + 0.0760	s.e.e. = 0.824 (9.64%)
76 men	
TBP = –6.793 – 0.0482A + 0.122H	s.e.e. = 1.630 (12.80%)
TBP = –7.312 – 0.0316A + 0.0655H + 0.128M	s.e.e. = 1.058 (8.31%)

Total body water (L)

86 women	
TBW = –41.990 + 0.0723A + 0.436H	s.e.e. = 3.233 (9.9%)
TBW = –18.821 + 0.0091A + 0.211H + 0.264M	s.e.e. = 2.738 (8.4%)
76 men	
TBW = –10.825 – 0.0323A + 0.321H	s.e.e. = 5.881 (13.3%)
TBW = –12.191 + 0.0112A + 0.173H + 0.337M	s.e.e. = 4.917 (11.1%)

SECTION IV
RESTING METABOLIC RATE REGRESSION FOR NORMAL SUBJECTS

RME (kcals/kg/day) = 13.6 [fat free body mass in kg] + 550

The average ratio of the measured RME for normals is 1.00 ± 0.951 (males and females) and so patients with a ratio of RME measured/RME predicted > 1.18 can be considered as having a raised RME and suffer from metabolic stress.

SECTION V
TECHNIQUE FOR IMMEDIATE ASSESSMENT OF NUTRITIONAL STATUS

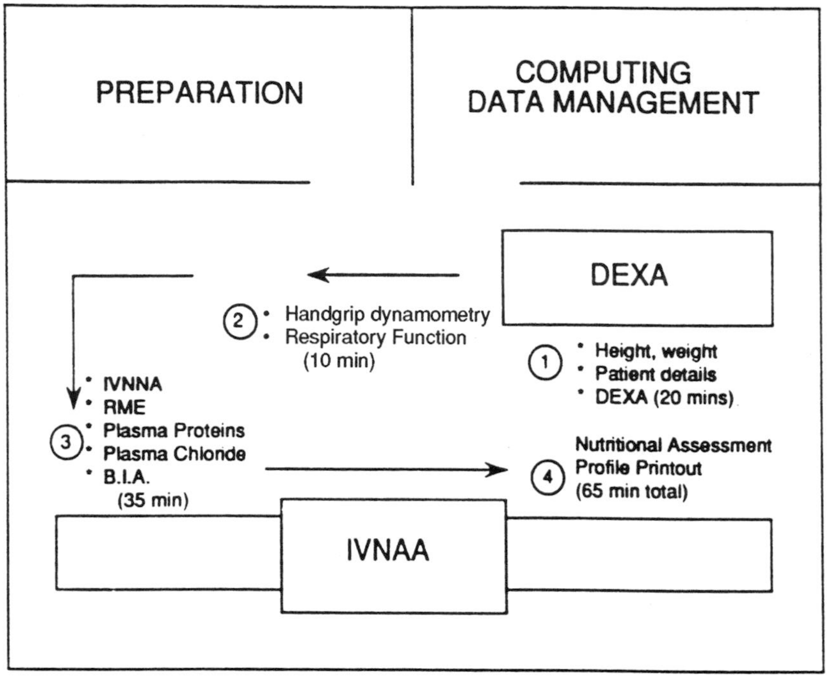

Fig. AI.1 Combined dual energy X-ray absorptiometry (DEXA) in vivo neutron activation (IVNAA) technique for the rapid assessment of body composition as used at the University of Auckland. Plasma proteins, physiological function, resting metabolic expenditure and bioelectrical impedance (BIA) are measured as well. The nutritional assessment profile printout is seen in Section VII.

SECTION VI
BODY COMPOSITION MODELS

MODELS

A Standard

M	=	TBF	+	TBP	+	TBM	+	TBG	+	TBW
↓		↓		↓		↓		↓		↓
direct weighing		by difference		IVNAA		Anthropometry				Tritium dilution

B Combined DEXA–IVNAA technique without using tritium

M	=	TBF	+	TBP	+	BM	+	NBM	=	TBG	+	TBW
↓		↓		↓		↓		↓		↓		↓
direct weighing		DEXA		IVNAA		DEXA		0.06TBP		Anthropometry		by difference

C Combined DEXA-IVNAA technique for the measurement of TBG

M	=	TBF	+	TBP	+	BM	+	NBM	+	TBG	+	TBW
↓		↓		↓		↓		↓		↓		↓
direct weighing		DEXA		IVNAA		DEXA		0.06TBP		by difference		Tritium dilution

Key: M = Body mass; TBF = Total body fat; TBP = Total body protein; TBM = Total body minerals; TBG = Total body glycogen; TBW = Total body water; BM = Bone mineral; NBM = Non bone mineral

SECTION VII
NUTRITIONAL ASSESSMENT PROFILE

Example

James Packer #058324, 54 years, adenocarcinoma gastric fundus. Measurement the day before total gastrectomy (21–10–90)

	Estimated value when well	Measured value	Change (%)
Body composition			
Body weight (kg)	63.0	52.0	−18
Total body fat (kg)	14.8	10.7	−28
Total body protein (kg)	9.8	6.3	−36
Total body water (L)	34.5	30.6	−11
Extracellular water (L)	17.0	15.3	−10
FFM (kg)	48.2	41.3	−14
TBW/FFM	0.72	0.74	+3
ECW/FFM	0.35	0.37	+6
ECW/ICW	0.97	1.0	+3
Vascular phase			
Haematocrit (%)	44	36	−9
Albumin (g/L)	38	36	−5
Transferrin (mg/dl)	230	176	−24
Prealbumin (mg/dl)	22	15.7	−29
Physiological function			
Grip strength (kg)	36	28	−22
Forced expiratory volume$_{1\ sec}$ (L)	3.6	3.2	−11
Vital capacity (L)	4.3	3.6	−17
Peak expiratory flow rate (L/min)	513	385	−25
Metabolic expenditure			
Resting metabolic expenditure (kcal/24 h)	1209	1140	−6
Activity energy expenditure (kcal/24 h)	1059	524	−34
Total energy expenditure (kcal/24 h)	2268	1664	−21
Stress index	1.0	1.02	+2

Diagnosis

Moderate protein energy malnutrition, nutritional marasmus
Not metabolically stressed

Appendix II

SECTION A
PARENTERAL NUTRITION

MACRONUTRIENTS
PROTEIN SOURCES

Standard protein products

Table A.1 Protein Products for Intravenous Use

Product (Manufacturer)	*Protein (%)*	*Nitrogen (g/100 ml)*	*Elecytrolytes (mEq/L)* Na^{+}	K^{+}	Mg^{++}	Cl^{-}	Acetate	Phosphate (mM/L^{-})	*Osmolality*	*Volume Supplied (ml)*
Crystalline amino acid infusions without electrolytes										
Aminosyn (5%) (Abbott)	5	0.786	—	5.4	—	—	60	—	500	250, 500, 1000
Travasol 5.5% (Clintec Nutrition)	5.5	0.924	—	—	—	22	35	—	520	500
Aminosyn 7% (Abbott)	7	1.1	—	5.4	—	—	88	—	700	500
Aminosyn 8.5% (Abbott)	8.5	1.34	—	5.4	—	35	90	—	850	500
Travasol 8.5% (Clintec Nutrition)	8.5	1.42	—	—	—	34	52	—	860	500
Aminosyn 10% (Abbott)	10	1.57	—	5.4	—	—	148	—	1000	500
Travasol 10% (Clintec Nutrition)	10	1.68	—	—	—	40	87	—	1000	500
Novamine 15% (Clintec Nutrition)	15	2.4	—	—	—	—	151	—	1388	500
Crystalline amino acid infusions with electrolytes										
Travasol 5.5% w/Electrolytes (Clintec Nutrition)	5.5	0.924	70	60	10	70	100	30	850	500
Aminosyn 7% w/Electrolytes (Abbott)	7	1.1	70	66	10	96	124	30	1013	500
Aminosyn 8.5% w/Electrolytes (Abbott)	8.5	1.14	70	66	10	98	142	30	1160	500
FreAmine III 8.5% (Kendall McGaw)	8.6	1.1	10	—	—	<2	74	10	810	500
Travasol 8.5% w/Electrolytes (Clintec Nutrition)	8.6	1.42	70	60	10	70	135	30	1160	500
Veinamine (Cutter)	8	1.71	40	30	6	50	50	—	950	500
Crystalline amino acid infusions for peripheral use										
FreAmine III 3% w/Electrolytes (Kendall McGaw)	3	0.46	15	24.5	5	40	44	3.5	405	1000
Aminosyn 3.5% (Abbott)	1.5	0.55	40	18.4	3	40	68	3.5	460	1000
3.5% Travasol M w/Electrolytes (Clintec Nutrition)	3.5	0.59	25	15	5	25	54	7.5	450	500, 1000
Procalamine (Kendall McGaw)	3	0.46	35	24	5	41	47	7	735	1000

* Reprinted from Blackburn G L, Bell S J, Mullen J L (eds) 1989 Nutritional medicine — a case management approach, with permission of the publishers, W B Saunders Company, Philadelphia

Specialized solutions

Table A.2 Specialized Amino Acid Solutions for Patients with Severe Stress and N_2 Retention Disorders*

	HepatAmine	***FreAmine HBC***	***BranchAmin***
Manufacturer	Kendall McGaw	Kendall McGaw	Clintec Nutrition
Supplied in (ml)	500	750	500
Protein concentration (%)	8.0	6.9	4.0
Nitrogen (g/100 ml)	1.25	0.650	0.441
Essential amino acids (mg/100 ml)			
Isoleucine	900	760	1380
Leucine	1100	1370	1380
Lycine	610	410	—
Methionine	100	250	—
Phenylalanine	100	320	—
Threonine	450	200	—
Tryptophan	66	90	—
Valine	840	880	1240
Nonessential amino acids (mg/100 ml)			
Alanine	770	400	—
Arginine	600	580	—
Histidine	240	160	—
Proline	800	630	—
Serine	500	330	—
Tyrosine	0	0	—
Glycine	900	300	—
Glutamic acid	0	0	—
Aspartic acid	0	0	—
Cysteine	<20	<20	—
Electrolytes (mEq/l)			
Sodium	10	10	—
Potassium	0	0	—
Magnesium	0	0	—
Chloride	<3	<3	—
Acetate	62	57	—
Phosphate (mM/l)	10	0	—
Osmolarity (mOsm/l)	785	620	316

* Compiled by David Driscoll, M.S., R.Ph., New England Deaconess Hospital, Boston, MA.

SECTION B
ENTERAL NUTRITION

CURRENTLY AVAILABLE ENTERAL FORMULAS

Table A.3 Currently Available

Formula	*Calories per ml*	*mOsm/kg water*	*Protein* Source	*Protein* gm per 1000 cal	*Protein* %	*Nonprotein Calories gm N*	*Carbohydrate* Source	*Carbohydrate* gm per, 1000 cal	*Carbohydrate* %
Fiber-Containing§									
Enrich (FC: 13)	1.1	480	SCC, SPI	36.2	14.5	148:1	HCS, sucrose, soy polysaccharide	143.3	55
Jevity (FC: 13.6)	1.06	310	SCC	42	16.7	125:1	HCS, soy polysaccharide	143.6	53.3
Profiber (FC: 12)	1.0	300	SCC	40	16	131:1	HCS, soy fiber	132	48
Sustacal with fiber (FC: 6)	1.06	450	CSC, SPI	43	17	120:1	Maltodextrin, sugar, soy fiber	133	53
1.0–1.4 cal/ml Lactose-Free									
Attain	1.0	300	SCC	40	16	131:1	Maltodextrin	120	48
Ensure	1.06	470	SCC, SPI	35.2	14	153:1	Corn syrup, sucrose	137.2	54.5
Ensure HN	1.06	470	SCC, SPI	42	16.7	125:1	Corn syrup, sucrose	133.6	53.2
Entralife	1.0	300	WP concentrate, soy protein	37	15	144:1	HCS	138	55
Entrition	1.0	300	SCC	35	14	154:1	Maltodextrin	136	54.4
Entrition HN	1.0	300	SCC, SPI	44	17.6	117:1	Maltodextrin	114	45.6
Isocal	1.06	300	CSC, SPI	32.5	13	167:1	Maltodextrin	125	50
Isocal HN	1.06	300	CSC, SPI	42.5	17	127:1	Maltodextrin	117.5	47
Isosource	1.25	300	SCC	35	14	155:1	Maltodextrin	140	56
Isosource HN	1.28	300	SCC	42.5	17	125:1	Maltodextrin	132.5	53
Nutren 1.0	1.0	300–380	Casein	40	16	131:1	Maltodextrin, corn syrup	127	51
Osmolite	1.06	300	SCC, SPI	35.2	14	153:1	HCS	137.2	54.6
Osmolite HN	1.06	300	SCC, SPI	42	16.7	125:1	HCS	133.6	53.3

Enteral Formulas*†

Fat			*Na*		*K*		*Free water*				
SOURCE	GM PER 1000 CAL	%	MEQ/L	MG/L	MEQ/L	MG/L	(%)	*Calories*‡	*Flavors*	*Form*	*Supplier*
Corn oil	33.8	30.5	36.7	845	40	1564	82.9	1530	Varied	Liquid	Ross
MCT, corn oil	34.8	30	40.4	930	40	1564	83.3	1400	Unflavored	Liquid	Ross
Corn oil	40	36	32	730	32	1250	84.5	1500	Unflavored	Liquid/KDS	Sherwood Medical
Corn oil	33.2	30	30.6	704	36	1408	76	1500	Vanilla	Liquid	Mead Johnson
Corn oil	40	36	30	680	29	1150	85.5	1600	Unflavored	Liquid/KDS	Sherwood Medical
Corn oil	35.2	31.5	36.7	845	40	1564	84.5	2000	Varied	Liquid	Ross
Corn oil	33.6	30.1	40.4	930	40	1564	83.9	1400	Varied	Liquid	Ross
Corn oil, MCT	33.6	30	31.3	720	25.6	1000		2000	Unflavored	Liquid	Corpak
Corn oil	35	31.5	31	700	30.8	1200	83	2000	Unflavored	Prefilled RTU pouch	Biosearch
Corn oil	41	36.8	36.7	845	40.5	1579	83	1300	Unflavored	Prefilled RTU pouch	Biosearch
Soy oil, MCT	41	37	22.9	527	33.8	1316	84	2000	Unflavored	Liquid	Mead Johnson
Soy oil, MCT	40	36	35	802	27	1055	84	1250	Unflavored	Liquid	Mead Johnson
MCT, corn oil	33.3	30	31	720	43	1700	80.4	1875	Vanilla	Liquid	Sandoz
MCT, corn oil, mono- and diglycerides	33.3	30	31	720	43	1700	80	1920	Vanilla	Liquid	Sandoz
MCT, corn oil	38	33	21.7	500	32.1	1252	85	2000	Unflavored, varied	Liquid	Clintec Nutrition
MCT, corn oil, soy oil	36.4	31.4	27.6	634	25.9	1014	84.4	2000	Unflavored	Liquid	Ross
MCT, corn oil, soy oil	34.8	30	40.5	938	40.1	1564	84.4	1400	Unflavored	Liquid	Ross

Table A.3 Currently Available (contd)

Formula	Calories per ml	mOsm/kg water	Protein Source	Protein gm per 1000 cal	Protein %	Nonprotein Calories gm N	Carbohydrate Source	Carbohydrate gm per, 1000 cal	Carbohydrate %
1.0–1.4 cal/ml Lactose-Free *Continued*									
Pre-Attain	0.5	150	Sodium caseinate	20	16	131:1	Maltodextrin	60	48
Replete	1.0	350	Casein	62	25	75:1	Maltodextrin, sucrose	113	45
Resource Instant Crystals	1.06	450	SCC, SPI	35	14	153:1	Maltodextrin, sucrose	136.3	54.5
Sustacal Liquid	1.0	625	Calcium caseinate, SPI, sodium caseinate	612	24	79:1	Sugar (sucrose), corn syrup	140	55
Travasorb MCT Powder	1.0	312	Lactalbumin, potassium & sodium caseinates	49.3	20	100:1	CSS	123	50
1.5–2.0 Cal/ml Lactose-Free									
Comply	1.5	410/600–650	CSC	40	16	131:1	HCS	120	48
Ensure Plus	1.5	690	SCC, SPI	36.6	14.7	146:1	Corn syrup, sucrose	133.2	53.3
Ensure Plus HN	1.5	650	SCC, SPI	41.7	16.7	125:1	Hydrolyzed corn starch, sucrose	133.2	53.3
Isocal HCN	2.0	690	CSC	37.4	15	145:1	Corn syrup	112	45
Magnacal	2.0	590	SCC	35	14	154:1	Maltodextrin, sucrose	125	50
Nutren 1.5	1.5	420–600	Casein	40	16	131:1	Maltodextrin, corn syrup	112.5	45
Nutren 2.0	2.0	800	Casein	40	16	131:1	CSS, sucrose, maltodextrin	98	39
Resource Plus	1.5	600	SCC, SPI	36.8	14.7	146:1	Maltodextrin, sucrose	133	53.3
Sustacal HC	1.5	650	CSC	40	16	134:1	CSS, sugar	125	50.3
Twocal	2.0	690	SCC	41.7	16.7	125:1	HCS, sucrose	108	43.2
Blenderized									
Compleat Modified	1.07	300	Beef, calcium caseinate	40	16	131:1	HC, fruit, vegetables	135	54
Compleat Regular	1.07	405	Beef, nonfat, milk	40	16	131:1	HC solids, fruits, vegetables, maltodextrin, lactose	120	48
Vitaneed	1.0	300	Purée beef, CSC	40	16	131:1	Maltodextrin, fruit, vegetables, soy fiber	128	48
Milk-Based									
Carnation Instant Breakfast‖	1.06	671/758	Nonfat dry milk, calcium caseinate, sweet dairy whey	55	22	92:1	Sugar, maltodextrin, lactose	125.5	50.2
Meritene Liquid	0.96	505 (Vanilla)	Concentrated sweet skim milk	60	24	79:1	Lactose, CSS, sucrose	115	46

Enteral Formulas*†

Fat			*Na*		*K*		*Free water*				
Source	gm per 1000 cal	%	mEq/L	mg/L	mEq/L	mg/L	(%)	*Calories*‡	*Flavors*	*Form*	*Supplier*
Corn oil	20	36	15	340	15	575	93	1600	Unflavored	Liquid/KDS	Sherwood Medical
Corn oil	33	30	21.7	500	40	1560	85	2000	Vanilla	Liquid	Clintec Nutrition
Hydrogenated soy oil	35	31.5	36.8	850	40	1560	73	2010	Varied	Instant crystals	Sandoz
PH soy oil	23.2	21	40.9	928	53	2067	84	1080	Varied	Liquid	Mead Johnson
MCT, sunflower oil	33	30	15.2	350	25.6	1000	64	2000	Unflavored	Powder	Clintec Nutrition
Corn oil	40	36	48	1100	47	1850	77.8	1500	Unflavored, varied	Liquid/KDS	Sherwood Medical
Corn oil	35.5	32	49.6	1141	54.1	2114	76.9	2130	Varied	Liquid	Ross
Corn oil	33.2	30	51.5	1184	46.5	1818	76.9	1420	Varied	Liquid	Ross
Soybean oil, MCT	45.4	40	34.7	798	35.8	1396	71	2000	Unflavored	Liquid	Mead Johnson
PH soy oil	40	36	43.5	1000	32	1250	69	2000	Vanilla	Liquid	Sherwood Medical
MCT, corn oil	43.3	39	32.6	752	48.2	1800	78	2000	Unflavored, varied	Liquid	Clintec Nutrition
MCT, corn oil	53	45	43.4	1000	64.1	2500	70	2000	Vanilla	Liquid	Clintec Nutrition
Corn oil	35.5	32	39.2	899	44.5	1740	65	2400	Varied	Liquid	Sandoz
PH soybean oil	37.7	34	36.7	844	37.6	1477	78	1800	Varied	Liquid	Mead Johnson
Corn oil, MCT	44.5	40.1	46	1057	59.6	2325	78.6	1600	Vanilla	Liquid	Ross
Beef, corn oil	33.3	40	29.1	670	35.9	1400	83.1	1605	Natural	Liquid	Sandoz
Beef, corn oil	40	36	56.5	1300	35.9	1400	78.1	1605	Natural	Liquid	Sandoz
Corn oil	40	36	30	680	32	1250	84.5	1500	Natural	Liquid/KDS	Sherwood Medical
Whole milk	29.2	26.3	42–52	969–1197	56.7–77.2	2212–3010	81.1	1124 (except biotin)	Varied	Powder	Clintec Nutrition
Corn oil	33.3	30	38.3	880	41	1600	84.8	1200	Varied	Liquid	Sandoz

Table A.3 Currently Available

Formula	Calories per ml	mOsm/kg water	Protein Source	Protein gm per 1000 cal	Protein %	Nonprotein Calories gm N	Carbohydrate Source	Carbohydrate gm per, 1000 cal	Carbohydrate %
Modular									
Casec	3.7/gm		Calcium caseinate		95				
High Fat Supplement	6.12/gm				3				26
MCT oil	8.3/gm								
Microlipid	4.5								
Moducal	3.8/gm						Maltodextrin		100
Nutrisource Carbohydrate	3.2						Deionized CSS		100
Nutrisource Lipid—Long Chain Triglycerides	2.2								
Nutrisource Lipid—Medium Chain Triglycerides	2								
Nutrisource Protein	4/gm		Delactosed lactal- bumin, egg white solids		75				6
Polycose Liquid	2						Glucose polymers		100
Polycose Powder	3.8 gm						Glucose polymers		100
Pro-Mix R.D.P.	3.6/mg		WP		83				6
Promod	4.2/gm		WP concent- rate		71.3				9.5
ProPAC	4/gm		WP concent- rate		76				6
Pure Carbohydrate Supplement	4						Glucose polymers		100
Sumacal	3.8 gm						Maltodextrin		100
Elemental									
Criticare HM	1.06	650	Enzymati- cally hydro- lyzed casein, free AA	35	14	148 : 1	Maltodextrin, modified corn starch	207.5	83
Peptamen	1.0	260	Hydrolyzed whey	40	16	131 : 1	Maltodextrin	127	51
Pepti-2000	1.0	490	Hydrolyzed lactal- bumin	40	16	131 : 1	Maltodextrin	189	75.5
Reabilan	1.0	350	Whey peptides, casein peptides	31.5	12.5	175 : 1	Maltodextrin, tapioca starch	131.5	52.5
Reabilan HN	1.33	490	Whey pep- tides, casein peptides	43.6	17.5	125 : 1	Maltodextrin, tapioca starch	118.6	47.5
Tolorex	1.0	550	Free AA	20.6	8.2	284 : 1	GO	231	92.4
Travasorb HN	1.0	560	Hydrolyzed lactal- bumin	45	18	114 : 1	GO	175	70
Travasorb Standard	1.0	560	Hydrolyzed lactal- bumin	30	12	184 : 1	GO	190	76

Table A.3 Currently Available (contd)

Formula	*Calories per ml*	*mOsm/kg water*	*Protein* Source	*Protein* GM PER 1000 CAL	*Protein* %	*Nonprotein Calories gm N*	*Carbohydrate* Source	*Carbohydrate* GM PER 1000 CAL	*Carbohydrate* %
***Elemental** Continued*									
Vital HN	1.0	460	PH whey & meat, soy, free essential AA	41.7	16.7	125:1	HCS, sucrose	185	73.9
Vivonex HN	1.0	810	Free AA	44.4	17.8	125:1	GO	210	81.5
Vivonex T.E.N.	1.0	630	Free AA (30% branched chain AA)	38.2	15.3	139:1	Maltodextrin, modified starch	206	82.2
Special									
Amin-Aid	2.0	700	Essential AA plus histidine	10	4	640:1	Maltodextrin, sugar	187	74.8
Citrotein	0.66	480 (punch)	Egg white solids	62.5	25	76:1	Sucrose, maltodextrin	182.5	73
Hepatic-Aid II	1.2	560	Essential & nonessential AA	37.5	15	340:1	Maltodextrin, sucrose	143.3	57.3
Pulmocare	1.5	490	SCC	41.7	16.7	125:1	Sucrose, HCS	70.4	28.1
Ross SLD	0.7	545	Egg white solids	53.6	21.4	92:1	HCS, sucrose	195	78
Stresstein	1.2	910	AA (44% branched chain AA)	57.5	23	97:1	Maltodextrin	142.5	57
Traumacal	1.5	550	Calcium caseinate	55	22	90:1	Corn syrup, sugar	100	40
Travasorb Hepatic	1.1	600	Crystalline L-AA	26.4	10.6	211:1	GO	193.6	77.5
Travasorb Renal	1.4	590	Crystalline L-AA	17.1	6.9	340:1	GO	202.9	81.1

* *Modified from* Enteral comparison chart; a handy guide to more than 70 currently available formulas. St. Louis, MO, Sherwood Medical, 1988. 'Note a comprehensive listing is not intended. The information herein concerning competing products was obtained from publications. Sherwood Medical disclaims any responsibility for the accuracy of the information, except with respect to its own products.

'† Abbreviations: AA = amino acids; CSC = calcium and sodium caseinates; CSS = corn syrup solids; GO = glucose oligosaccharides; HC = hydrolyzed cereal; HCS = hydrolyzed corn starch; HL = hydrolyzed lactalbumin; KDS = kangaroo delivery system; MCT = medium chain triglycerides; N/A = not applicable; PH = partially hydrogenated; RTU = ready to use; SPI = soy protein isolate; WP = whey protein.

‡ To meet 100% U.S. RDA vitamins and minerals.

§ FC = fiber content in grams per 1000 calories.

|| With 8 oz whole milk.

Enteral Formulas*†

Fat			*Na*		*K*						
SOURCE	GM PER 1000 CAL	%	MEQ/L	MG/L	MEQ/L	MG/L	*Free water (%)*	*Calories‡*	*Flavors*	*Form*	*Supplier*
		5								Powder	Mead Johnson
PH coconut oil		70								Powder	Corpak
Coconut oil		100								Liquid	Mead Johnson
Safflower oil		100								Liquid	Sherwood Medical
										Powder	Mead Johnson
										Liquid	Sandoz
Soybean oil		100								Liquid	Sandoz
Coconut oil		100								Liquid	Sandoz
		19	29	670	36	1414				Powder	Sandoz
										Liquid	Ross
										Powder	Ross
		11		230 mg/ 100 gm		828 mg/ 100 gm				Powder	Corpak
		19.2	8.6 mEq/ 100 gm	196 mg/ 100 gm	25.1 mEq/ 100 gm	985 mg/ 100 gm				Powder	Ross
		18	9.8 mEq/ 100 gm	22.5 100 gm	12.8 mEq/ 100 gm	500 mg/ 100 gm				Powder	Sherwood Medical
										Powder	Corpak
										Powder	Sherwood Medical
Safflower oil	3.2	3	27.5	632	33.9	1320	83.1	2000	Unflavored	Liquid	Mead Johnson
MCT, Sunflower oil	39	33	21.7	500	32.1	1250	85	2000	Unflavored	Liquid	Clintec Nutrition
MCT, corn oil	10	8.5	29	680	29	1150	83.5	1600	Vanilla	Powder	Sherwood Medical
MCT, *Oenothera biennis* oil, soya oil	39	35	30.4	699.2	32	1248	85.1	2250	Unflavored	Liquid	O'Brien Pharmaceuticals
MCT, *Oenothera biennis* oil, soya oil	39	35	43.4	998.2	42.3	1649.7	79.8	2494	Unflavored	Liquid	O'Brien Pharmaceuticals
Safflower oil	1.4	1.3	20.4	468	30	1169	86.7	1800	Unflavored	Powder	Norwich Eaton
MCT, sunflower	13.5	12	40.1	922	30	1171	85.5	2000	Unflavored	Powder	Clintec Nutrition
MCT, sunflower	13.5	12	40.1	922	30	1171	85.5	2000	Unflavored	Powder	Clintec Nutrition

Enteral Formulas*†

Fat			Na		K		Free water				
Source	gm per 1000 cal	%	mEq/L	mg/L	mEq/L	mg/L	(%)	Calories‡	Flavors	Form	Supplier
Safflower oil, MCT	10.8	9.4	20.3	467	34.2	1334	86.7	1500	Mild vanilla	Powder	Ross
Safflower oil	0.9	0.8	23	530	30	1174	86.7	3000	Unflavored	Powder	Norwich Eaton
Safflower oil	2.8	2.5	20	461	20	782	84.6	2000	Unflavored	Powder	Norwich Eaton
PH soybean oil	23.5	21.2	<15		Negligible			N/A	Varied	Powder	Kendall McGaw
PH soybean oil	2.2	2	31	710	18.2	710	94.5	891	Varied	Powder	Sandoz
PH soybean oil	30.7	27.7	<15		Negligible			82.4	Varied	Powder	Kendall McGaw
Corn oil	61.4 0.7	55.2 0.6	57 36.3	1310 835	48.6 21.4	1902 835	78.6 82	1420 840	Vanilla Fruit punch	Liquid Powder	Ross Ross
MCT, soybean oil	22.2	20	28.3	650	28.2	1100	81.8	2400	Unflavored	Powder	Sandoz
Soybean oil, MCT	42.2	38	51	1176	35.7	1386	78	3000	Vanilla	Liquid	Mead Johnson
MCT, sunflower	13.3	11.9	10.1	233	22.4	873	77		Varied	Powder	Clintec Nutrition
MCT, sunflower	13.3	11.9					70		Varied	Powder	Clintec Nutrition

Table A.4 Vitamin and Mineral Preparations Available for Tube Feeding Formulas

	Chemical Form	*Structural Form; M'f'turer*	*Contents*	*Daily Dose*
Vitamins				
Multiples				
MVI module® NutriSource	Multivitamins	Powder; Sandoz (Minneapolis, MN)	Contains 100% of RDA	1 pkt
Single				
Folic Acid	Folate	Tablet: United Research Labs (Philadelphia, PA)	1 mg/tablet (NRC-RDA = 400 mcg)	Variable
Ascorbic Acid	Vitamin C	Liquid	100 mg/ml (NRC-RDA = 60 mg)	Variable
Vitamin D	Vitamin D	Liquid; Winthrop-Bream (New York, NY)	2000 IU/drop (2 drops = NRC-RDA × 10)	Variable
Vitamin D	Vitamin D	Capsule; United Research Labs (Philadelphia, PA)	50,000 units/capsule 1.25 mg)	Variable
Vitamin B_{12}	Vitamin B_{12}	Tablet	25 mcg/tablet (3.0 mcg = NRC-RDA)	Variable
Trace Elements				
Multiples				
Trace Minerals Parenteral Patramin-6A [8]	Trace elements	Liquid; Pentcal, Inc. (Allston, MA)	Zinc 1.5 mg/ml; Copper 0.5 mg/ml; Manganese 0.2 mg/ml; Iron 28 μcg/ml; Chromium 5 μcg/ml; Selenium 25 μcg/ml	5 ml
Single				
Zinc	$ZnSO_4$	Capsule	1 capsule = 220 mg $ZnSO_4$ (50 mg Zn^{++}) (US RDA = 15 mg)	1
Minerals				
Multiples				
Mineral module Nutri-Source®	Minerals with trace elements and electrolytes (Osmolality 290 mOsm/kg)	Powder; Sandoz (Minneapolis, MN)	Contains 100% of RDA for minerals with Na^+ 56 mEq; K^+ 56 mEq; Cl^- 56 mEq	1 pkt
Mineral module Nutri-Source® (Osmolality 100 mOsm/kg)	Minerals with trace elements and electrolytes	Powder; Sandoz (Minneapolis, MN)	Contains 100% RDA for minerals and trace elements with no electrolytes (0 mEq of Na^+, K^+, and Cl^-)	1 pkt
Single				
Sodium Chloride (Table Salt)	NaCl	Powder	1 tsp = 85.5 mEq Na^+ and 85.5 mEq Cl^-	Variable
Sodium Bicarbonate	$NaHCO_3$	Tablet; Eli Lilly (Indianapolis, IN)	7.7 mEq Na^+ and 7.7 mEq HCO_3 per tablet	Variable
Potassium Chloride	KCl	Elixir; Roxane (Columbus, OH)	15 ml = 20 mEq K^+	Variable
Salt Substitute	KCl	Powder; Neocurtasal (New York, NY)	5 g KCl = 12 mEqK^+ (1 tsp.)	Variable
K-Lyte	$KHCO_3$	Tablet; Mead Johnson (Evansville, IN)	1 tablet contains 25 mEqK^+ and 25 mEq HCO_3	Variable
Calcium Neo-Calglucon®	Calcium gluconate	Red liquid; Sandoz (E. Hanover, NJ)	5 ml = 115 mg Ca^{++} (US RDA = 1000 mg)	45 ml
Magnesium Uro-Mag®	MgO	Capsule; Blaine Co. Inc. (Ft. Mitchell, KY)	140 mg MgO = 84 mg Mg^{++} (US RDA = 400 mg)	4 capsules
Phosphorus Neutraphos®	Sodium & Potassium phosphorus	Capsule; Willen Drug Co. (Baltimore, MD)	1 capsule = 250 mg P, 7 mEqNa^+, and 7 mEqK^+ (US RDA = 1000 mg	4 capsules
Iron	$FeSO_4$	Feosol elixir; Barre Drug Co. (Baltimore, MD)	5 ml $FeSO_4$ = 44 mg Fe^{+++} (US RDA = 18 mg)	2 ml

References

Abad-Lacruz A, Gonzalez-Huix F, Esteve M et al 1990 Liver function tests abnormalities in patients with inflammatory bowel disease receiving artificial nutrition: a prospective randomised study of total enteral nutrition vs total parenteral nutrition. J Parenter Enter Nutr 14: 618–621

Able R M, Beck C H Jr, Abbott W M et al 1973 Improved survival from acute renal failure after treatment with intravenous essential L-amino acids and glucose: results of a prospective double blind study. N Engl J Med 288: 695–699

Abouna G M, Veazey P R, Terry D B Jr 1974 Intravenous infusion of hydrochloric acid for treatment of severe metabolic alkalosis. Surgery 75: 194–202

Aggett P J, Thorn J M, Delves H T et al 1979 Trace element malabsorption in exocrine pancreatic insufficiency. Monogr Paediatr 10: 8–11

Albers S Wernerman J, Stehle P et al 1989 Availability of amino acids supplied by constant intravenous infusion of synthetic dipeptides in healthy man. Clinical Science 76: 643–648

Alexander J W 1990 Nutrition and translocation. J Parenter Enter Nutr 12: 170S–174S

Alexander J W, Fischer J E 1990 The Snowbird Conference on nutritional pharmacology. J Parenter Enter Nutr 14 no 5 (suppl.) 14(5): 15–259S

Alexander-Williams J 1984 Complications of gastric surgery. In: Bouchier I A D, Allan R N, Hodgson H J F, Keighley M R B (eds) The text book of gastroenterology. Baillière Tyndall, London, p 209

Alexander-Williams J, Haynes I 1985 Conservative operations for Crohn's disease of the small bowel. World J Surg 9: 945–951

Alverdy J C, Aoys E, Moss G S 1988 Total parenteral nutrition promotes bacterial translocation from the gut. Surgery 104: 185–190

Alvolio A P, Chen S G, Wang R P et al 1983 Effects of aging on changing arterial compliance and left ventricular load in a northern Chinese urban community. Circulation 68: 50–58

American Society of Parenteral and Enteral nutrition Board of Directors 1986 Guidelines for use of total parenteral nutrition in the hospitalized adult patient. J Parenter Enter Nutr 10: 441

Andersson H, Filipsson S, Hulten L 1978 Urinary oxalate excretion related to ileocolic surgery in patients with Crohn's disease. Scand J Gastroenterol 13: 465–469

Aoki T T, Finlay R J 1986 The metabolic response to fasting. In: Rombeau J L, Caldwell M D I (eds) Clinical nutrition. W B Saunders, Philadelphia, vol 2, p 11

Apelgren K N 1987 Triple lumen catheters, technological advance or setback? Am Surg 53: 113–116

Apuzzo J L, Weiss N H, Petersons V 1977 Effect of positive end expiratory pressure ventilation on intracranial pressure in man. J Neurosurg 46: 227–32

Arora N S, Rochester D F 1982 Respiratory muscle strength and maximal voluntary ventilation in undernourished patients. Am Rev Resp Dis 126: 5–8

Askanazi J, Elwyn D H, Silverberg P A et al 1980 Respiratory distress secondary to a high carbohydrate load. Surgery 87: 596–598

Backman L, Hallberg D 1974 Small-intestinal length. An intraoperative study in obesity. Acta Chir Scand 140: 57–63

Baker S P, O'Neill B, Haddon W Jr et al 1974 The injury severity score: a method for describing patients with multiple injuries and evaluating emergency care. J Trauma 14: 187–196

Baldwin E D, Cournand A, Richards D W 1958 Pulmonary insufficiency: physiological classification, clinical methods of analysis, standard values in normal subjects. Medicine 27: 243–278

Balldin G, Ohlsson K 1979 Demonstration of pancreatic protease–antiprotease complexes in the peritoneal fluid of patients with acute pancreatitis. Surgery 85: 451–456

Bambach C P, Hill G L 1982 Long term nutritional effects of extensive resection of the small intestine. Aust NZ J Surg 52: 500–506

Bambach C P, Robertson W G, Peacock M, Hill G L 1981 Effect of intestinal surgery on the risk of urinary stone formation. Gut 22: 257–263

Barbul A 1986 Arginine: biochemistry, physiology and therapeutic implications. J Parenter Enter Nutr 10: 227–238

Barbul A 1990 Arginine and immune function. Nutrition 6: S53–S58

Barbul A, Lazarou S A, Efron D T et al 1990 Arginine enhances wound healing and lymphocyte immune response in humans. Surgery 108: 331–337

Barot L R, Rombeau J L, Steinberg J J et al 1981 Energy expenditure in patients with inflammatory bowel disease. Arch Surg 116: 460–462

Barot L R, Rombeau J L, Feurer I D et al 1982 Caloric requirements in patients with inflammatory bowel disease. Ann Surg 195: 214–218

Barros D'Sa A A, Parks T G, Roy A D 1978 The problems of massive small bowel resection and difficulties encountered in management. Postgrad Med J 54: 323–7

Bartlett R H, Dechert R E, Mault J R et al 1982 Measurement of metabolism in multiple organ failure. Surgery 92: 771–9
Beach J E, Smallridge R C, Kinzer C A et al 1989 Rapid release of multiple hormones from rat pituitaries perfused with recombinant interleukin-1. Life Sci 44: 1–7
Beddoe A H, Streat S J, Hill G L 1984 Evaluation of an in vivo prompt gamma neutron activation analysis facility for body composition studies in critically ill intensive care patients: results on 41 normals. Metabolism 33: 270–280
Beddoe A H, Streat S J, Hill G L 1985 Hydration of fat free body in protein depleted patients. Am J Physiol 249 (Endocrinol Metab 12): E227–E233
Beisel W R, Sawyer W D, Ryll E D et al 1967 Metabolic effects of intracellular infections in man. Ann Intern Med 67: 744–779
Bell R C, Coalson J J, Smith J D et al 1983 Multiple organ system failure and infection in adult respiratory distress syndrome. Ann Intern Med 99: 293–298
Berg R D 1983 Translocation of indigenous bacteria from the intestinal tract. In: Hentges D J (ed) Human intestinal microflora in health and disease. Academic Press, New York
Berlin J A, Chalmers T C 1989 Meta-analysis of branched-chain amino acids in hepatic encephalopathy. Gastroenterology 97: 1043–5
Bernardier C D 1988 Role of membrane lipids in metabolic regulation. Nutr Reviews 46: 145–149
Bernstein L H, Leukhardt-Fairfield C J, Pleban W et al 1989 Usefulness of data on albumin and prealbumin concentrations in determining effectiveness of nutritional support. Clin Chem 35: 271–274
Bessey P Q 1989 Metabolic response to critical illness. In: Wilmore D W, Brennan M F, Harken A H et al (eds) Care of the surgical patient. Scientific American, New York, II: 111–23
Bessey P Q, Brooks D C, Black P R et al 1983 Epinephrine acutely mediates skeletal muscle resistance. Surgery 94: 172–9
Bessey P Q, Watters J M, Aoki T T et al 1984 Combined hormonal infusion stimulates the metabolic response to injury. Ann Surg 200: 264–281
Best W R, Becktel J M, Singleton J W et al 1976 Development of a Crohn's disease activity index. National Cooperative Crohn's disease study Gastroenterology 70: 439–44
Bianchi A 1980 Intestinal loop lengthening. A technique for increasing small intestinal length. J Pediat Surg 15: 145–51
Binder H J 1973 Fecal fatty acids: mediators of diarrhoea. Gastroenterology 65: 847–50
Birke H J, Thorlacus-Ussing O, Hesov I 1990 Trophic effect of dietary peptides on mucosa in the rat small bowel. J Parenter Enter Nutr 14: 26S
Birkhahn R H, Long C L, Fitkin B S et al 1980 Effects of major skeletal trauma on whole body protein turnover in man measured by L-14 leucine. Surgery 88: 294–300
Bistrian B R 1977 Nutritional assessment and therapy of protein calorie malnutrition in the hospital. J Am Dietet Assoc 71: 393–7
Bistrian B R 1979 A simple technique to estimate severity of stress. Surg Gynaec Obstet 148: 675–678
Bistrian B R 1990 Recent advances in parenteral and enteral nutrition: a personal perspective. J Parenter Enter Nutr 14: 329–334
Bistrian B R, Sherman M, Blackburn G L et al 1972 Cellular immunity in adult marasmus. Arch Intern Med 137: 1408–1411
Bistrian B R, Blackburn G L, Hallowell E et al 1974 Protein nutritional states of general surgical patients. JAMA 230: 838–860
Bistrian B R, Blackburn G L, Scrimshaw N J et al 1975 Cellular immunity in semistarved states in hospitalized adults. Am J Clin Nutr 28: 1148–1155
Blackburn G L, Flatt J P, Clowes G H et al 1973 Peripheral intravenous feeding with isotonic amino acid solutions. Am J Surg 125: 447–454
Blackburn G L, Williams L F, Bistrian B R et al 1976 New approaches to the management of severe acute pancreatitis. Am J Surg 131: 114–124
Bloom W 1967 Carbohydrates and water balance. Am J Clin Nutr 20: 157–162
Bonadimani B, Sperti C, Stevanin A et al 1987 Central venous catheter guidewire replacement according to the seldinger technique: usefulness in the management of patients on total parenteral nutrition. J Parenter Enter Nutr 11: 267–270
Bone R C 1991 Sepsis, the sepsis syndrome, multiorgan failure: a plea for comparable definitions. Ann Intern Med 114: 332–333
Boop F A, Andrassy R J, Brown W E et al 1985 Excessive nitrogen losses in severe brain injury. Neurosurgery 16: 725
Border J, Hassett J, La Duca J et al 1987 The gut origin septic states in blunt multiple trauma (ISS = 40) in the ICU. Ann Surg 206: 427–448
Borgstrom B, Dahlquist A, Lundh G, Sjovall J 1957 Studies of intestinal digestion and absorption in the human. J Clin Invest 36: 1521
Bounous G 1990 The intestinal factor in multiple organ failure and shock. Surgery 107: 118–119
Bower R H 1990a A unique enteral formula as adjunctive therapy for septic and critically ill patients. Multicentre study design and rationale. Nutrition 16: 92–95
Bower R H 1990b Nutritional and metabolic support in critically ill patients. J Parenter Enter Nutr 14: 257S–259S
Bower R H, Muggia Sullam M, Vallgren S et al 1986a Branched chain amino acid-enriched solutions in the septic patient: a randomised prospective trial. Ann Surg 203: 13–21
Bower R H, Talamini M A, Sax H C et al 1986b Postoperative enteral vs parenteral nutrition. Arch Surg 121: 1040–5
Boyd J B, Bradford B Jr, Watne A L 1980 Operative risk factors of colon resection in the elderly. Ann Surg 192: 743–746
Bradley J A, King R F J G, Schorah C J, Hill G L 1978 Vitamins in intravenous feeding — a study of water soluble vitamins and folate in critically ill patients receiving intravenous nutrition. Br J Surg 65: 492–494
Branicki F J, Coleman S Y, Fok P J et al 1990 Bleeding peptic ulcer: a prognostic evaluation of risk factors for rebleeding and death. World J Surg 14: 262–270
Brennan M F 1977 Uncomplicated starvation versus cancer cachexia. Cancer Res 37: 2359–2364
Brennan M F, Cerra F, Daly J M et al 1986 Report of a workshop: branched-chain amino acids in stress injury. J Parenter Enter Nutr 10: 446

Brinson R R, Curtis W D, Singh M 1987 Diarrhoea in the intensive care unit: the role of hypoalbuminaemia and the response to a chemically defined diet (case reports and review of the literature). J Am Coll Nutr 6: 517–523

Bristol J B, Williamson R C 1985 Postoperative adaptation of the small intestine. World J Surg 9: 825–832

British Medical Journal Editorial 1980 Corticosteroids and hypothalmic pituitary adrenocortical function. Br Med J 1: 813–814

Brooke B N, Cave D R, Gurry J F et al 1977 Crohn's disease. Macmillan, London.

Browning J A, Linberg S E, Turney S Z et al 1982 The effects of a fluctuating FIO_2 on metabolic measurements in mechanically ventilated patients. Crit Care Med 10: 82

Burke D J, Alverdy J C, Aoys E, Moss G S 1989 Glutamine-supplemented TPN improves gut immune function. Arch Surg 124: 1396–1399

Buzby G P 1990 Perioperative nutritional support. J Parenter Enter Nutr 14: 197S–199S

Buzby G P, Mullen J L, Mathews D C et al 1980 Prognostic nutritional index in gastrointestinal surgery. Am J Surg 139: 160–167

Buzby G P, Knox L S, Crosby O et al 1988 Study protocol: a randomized clinical trial of total parenteral nutrition in malnourished surgical patients. Am J Clin Nutr 47: 366–381

Buzby G P and the *Veterans Affairs* Total Parenteral Nutrition Co-operative Study Group 1991 Perioperative total parenteral nutrition in surgical patients. N Engl J Med 325: 525–532

Byrne W J, Ament M E, Burke M et al 1979 Home parenteral nutrition. Surg Gynaec Obstet 149: 593–599

Cahill G F 1970 Starvation in man. N Engl J Med 282: 668–675

Canizaro P C, Prager M D, Shires G T 1971 The infusion of Ringer's lactate solution during shock: changes in lactate, excess lactate, and pH. Am J Surg 122: 494

Carlsson M, Nordenstrom J, Hedenstierna G 1984 Clinical implications of continuous measurement of energy expenditure in mechanically ventilated patients. Clin Nutr 3: 103

Carpentier Y A 1988 Carbohydrate and fat metabolism. In: Kinney J M, Jeejeebhoy K N, Hill G L, Owen O E (eds) Nutrition and metabolism in patient care. W B Saunders, Philadelphia, p 666–671

Carpentier Y A 1990 Intravascular metabolism of fat emulsions. Clin Sci

Carr N D, Pullen B R, Hasleton P S et al 1984 Microvascular studies in human radiation bowel disease. Gut 25: 448–454

Celli B R, Rodriguez K S, Snider G L 1984 A controlled trial of intermittent positive pressure breathing, incentive spirometry and deep breathing exercises in preventing pulmonary complications. Am Rev Resp Dis 130: 12

Cerra F B 1990 How nutrition intervention changes what getting sick means. J Parenter Enter Nutr 14: 164S–169S

Cerra F B, Lehman S, Konstantinidis N et al 1990 Effect of enteral nutrient on in vitro tests of immune function in ICU patients: a preliminary report. Nutrition 6: 84–87

Charlson M E, MacKenzie C R, Gold J P et al 1990 Preoperative blood pressure: what patterns identify patients at risk of postoperative complications? Ann Surg 212: 567–580

Chen M K, Salloum R M, Austgen T R et al 1991 Tumour regulation of hepatic glutamine metabolism. J Parenter Enter Nutr 15: 159–164

Christenson T, Bendix T, Kehlet H 1982 Fatigue and cardiorespiratory function following abdominal surgery. Br J Surg 69: 417–419

Christiansen T, Kehlet H 1984 Postoperative fatigue and changes in nutritional status. Br J Surg 71: 473

Christie P M, Hill G L 1990a Effect of intravenous nutrition and function in acute attacks of inflammatory bowel disease. Gastroenterology 99: 730–736

Christie P M, Hill G L 1990b Return to normal body composition after ileo-anal J pouch anastomosis for ulcerative colitis. Dis Colon and Rectum 33: 584–586

Christie P M, Knight G S, Hill G L 1990 Metabolism of body water and electrolytes after surgery for ulcerative colitis: conventional ileostomy versus J pouch. Br J Surg 77: 149–151

Church J M, Hill G L 1987 Assessing the efficacy of intravenous nutrition in general surgical patients — dynamic nutritional assessment with plasma proteins. J Parenter Enter Nutr 11: 135–139

Church J M, Choong S Y, Hill G L 1984 Abnormalities of muscle metabolism and histology in malnourished patients awaiting surgery: effects of a course of intravenous nutrition. Br J Surg 71: 563–569

Clague M B, Keir M J, Wright P D et al 1983 The effects of nutrition and trauma on whole body protein metabolism in man. Clin Sci 65: 165

Clark J, Walker W F 1983 Acid-base problems in surgery. World J Surg 7: 590–598

Clifton G L, Robertson C S, Grossman R G et al 1984 The metabolic response to severe head injury. J Neurosurg 60: 687

Cogen R, Weinrijb J 1989 Aspiration pneumonia in nursing home patients fed via gastrostomy tubes. Am J Gastro 84: 1509–1512

Cohen J, Glauser M P 1991 Septic shock-treatment. Lancet 338: 736–739

Cohn S H, Vaswani A, Zanzi I et al 1976 Changes in body chemical composition with age measured by total body neutron activation. Metabolism 25: 85–95

Cohn V H 1975 Vitamin K and vitamin E. In: Goodman L S, Gillman A (eds) The pharmacological basis of therapeutics. MacMillan, New York, p 1591–1600

Collins J P, Oxby C B, Hill G L 1978 Intravenous amino acids and intravenous hyperalimentation as protein-sparing therapy after major surgery. A controlled clinical trial. Lancet 1: 788–799

Collins J P, McCarthy I D, Hill G L 1979 Assessment of protein nutrition in surgical patients — the value of anthropometrics. Am J Clin Nutr 32: 1527–1530

Compston J E, Ayers A B, Horton L W L et al 1978 Osteomalacia after small-intestinal resection. Lancet 1: 9–12

Copeland E M 1990 Total parenteral nutrition in the cancer patient: the present as viewed from the past. J Parenter Enter Nutr 6: 25–35

Covelli H D, Black J W, Olsen M S et al 1981 Respiratory failure precipitated by high carbohydrate loads. Ann Intern Med 95: 579–581

Craig R P, Tweedle D, Davidson H A et al 1977 Intravenous glucose, amino acids, and fat in the postoperative period. A controlled evaluation of each substrate. Lancet II: 8–11

Crane M G, Harris J J 1976 Effect of aging on renin activity and aldosterone excretion. J Lab Clin Med 87: 947–959

Crass R A, Meyer A A, Jeffrey R B et al 1985 Pancreatic abscess: impact of computerized tomography on early diagnosis and surgery. Am J Surg 150: 127–131

Cruickshank A M, Fraser W D, Burns H J G et al 1990 Response of serum interleukin-6 in patients undergoing elective surgery of varying intensity. Clin Sci 79: 161–165

Cunningham J N Jr, Carter N W, Rector F C et al 1971 Resting transmembrane potential difference of skeletal muscle in normal subjects and severely ill patients. J Clin Invest 50: 49

Curran F T, Hill G L 1990 Failure of nutritional therapy after total gastrectomy. Br J Surg 77: 1015–1017

Curran F T, Stokes M A, Hill G L 1990 Long term changes in body composition after pancreaticoduodenectomy. J Roy Col Surg Edin 36: 32–34

Cuschieri A 1991 Personal communication

Cuthbertson D P 1932 Observations on the disturbance of metabolism produced by injury to the limbs. Q J Med 1: 233–246

Daly J M, Lieberman M, Goldfine M S et al 1992 Enteral nutrition with supplemental arginine, RNA and omega-3 fatty acids — a prospective clinical trial. Surgery (in press)

Daly J M, Reynolds J, Thom A et al 1982 Immune and metabolic effects of arginine in the surgical patient. Ann Surg 208(4): 512–523

Daly J M, Shearer J D, Mastrofrancesco B et al 1990 Glucose metabolism in injured tissue: a longitudinal study. Surgery 107: 187–192

Darmaun D, Messing B, Just B et al 1991 Glutamine metabolism after small intestinal resection in humans. Metabolism 40: 42–44

Debongnie J C, Phillips S F 1978 Capacity of the human colon to absorb fluid. Gastroenterology 74: 698–703

D'Egidio A, Schein M 1991 Surgical strategies in the treatment of pancreatic necrosis and infection. Br J Surg 78: 133–137

Deitch E A, Berg R, Specian R 1987 Endotoxin promotes the translocation of bacteria from the gut. Arch Surg 122: 185–190

Del Guercio L R, Cohn J D 1980 Monitoring operative risk in the elderly. JAMA 243: 1350–1355

Derogatis L R 1978 SCL-90. Administration, scoring and procedures manual. Johns Hopkins University, Baltimore

Detsky A S, Baker J P, O'Rourke K et al 1987a Perioperative nutrition: a meta-analysis. Ann Intern Med 107: 195–203

Detsky A S, McLaughlin J R, Baker P et al 1987b What is subjective global assessment of nutritional status? J Parenter Enter Nutr 11: 7

Dickhaut S C, DeLee J C, Page C R 1984 Nutritional status: importance in predicting wound healing after amputation. J Bone Joint Surg 66A: 71–75

Dickinson R J, Ashton M G, Axon A T R et al 1980 Controlled trial of intravenous hyperalimentation and total bowel rest as an adjunct to the routine therapy of acute colitis. Gastroenterology 79: 1199–1204

DiMagno E P, Go V L W, Summerskill W H 1973 Relations between pancreatic enzyme outputs and malabsorption in severe pancreatic insufficiency. N Engl J Med 288: 813–15

Dobb G, Towler S 1990 Diarrhoea during enteral feeding in the critically ill; a comparison of the feeds with and without fibre. Intensive Care Med 16: 252–255

Donahue S P, Phillips L S 1989 Response of IGF-I to nutritional support in malnourished hospital patients. A possible indicator of short term changes in nutritional status. Am J Clin Nutr 50: 962–969

Douglas R G, Humberstone D A, Haystead A et al 1990 Metabolic effects of recombinant human growth hormone: isotopic studies in the post absorptive state during total parenteral nutrition. Br J Surg 77: 785–790

Douglas R G, Shaw J H F 1989 Metabolic response to sepsis and trauma. Br J Surg 76: 115–122

Douglas R G, Shaw J H F 1990 Metabolic effects of cancer. Br J Surg 77: 246–254

Doweiko J P, Nompleggi D J 1991 Role of albumin in human physiology and pathophysiology. J Parenter Enter Nutr 15: 207–211

Dowling R H 1982 Small bowel adaptation and its regulation. Scand J Gastroenterol 74: 53–74

Downs J B, Douglas M E 1982 Applied physiology and respiratory care. In: Shoemaker W C, Thompson W L (eds) Critical care — state of the art. Society of Critical Care Medicine, Fullerton, California, vol 3

Driscoll R H Jr, Rosenberg I H 1978 Total parenteral nutrition in inflammatory bowel disease. Med Clin North Am 62: 185–201

Drucker W R, Chadwick C D, Gann D S 1981 Transcapillary refill in haemorrhage and shock. Arch Surg 116: 1344–53

Dudrick S J, Copeland E M 1973 Parenteral hyperalimentation. In: Nyhus L M (ed) Surgery annual. Appleton-Century-Crofts, New York

Dudrick S J, Wilmore D W, Vars H M et al 1968 Long-term total parenteral nutrition with growth development and positive nitrogen balance. Surgery 64: 134–141

Dudrick S J, O'Donnell J J, Englert D M et al 1984 100 patient years of ambulatory home total parenteral nutrition. Ann Surg 199: 770–781

Dunn D L 1988 Antibody immunotherapy of Gram-negative bacterial sepsis in an immunosuppressed animal model. Transplantation 45: 424–429

Durnin J G V A, Passmore R 1967 Energy, work and leisure. Heinemann Educational Books, London

Durnin J G V A, Womersley J 1974 Body fat assessed from total body density and its estimation from skinfold thickness — measurements on 481 men and women aged from 16–72 years. Br J Nutr 32: 77–97

Dutta S K, Bustin M T, Russel R M et al 1982 Deficiency of fat soluble vitamins in treated patients with pancreatic insufficiency. Ann Intern Med 97: 549–552

Edelman I S, Leibman J, O'Meara M P et al 1958 Interrelations between serum sodium concentration, serum osmolarity and total exchangeable sodium, total exchangeable potassium and total body water. J Clin Invest 37: 1236–56

Edelman I S, Leibman J 1959 Anatomy of body water and electrolytes. Am J Med 27: 256–277

Edes T E, Walk B E, Austin J L 1990 Diarrhoea in tube-fed patients: feeding formula not necessarily the cause. Am J Med 88: 91–93

Edgahl R H 1959 Pituitary response following trauma to the isolated leg. Surgery 46: 9

Egbert L D, Battit G E, Welch C E et al 1964 Reduction of postoperative pain by encouragement and instruction of patients — a study of doctor–patient rapport. N Engl J Med 270: 825–7

Ellis H 1986 Pyloric stenosis. In: Nyhus L M, Wastell C (eds) Surgery of the stomach and duodenum. 4th edn. Little Brown, Boston, p 475–490

Elmore M F, Gallagher S C, Jones J G et al 1989 Esophagogastric decompression and enteral feeding following cholecystectomy: a controlled randomised prospective trial. J Parenter Enter Nutr 13: 377–381

Elwyn D H 1980 Nutritional requirements of adult surgical patients. Crit Care Med 8: 9–20

Endres S, Ghorbani R, Kelley V E et al 1989 The effect of dietary supplementation with n-3 polyunsaturated fatty acids on the synthesis of Interleukin-1 and tumour necrosis factor by mononuclear cells. N Engl J Med 320: 256–271

Espevik T, Brockhaus M, Loetscher H et al 1990 Characterization of binding and biological effects of monoclonal antibodies against a human tumor necrosis factor receptor. J Exp Med 171: 415–426

Exley A R, Cohen J, Bourman W A et al 1990 Monoclonal antibody to TNF in severe septic shock. Lancet 335: 1275–1277

Fagerman K E 1988 Drug compatibilities with enteral feeding solutions coadministered by tube. Nutr Supp Serv 8: 31–32

Falchuk K H, Peterson L, McNeil B J 1985 Microparticulate-induced phlebitis. Its prevention by in-line filtration. N Engl J Med 312: 78–82

Fauci A S, Dale D C, Balow J E 1976 Glucocorticoid therapy: mechanisms of action and clinical considerations. Ann Intern Med 84: 304–315

Feinstein E I, Blumenkrantz M J, Healy M et al 1981 Clinical and metabolic responses to parenteral nutrition in acute renal failure: a controlled double-blind study. Medicine (Baltimore) 60: 124–37

Fekete F, Belghiti J 1988 Nutritional factors and oesophageal resection. In: Jamieson G G (ed) Surgery of the oesophagus. Churchill Livingstone, Edinburgh, p 119–124

Feller A, Rudman D, Caindec N 1989 Comparison of nutritional efficacy of peptamin and vivonex TEN elemental diets in elderly tube fed subjects. J Parenter Enter Nutr 13: 12S

Fischer J E 1984 Adjuvant parenteral nutrition in the patient with cancer. Surgery 96: 578–80

Fisher C J Jr, Zimmerman J, Khazaeli M B et al 1990 Initial evaluation of human monoclonal antilipid A antibody (HA-1A) in patients with sepsis syndrome. Crit Care Med 18: 1311–1315

Flear C T, Bhattacharya S S, Singh C M 1980 Solute and water exchanges between cells and extracellular fluids in health and disturbances after trauma. J Parenter Enter Nutr 4: 98–120

Flint J M 1912 The effect of extensive resection of the small intestine. Johns Hopkins Hosp Bull Balt 23: 127–144

Flint L M, Cryer H M, Simpson C J et al 1984 Microcirculatory norepinephrine constrictor response in hemorrhagic shock. Surgery 96: 240–7

Flores E A, Bistrian B R, Pomposelli J J et al 1989 Infusion of tumour necrosis factor/cachectin promotes muscle catabolism in the rat. A synergistic effect with interleukin. J Clin Invest 83: 1614–1622

Foley E F, Borlase B C, Dzik W H et al 1990 Albumin supplementation in the critically ill. A prospective randomized trial. Arch Surg 125: 739–742

Fong Y, Marano M A, Barber A et al 1989a Total parenteral nutrition and bowel rest modify the metabolic response to endotoxin in humans. Ann Surg 210: 449–457

Fong Y, Moldawer L L, Marano M et al 1989b Endotoxaemia elicits increased circulating beta 2-IFN/IL-6 in man. J Immunol 142: 2321–2324

Fong Y, Lowry S F 1990a Cytokines and the cellular response to injury and infection. In: Care of the surgical patient — part iv. American College of Surgeons, vol I, ch 7: 1–17

Fong Y, Lowry S F 1990b Tumor necrosis factor in the pathophysiology of infection and sepsis. Clin Immunol Immunopathol 55: 157–170

Foschi D, Cavagna G, Callioni F et al 1986 Hyperalimentation of jaundiced patients on percutaneous transhepatic biliary drainage. Br J Surg 73: 716–719

Fox A D, Kripke S A, De Paula J et al 1988 Effect of a glutamine-supplemented enteral diet on methotrexate-induced enterocolitis. J Parenter Enter Nutr 12: 325–331

Freeman J B, Fairful-Smith R J 1983 Physical approach to peripheral parenteral nutrition. In: Fischer J G (ed) Surgical nutrition. Little Brown, Boston, p 703–717

French J M, Crane C W 1963 Undernutrition, malnutrition and malabsorption after gastrectomy. In: Stammers F A R, Alexander-Williams J Postgastrectomy complications and metabolic consequences. Butterworths, London

Frenk S, Metcoff J, Gonez F et al 1957 Intracellular composition and hemostatic mechanisms in severe chronic infantile malnutrition. Paediatrics 20: 105–20

Fried G M, Odgen W D, Rhea A et al 1982 Pancreatic protein secretion and gastrointestinal hormone release in response to parenteral amino acids and lipids in dogs. Surgery 92: 902–905

Fried R C, Mullen J, Stein T P et al 1985 The effects of glucose and amino acids on tumour and host DNA synthesis. J Surg Res 39: 461–469

Friedberg C E, Koomans H A, Bijlsma J A et al 1991 Sodium retention by insulin may depend on decreased plasma potassium. Metabolism 40: 201–204

Furst P, Albers S, Stehle P et al 1989 Availability of glutamine supplied intravenously as alanylglutamine. Metabolism 38: 67–72

Galland R B, Spencer J 1986 Surgical management of radiation enteritis. Surgery 99: 133–138

Gann D S, Lilly M P 1983 The neuroendocrine response to multiple trauma. World J Surg 7: 101–118

Gann D S, Lilly M P 1984 Prog Crit Care Med 1, 17

Gauderer M W L, Ponsky J L 1980 A simplified technique for constructing a tube feeding gastrostomy. Surg Gynaec Obstet 152: 83–85

Gerson M C, Hurst J M, Hertzberg V S et al 1985 Cardiac prognosis in noncardiac geriatric surgery. Ann Intern Med 103: 832–837

Gil R T, Kruse J A, Thill-Baharozian M D et al 1989 Triple vs single lumen central venous catheters. A prospective study in a critically ill population. Arch Intern Med 149: 1139–1143

Glauser M P, Zanetti G, Baumgartner J-D, Cohen J 1991 Septic shock: pathogenesis. Lancet 338: 732–736

Goligher J C 1971 Resection and exteriorisation in the management of faecal fistulas originating in the small intestine Br J Surg 58: 163–7

Goligher J C 1984 Surgery of the anus, rectum and colon. 5th edn. Baillière Tindall, London, p 971–1017

Gorey T F 1980 The recovery of intestine after ischaemic injury. Br J Surg 67: 699—702

Gough D B 1991 Educate the phagocyte. Br J Surg 78: 1–2

Grant J P, James S, Grabowski V et al 1984 Total parenteral nutrition in pancreatic disease. Ann Surg 200: 627–631

Greenberg G R, Wolman S L, Christofides N D et al 1981 Effect of total parenteral nutrition on gut hormone release in humans. Gastroenterology 80: 988–993

Greenberg G R, Fleming C R, Jeejeebhoy K N et al 1988 Controlled trial of bowel rest and nutritional support in the management of Crohn's disease. Gut 29: 1309–1315

Griffen G E, Fagan E F, Hodgson H J et al 1982 Enteral therapy in the management of massive gut resection complicated by chronic fluid and electrolyte depletion. Dig Dis Sci 27: 902–908

Grube B J, Gamelli R L, Foster R S 1985 Refeeding differentially affects tumour and host cell proliferation. J Surg Res 339: 535–542

Hack C E, Nuijens J H, Strack van Schijndel R J M et al 1990 A model for the interplay of inflammatory mediators in sepsis: a study in 48 patients. Intens Care Med (suppl. 3) 16: S187–S191

Hackett A F, Yeung C K, Hill G L 1979 Eating patterns in patients recovering from major surgery: a study in voluntary food intake and energy balance. Br J Surg 66: 415–418

Hadley S A, Fitzsimmons L 1990 Nutrition and wound healing. Top Clin Nutr 5: 72

Hamamoui E, Lefkowitz R, Olender L et al 1990 Enteral nutrition in the early postoperative period: a new semi elemental formula versus total parenteral nutrition. J Parenter Enter Nutr 14: 501–507

Hammarquist F, Wernerman J, Ali R et al 1989 Addition of glutamine to total parenteral nutrition after elective abdominal surgery spares free glutamine in muscle, counteracts the fall in muscle protein synthesis and improved nitrogen balance. Ann Surg 209: 455–461

Harris P E, Kendall-Taylor P 1989 Steroid therapy and surgery. Current Practice in Surgery 1: 165–169

Hartwell J A, Hoguet J P 1912 Experimental intestinal obstruction in dogs with special reference to the cause of death and the treatment by large amounts of normal saline solution. J Am Med Assn 59: 82–87

Hauer-Jensen M 1990 Later radiation injury of the small intestine. Clinical pathophysiological and radiological aspects — a review. Acta Oncol 29: 401–415

Hawker P C, Givel J C, Keighley M R B et al 1983 Management of enterocutaneous fistulas in Crohn's disease. Gut 24: 284–7

Haydock D A, Hill G L 1986 Impaired wound healing in surgical patients with varying degrees of malnutrition. J Parenter Enter Nutr 10: 550–554

Haydock D A, Hill G L 1987 Improved wound healing response in surgical patients receiving intravenous nutrition. Br J Surg 74: 320–323

Haydock D A, Flint M H, Hyde K F et al 1988 The efficacy of subcutaneous Goretex implants in monitoring wound healing response in experimental protein deficiency. Connective Tissue Research 17: 159–169

Haymond H E 1935 Massive resection of the small intestine. Analysis of 257 collected cases Surg Gynaec Obstet 61: 693–701

Hedderich G S, Wexler M J, McLean A P et al 1986 The septic abdomen: open management with Marlex mesh with a zipper. Surgery 99: 399–408

Helderman J H, Vestal R E, Rowe J W et al 1978 The response of arginine vasopressin to intravenous ethanol and hypertonic saline in man: the impact of aging. J Gerontol 33: 39–47

Herskowitz K, Souba W W 1990 Intestinal glutamine metabolism during critical illness: a surgical perspective. Nutrition 6: 199–206

Hessov I, Allen J, Arendt K, Gravhort L 1977 Infusion thrombophlebitis in a surgical department. Acta Chir Scand 143: 151–154

Heymsfield S B, Williams P J 1988 Nutritional assessment by clinical and biochemical methods. In: Shils M E, Young V R (eds) Modern nutrition in health and disease, 7th edn. Lea & Febiger, Philadelphia, ch 45: 823–824

Heymsfield S B, Bethel R A, Ansley J D et al 1978 Cardiac abnormalities in cachetic patients before and during nutritional repletion. Am Heart J 95: 584–594

Heymsfield S B, Wang J, Heshka S et al 1989 Dual photon absorptiometry: comparison of bone mineral and soft tissue mass measurements in vivo with established methods. Am J Clin Nutr 49: 1283–89

Heys S D, Park K G M, McNurlan M A et al 1991 Stimulation of protein synthesis in human tumours by parenteral nutrition: evidence for modulation of tumour growth. Br J Surg 78: 483–487

Hiatt J R, Fink A S, King W et al 1985 Percutaneous aspiration of peripancreatic fluid collections: a safe and effective diagnostic technique. Dig Dis Sci 30: 974

Hill G L 1976 Ileostomy, surgery, physiology and management. Grune & Stratton, New York

Hill G L 1986 Massive enterectomy: indications and management. World J Surg 9: 833–841

Hill G L 1988 A transhiatal subdiaphragmatic distal oesophageal resection. In: Jamieson G G (ed) Surgery of the oesophagus. Churchill Livingstone, Edinburgh, ch 72: 659–663

Hill G L, Bambach C P 1981 A technique for operative closure of persistent external small-bowel fistulas. Aust NZ J Surgery 51: 477–485

Hill G L, Bambach C P 1983 Metabolic consequences of ileostomies in: Williams J A, Binder H J (eds) Large intestine. Gastroenterology. Butterworths, London, p 121–134

Hill G L, Mair W S J, Goligher J C 1975a Cause and management of high volume output salt depleting ileostomy. Br J Surg 62: 720–726

Hill G L, Mair W S J, Goligher J C 1975b Gallstones after ileostomy and ileal resection. Gut 16: 932–936

Hill G L, Mair W S J, Edwards J P, Morgan D B, Goligher J C 1975c Effect of a chemically defined liquid elemental diet on composition and volume of ileal fistula drainage. Gastroenterology 68: 676–682

Hill G L, Mair W S J, Edwards J P, Goligher J C 1976 Decreased trypsin and bile acids in ileal fistula drainage during the administration of a chemically defined liquid elemental diet. Br J Surg 63: 133–136

Hill G L, Blackett R L, Pickford I R, Bradley J A 1977a A survey of protein nutrition in patients with inflammatory bowel disease — a rational basis for nutritional therapy. Br J Surg 64: 894–896

Hill G L, Blackett R L, Pickford I et al 1977b Malnutrition in surgical patients. An unrecognized problem. Lancet I: 689–692

Hill G L, King R F G J, Smith R C et al 1979a

Multielement analysis of the living body by neutron activation analysis — application to critically ill patients receiving intravenous nutrition. Br J Surg 66: 868–872
Hill G L, Millward S F, King R F G J, Smith R C 1979b Normal ileostomy output: close relation to body size. Br Med J 2: 831–832
Hill G L, Pickford I R 1979 A new appliance for collecting ileostomy and jejunostomy fluid in the postoperative period Br J Surg 66: 203–206
Hill G L, Bourchier R G, Witney G B 1988 Surgical and metabolic management of patients with external fistulas of the small intestine associated with Crohn's disease. World J Surg 12: 191–197
Hill G L, Witney G B, Christie P M, Church J M 1991 Protein status and metabolic expenditure determine the response to intravenous nutrition — a new classification of surgical malnutrition. Br J Surg 78: 109–113
Hill G L, Douglas R G, Schroeder D S 1992 Metabolic basis of management of patients undergoing uncomplicated major surgery. World J Surg (in press)
Hoare A M, McLeish A, Thompson H et al 1977 Hydrotalcite in the treatment of bile vomiting. Br J Surg 64: 849–850
Hoffer L J 1988 Starvation. In: Shils M E, Young V R (eds) Modern nutrition in health and disease. Lea & Febiger, Philadelphia, p 774–794
Hofman A F, Poley J R 1972 Role of bile acid malabsorption in the pathogenesis of diarrhoea and steatorrhoea in patients with ileal resection. I. Response to cholestyramine or replacement of dietary long chain triglycerides by medium chain triglycerides. Gastroenterology 62: 918–934
Hogan R B, De Marco D C, Hamilton J K et al 1986 Percutaneous endoscopic gastrostomy — to push or pull, a prospective randomised trial. Gastrointest Endosc 32: 253
Holbling N, Funovics J, Rothe et al 1982 Amino acid metabolism in acute necrotising pancreatitis. Aspects of parenteral nutrition. In: Hollander L F (ed) Controversies in acute pancreatitis. Springer-Verlag, Berlin, p 297–301
Hudson-Goodman P, Girard N, Jones M B 1990 Wound repair and potential use of growth factors. Heart Lung 19: 379–386
Humberstone D A, Shaw J H F 1988 Metabolism in haematologic malignancy. Cancer 62: 1619–1624
Hume D M, Egdahl R H 1959 The importance of the brain in the endocrine response to injury. Ann Surg 150: 697–712
Hyde D, Floch M H 1984 The effect of peripheral nutritional support and nitrogen balance in acute pancreatitis. Gastroenterology 86: 1119
Imrie C W, Blumgart L 1975 Acute pancreatitis: a prospective study on some factors in mortality. Bulletin de la Societé Internationale de Chirurgie 6: 601–603
Imrie C W, Shearer M G 1986 Diagnosis and management of severe acute pancreatitis. In: Russell R C G (ed) Recent advances in surgery 12. Churchill Livingstone, Edinburgh, p 143–154
Inculet R I, Finlay R I, Duff J H et al 1986 Insulin decreases muscle protein loss after operative trauma in man. Surgery 99: 752–8
Irving M 1983 Assessment and management of external fistulas in Crohn's disease. Br J Surg 70: 233–6
Isaksson B, Edlund Y, Gelin L E et al 1959 The value of protein enriched diet in patients with peptic ulcer. Acta Chir Scand 118: 418–427
Iwaki Y, Starzl T E, Yagihashi A et al 1991 Replacement of donor lymphoid tissue in small bowel transplants. Lancet 337: 818–819
Jeejeebhoy K N 1983 Therapy of the short gut syndrome. Lancet I: 1427–1430
Jeejeebhoy K N 1986 Muscle function and nutrition. Gut 27: 25–39
Jeejeebhoy K N 1988 Bulk or bounce — the object of nutritional support. J Parenter Enter Nutr 12: 539–549
Jensen G L, Mascioli E A, Seidner D L et al 1990 Parenteral infusion of long and medium chain triglycerides and reticuloendothelial system function in man. J Parenter Enter Nutr 14: 467–471
Jiang Z-M, He G Z, Zhang S-Y et al 1989 Low dose growth hormone and hypocaloric nutrition attenuate the protein catabolic response after major operation. Ann Surg 210: 513–24
Johnson C D, Ellis H 1990 Gastric outlet obstruction now predicts malignancy. Br J Surg 77: 1023–1024
Johnston I D A, Welbourne R, Acheson K 1958 Gastrectomy and loss of weight. Lancet I: 1242–1245
Jones M, Santanello S O, Falconer R E 1990 Percutaneous endoscopic vs surgical gastrostomy. J Parenter Enter Nutr 14: 533–534
Jones N J M, Lees R, Andrews J et al 1983 Comparison of an elemental and polymeric enteral diet in patients with normal gastrointestinal function. Gut 24:78–84
Jones P F 1987 Intraoperative techniques in small bowel obstruction without associated vascular impairments. In: Fielding L P, Welch J P (eds) Intestinal obstruction. Churchill Livingstone, Edinburgh, p 110
Katz A I, Hollingsworth D R, Epstein F H 1968 Influence of carbohydrate and protein on sodium excretion during fasting and refeeding. J Lab Clin Med 72: 93–104
Keck Jones L, Claxton B, Concepcion J et al 1991 Measured versus predicted energy expenditure in adults receiving TPN. Abstract ASPEN, Clinical Conference Proceedings 93: 384
Kehlet H 1975 A rational approach to dosage and preparation of parenteral glucocorticoid substitution therapy during surgical procedures: a short review. Acta Anaesthesiol Scand 19: 260–264
Kehlet H 1987 Modification of responses to surgery and anaesthesia by neural blockade. In: Cousins M J, Bridenhagh P O (eds) Clinical anaesthesia and management of pain. J B Lippincott, Philiadelphia
Kehlet H, Binder C 1973 Adrenocortical function and clinical course during and after surgery in unsupplemented glucocorticoid-treated patients. Br J Anaesth 45: 1043–1048
Kelly G A, Nahrwold D L 1976 Pancreatic secretion in response to an elemental diet and intravenous hyperalimentation. Surg Gynaec Obstet 143: 87–91
Keys A, Brozek J, Henschel A et al 1950 The biology of human starvation. University of Minnesota Press, Minneapolis vol I: 129
Khazaeli M B, Wheeler R, Rogers K et al 1990 Initial evaluation of a human immunoglobulin M monoclonal antibody (HA-1A) in humans. J Biol Response Mod 9: 178–184
King R F G J, Collins J P, Morgan D B, Hill G L 1978 Muscle chemistry of critically ill surgical patients and the effects of a course of intravenous nutrition. Br J Surg 65: 495–498

King R F G J, MacFie J, Hill G L, Smith R C 1981 Effect of intravenous nutrition, with glucose as the only calorie source, on muscle glycogen. J Parenter Enter Nutr 5: 226–229

Kingsworth A N, Slavin J 1991 Peptide growth factors and wound healing. Br J Surg 78: 1286–1290

Kinney J M, Lister J, Moore F D 1963 Relationship of energy expenditure to total exchangeable potassium. Ann N Y Academy Sci 110: 711–722

Kinney J M, Long C L, Gump F E et al 1968 Tissue composition of weight loss in surgical patients I: Elective operation. Ann Surg 168: 459–74

Kinney J M, Furst P 1988 The intensive care patient — energy metabolism. In: Kinney J M, Jeejeebhoy K M, Hill G L, Owen O E (eds) Nutrition and metabolism in patient care, p 657–661

Kinney J M 1990 Clinical biochemistry: implications for nutritional support. J Parenter Enter Nutr 14: 148S–156S

Kirby R R, Downs J B, Civetta J M et al 1975 High level positive end expiratory pressure (PEEP) in acute respiratory insuffiency. Chest 67: 156–63

Klidjian A M, Archer T J, Foster K J et al 1982 Detection of dangerous malnutrition. J Parenter Enter Nutr 6: 119–121

Klimberg V S, Souba W W, Dolson D et al 1990 Prophylactic glutamine protects the intestinal mucosa from radiation injury. Cancer 66(1): 62–68

Knaus W A, Draper E A, Wagner D P et al 1985 APACHE II: a severity of disease classification system. Crit Care Med 13: 818–829

Knight G S, Beddoe A H, Streat S J, Hill G L 1986 Body composition of two human cadavers by neutron activation and chemical analysis. Am J Physiol 250 (Endocrinol Metab 13): E179–E185

Kobayashi T, Kesselly B, Wilmore D et al 1991 Starvation reduces high energy phosphate stores, work efficiency and oxidative capacity in skeletal muscle. Scientific Abstract 11, 15th Clinical Congress American Society of Parenteral and Enteral Nutrition, p 402

Konstantinides F N, Konstantinides N N, Li J C et al 1991 Urinary urea nitrogen: too insensitive for calculating nitrogen balance studies in surgical clinical nutrition. J Parenter Enter Nutr 15: 189–193

Kozarek R A, Patterson D J, Gelfund M D et al 1989 Methotrexate induces clinical and histologic remission in patients with refractory inflammatory bowel disease. Ann Intern Med 110: 353–356

Krieger M 1929 Ueber die Atrophie der menschlichen Organe bei inanition. Zeitsch ang Anat 7: 87–134

Krook S S 1947 Obstruction of the small intestine due to adhesions and bands. Acta Chir Scand (suppl. 125) 95: 1–200

Kudsk K A, Campbell S M, O'Brian T et al 1990 Postoperative jejunal feeding following complicated pancreatitis. Nutrition in Clinical Practice 5: 14–17

Kumar A, Falke J, Geffin B et al 1970 Continuous positive-pressure ventilation in acute respiratory failure — effects on haemodynamics and lung function. N Engl J Med 283: 1430–6

Ladefoged K, Christensen K, Hegnhoj J et al 1989 Effect of a long acting somatostatin analogue SMS 201–995 on jejunostomy effluent in patients with severe short bowel syndrome. Gut 30: 943–949

Lancet 1979 Editorial: Postoperative fatigue. Lancet I: 84–85

Lancet 1990 Editorial: Severe symptomatic hyponatraemia: dangers of lack of therapy. Lancet 335: 825–826

Lancet 1990a Editorial: All aboard for octreotide! Lancet 336: 909–910

Lancet 1990 Editorial: Endotoxin bound and gagged. Lancet 337: 588–590

Larrick J W, Bourla J M 1986 Prospects for the therapeutic use of human monoclonal antibodies. J Biol Response Mod 5: 379–393

Larsson L, Grimby G, Karlsson J 1979 Muscle strength and speed of movement in relation to age and muscle morphology. J Appl Physiol 46: 451–456

Layzer R B 1991 How muscles are fuel. N Engl J Med 324: 411–412

Law D K, Dudrick S J, Abdou N I 1973 Immunocompetence of patients with protein calorie malnutrition. The effect of nutritional repletion. Ann Intern Med 79: 545–550

Lewis M I, Belman M J 1988 Nutrition and the respiratory muscles. Clin Chest Medicine 9: 337–348

Liljedahl S O, Gemzell C A, Plantin L O et al 1961 Effect of human growth hormone in patients with severe burns. Acta Chir Scand 122: 1–14

Lim S T, Choa R G, Lam K H et al 1981 Total parenteral nutrition versus gastrostomy in the preoperative preparation of patients with carcinoma of the oesophagus. Br J Surg 68: 69–72

Livesey G, Elia M 1988 Estimation of energy expenditure, net carbohydrate utilization and net fat oxidation and synthesis by indirect calorimetry: evaluation of errors with special reference to the detailed composition of fuels. Amer J Clin Nutr 47: 608–628

Long C L, Lowry S F 1990 Hormonal regulation of protein metabolism. J Parenter Enter Nutr 14: 555–562

Long C L, Schaffel N, Geiger J W et al 1979 Metabolic response to injury and illness: estimation of energy and protein needs from indirect calorimetry and nitrogen balance. J Parenter Enter Nutr 3: 452–456

Long C L, Birkhahn R H, Geiger J W et al 1981 Urinary excretion of 3-methylhistidine: an assessment of muscle protein catabolism in adult normal subjects and during malnutrition, sepsis, and skeletal trauma. Metabolism 30: 765–776

Lopes J, Russle D M, Whitwell J et al 1982 Skeletal muscle function in malnutrition. Am J Clin Nutr 36: 602–610

Louyot P, Mathieu J, Gaucher A 1961 L'osteose rareficante des gastrectomies. Archives des Maladies de l'Appareil Digestif et des Maladies de la Nutrition 50: 220–238

Lukaski H C, Bolonchuk W W 1988 Estimation of body fluid volumes using tetrapolar bioelectrical impedance measurements. Aviat Space Environ Med 59: 1163–1169

MacFie J, Holmfield J H M, King R F G, Hill G L 1983 Effect of the energy source on changes in energy expenditure and respiratory quotient during total parenteral nutrition. J Parenter Enter Nutr 7: 1–5

MacFie J, Burkinshaw L, Oxby C, Holmfield J H M, Hill G L 1982 The effect of gastrointestinal malignancy on resting metabolic expenditure. Br J Surg 69: 443–446

McIntyre P B, Powell-Tuck J, Wood S R et al 1986 Controlled trial of bowel rest in the treatment of severe acute colitis. Gut 27: 481–485

McIntyre P B, Wood S R, Powell-Tuck J et al 1983 Nocturnal nasogastric tube feeding at home. Postgrad Med J 59: 767–769

Macklem P T 1986 Muscular weakness and respiratory function. Editorial. N Engl J Med 314: 775–6

McMahon M J 1988 Diseases of the exocrine pancreas. In: Kinney J M, Jeejeebhoy K N, Hill G L, Owen J O E (eds) Nutrition and Metabolism in Patient Care. W B Saunders, Philadelphia pp 386–404

McNair D M, Lorr M, Droppleman L F 1971 Profile of mood states. Manual 1971. Education and Industrial Testing Services, San Diego

Madden H P, Breslin R J, Wasserkrug H L et al 1988 Stimulation of T cell immunity by arginine enhances survival in peritonitis. J Surg Res 44: 658–663

Marano M A, Fong Y, Moldawer L L et al 1990 Serum cachectin/TNF in critically ill patients with burns correlates with infection and mortality. Surg Gynaec Obstet 170: 32–38

Mason W, Wenberg B G, Welsch P 1977 The dynamics of clinical dietetics. J Waley & Sons, New York

Matthews D E, Heymsfield S B 1991 ASPEN 1990 research workshop on energy metabolism. J Parenter Enter Nutr 15: 3–14

Mayer A D, McMahon M J, Corfield A et al 1985 A randomized trial of peritoneal lavage for the treatment of severe acute pancreatitis. NEMJ 312: 399–404

Mazess R B, Barden H S, Bisek J P et al 1990 Dual energy X-ray absorptiometry for total body and regional bone mineral and soft tissue composition. Am J Clin Nutr 51: 1106–1121

Metheny N, Eisenberg P, McSweeney M 1988 Effect of feeding tube properties and three irrigants on clogging rates. Nurs Res 37: 165–169

Michie H R, Eberlein T J, Spriggs D R et al 1988a Interleukin-2 initiates metabolic responses associated with critical illness in humans. Ann Surg 208: 493–503

Michie H R, Manogue K R, Spriggs D R et al 1988b Detection of circulating tumour necrosis factor after endotoxin administration. N Engl J Med 318: 148–186

Michie H R, Spriggs D R, Manogue K R et al 1988c Tumour necrosis factor and endotoxin induce similar metabolic responses in human beings. Surgery 104: 280–286

Michie H R, Wilmore D W 1990 Sepsis and tumor necrosis factor — bed fellows that cannot be ignored. Ann Surg 212: 653–654

Minuto F, Barreca A, Adami G F 1989 Insulin like growth factor-I in human malnutrition. Relationship with some body composition and nutritional parameters. J Parenter Enter Nutr 13: 392–396

Mirtallo J M, Schneider P J, Mavko K et al 1982 I A comparison of essential and general amino acid infusions in the nutritional support of patients with compromised renal function. J Parenter Enter Nutr 6: 109–113

Mitchell A, Watkins R M, Collin J 1984 Surgical treatment of the short bowel syndrome. Br J Surg 71: 329

Mochizuki H, Trocki O, Dominioni L et al 1984 Mechanism of prevention of post burn hypermetabolism and catabolism by early enteral feeding. Ann Surg 200: 297–310

Moghissi K, Hornshaw J R, Teasdale P R, Dawes E A 1977 Parenteral nutrition in carcinoma of the oesophagus treated by surgery: nitrogen balance and clinical studies. Br J Surg 64: 125–128

Moore F A, Moore E E, Jones T N et al 1989 TEN versus TPN following major abdominal trauma. Reduced septic morbidity. J Trauma 29: 916–923

Moore F D 1959a Metabolic care of the surgical patient. W B Saunders, Philadelphia, p 25–48

Moore F D 1959b Septic starvation. In: Metabolic care of the surgical patient. W B Saunders, Philadelphia, ch 29: 452–456

Moore F D, Ball M R 1952 The metabolic response to surgery. American Lecture Seminars no. 32. Charles C Thomas, Springfield, III

Moore F D, Boyden C M 1963 Body cell mass and limits of hydration of the fat free body: their relation to estimated skeletal weight. Ann N Y Acad Sci 110: 62–71

Moore R, Najarian M P, Konvolinka C 1989 Measured energy expenditure in severe head trauma. J Trauma 29: 1633–1636

Morgan D B, Hill G L, Burkinshaw L 1980 The assessment of weight loss from a single measurement of body weight — the problems and limitations. Am J Clin Nutr 33: 2101–2105

Morgan R W, Jain M, Miller A B et al 1978 A comparison of dietary methods in epidemiological studies. Am J Epidemiol 107: 488–498

Morris D L, Hawker P C, Brearley S et al 1984 Optimal timing of operation for bleeding peptic ulcer. A prospective randomised trial. Br Med J 288: 1277–80

Mosca R, Curtas S, Forbes B, Meguid M M 1987 The benefits of isolator cultures in the management of suspected catheter sepsis. Surgery 102: 718–723

Moss G 1984 Efficient gastroduodenal decompression with simultaneous full enteral nutrition: a new gastrostomy catheter technique. J Parenter Enter Nutr 8: 203–207

Moss G, Greenstein A, Levy S et al 1980 Maintenance of GI function after bowel surgery and immediate full nutrition. I Doubling of canine colorectal anastomotic bursting pressure and intestinal wound mature collagen content. J Parenter Enter Nutr 4: 435–538

Muggia-Sullam M, Bower R H, Murphy F et al 1985 Postoperative enteral vs parenteral nutritional support in gastrointestinal surgery: a matched prospective study. Am J Surg 149: 106–112

Mughal M, Irving M H 1986 Home parenteral nutrition in the United Kingdom and Ireland. Lancet II: 383–387

Mullen J L, Buzby G P, Gertner M H et al 1980 Protein synthesis dyamics in human gastrointestinal malignancies. Surgery 87: 331–338

Murphy L M, Lipman T O 1987 Central venous catheter care in parenteral nutrition: a review. J Parenter Enter Nutr 11: 190–200

Nanni G, Siegel J H, Coleman B 1984 Increased lipid fuel dependence in the critically ill septic patient. J Trauma 24: 14–30

Neugebauer E, Troidl H, Spangenberger W et al 1991 Conventional versus laparascopic cholecystectomy and the randomised controlled trial. Br J Sur 78: 150–154

Newsholme E A, Parry-Billings M 1990 Properties of glutamine release from muscle and its importance for the immune system. J Parenter Enter Nutr 14: 63S–67S

Newsholme E A, Newsholme P, Curi R et al 1988 A role for muscle in the immune system and its importance in surgery, trauma, sepsis and burns. Nutrition 4: 261–268

Nichols B L, Alvarado J, Hazlewood C F et al 1972 Clinical significance of muscle potassium depletion in protein calorie malnutrition. J Paediatr 80: 319–30

NIH 1988 National Institute of Health consensus development statement on perioperative red cell transfusion. US Department of Health and Human Sciences, Bethesda, Maryland, vol 7

Nohr C 1989 Non-AIDS immunosuppression. In: Wilmore D W, Brennan M F, Harken A H et al (eds) The special problems in perioperative care in care of the surgical patient. Scientific American, New York, part 7, ch 3, p 14

Nordenstrom J, Jeevanandam M, Elwyn D H 1981 Increasing glucose intake during total parenteral nutrition increases norepinephrine excretion in trauma and sepsis. Clin Physiol 1: 525–534

Nordenstrom J, Jeppson B, Loven L et al 1991 Peripheral parenteral nutrition: Effect of a standardised compounded mixture on infusion phlebitis. Br J Surg 78: 1391–1394

Nubiola P, Badia J M, Martinez-Rodenas F et al 1989 Treatment of 27 postoperative enterocutaneous fistulas with the long half life somatostatin analogue SMS 201–995. Ann Surg 210: 56–58

Nyhus L M 1990 Invited commentary. W J Surg 14: 269–270

Oates J A, Fitzgerald G A, Branch R A et al 1988 Clinical implications of prostaglandins and thromboxane A_2 formation. New Engl J Med 319: 689–798

O'Dwyer S, Michie H, Ziegler T et al 1988 A simple dose of endotoxin increases intestinal permeability in humans. Arch Surg 123: 1459–1464

Ohlsson K, Björk P, Bergenfeldt M et al 1990 Interleukin-1 receptor antagonist reduces mortality from endotoxin shock. Nature 348: 550–552

Orgill D, Demling R H 1988 Current concepts in approaches to wound healing. Crit Care Med 16: 899–908

O'Rourke M F 1982 Vascular impedance in studies of arterial and cardiac function. Physiol Rev 62: 570–623

Ota D M, Frasier P, Guevara J et al 1985 Plasma proteins as indices of response to nutritional therapy in cancer patients. J Surg Onc 29: 160–165

Park K G M, Hayes P D, Garlick P J et al 1991 Stimulation of lymphocyte natural cytoxicity by L-arginine. Lancet 337: 645–646

Parks A G, Allen C L O, Frank J D et al 1978 A method of treating post irradiation rectovaginal fistulas. Br J Surg 65: 417–421

Parry B 1989 Energy requirements of surgical patients. MD Thesis, Otago University

Paterson-Brown S, Garden O J, Carter D C 1991 Laparascopic cholecystectomy. Br J Sur 78: 131–132

Payne-James J J, Silk D B 1988 Total parenteral nutrition as primary treatment in Crohn's disease–RIP? Gut 29: 1304–1308

Peck M, Ogle C, Alexander J W 1991 Composition of fat and enteral diets can influence outcome in experimental peritonitis. Ann Surg 214: 74–82

Person J L, Brower R A 1986 Necrotizing fasciitis/myositis following percutaneous endoscopic gastrostomy. Gastrointest Endoscop 32: 309

Petrakos A, Myers M L, Holliday R L et al 1981 A systemic increase in capillary permeability in septicaemia. Crit Care Med 9: 214

Petrosino B, Becker H, Christian B 1988 Infection rates in central venous catheter dressings. Oncol Nurs Forum 15: 709–717

Pettigrew R A, Hill G L 1986 Indicators of surgical risk and clinical judgment. Br J Surg 73: 47–51

Pettigrew R A, Charlesworth P M, Farmilo R W, Hill G L 1984 Assessment of nutritional depletion and immune competence: a comparison of clinical examination and objective measurements. J Parenter Enter Nutr 8: 21–24

Pettigrew R A, Lang S D, Haydock D A et al 1985 Catheter related sepsis in patients on intravenous nutrition: a prospective study of quantitative catheter cultures and guidewire changes for suspected sepsis. Br J Surg 72: 52–55

Phillips L S 1986 Nutrition, somatomedins and the brain. Metabolism 35: 78–87

Pillar B, Perry S 1990 Evaluating total parenteral nutrition: final report and statement of the technology. Assessment and Practice Guidelines Forum. Nutrition 6: 314–318

Pizzini R P, Kumar S, Kulkarni A D et al 1990 Dietary nucleotides reverse malnutrition and starvation induced immunosuppression. Arch Surg 125: 86–90

Ponsky J, Gauderer M W 1989 Percutaneous endoscopic gastrostomy: indications, limitations, techniques and results. World J Surg 13: 165–170

Present D I J, Korelitz B I, Wisch N et al 1980 Treatment of Crohn's disease with 6-mercaptopurine. N Engl J Med 302: 981

Pullan J M 1959 Massive intestinal resections. Proc R Soc Med 52: 31

Pullicino E, Goldberg G R, Elia M 1991 Energy expenditure and substrate metabolism measured by 24 hour whole body calorimetry in patients receiving cyclic and continuous total parenteral nutrition. Clin Sci 80: 571–582

Purdum P P, Kirby D F 1991 Short bowel syndrome: a review of the role of nutrition support. J Parenter Enter Nutr 15: 93–101

Quayle A R, Mangnall D, Clarke R G 1984 A comparison of immediate postoperative enteral and parenteral nutrition in patients with gastric carcinoma. Clinical Nutrition 3: 35–39

Ranson J H C, Pasternack B S 1977 Statistical methods for quantifying the severity of clinical acute pancreatitis. J Surg Res 22: 79–91

Ranson J H C, Spencer F C 1978 The role of peritoneal lavage in severe acute pancreatitis. Ann Surg 187: 565–574

Ranson J H C, Rifkind K M, Roses D F et al 1974 Prognostic signs and the role of operative management in acute pancreatitis. Surg Gynaec Obstet 139: 69–81

Ranson J H C, Balthazar E, Caccavale R et al 1985 Computed tomography and the prediction of pancreatic abscess in acute pancreatitis. Ann Surg 201: 656–665

Reber H A, Roberts L, Way L W, Dunphy J E 1978 Management of external gastrointestinal fistulas. Ann Surg 188: 460–467

Reid D J, Brown R O, Vehe K L et al 1988 Predicting human-albumin replacement dosages in hyperalbuminaemic patients receiving total parenteral nutrition. Clin Pharm 7: 894–897

Revhaug A, Michie H R, Manson J M et al 1988 Inhibition of cyclooxygenase attenuates the metabolic response to endotoxin in humans. Arch Surg 123: 162–170

Rhoades R A 1975 Influence of starvation on the lung: effect on glucose and palmitate utilization. J Appl Physiol 38: 513–516

Ritchie J K 1972 Ulcerative colitis treated by ileostomy and excisional surgery: 15 years experience at St Mark's Hospital. Br J Surg 59: 345–351

Roberts J P, Roberts J D, Skinner C et al 1985 Extracellular fluid deficit following operation and its

correction with Ringer's lactate. Ann Surg 202: 1–8
Roe C F, Kinney J 1962 The influence of growth hormone on energy sources in convalescence. Surg Forum 13: 369–371
Rombeau J L, Kripke S A 1990 Metabolic and intestinal effects of short chain fatty acids. J Parenter Enter Nutr 14: 181S–185S
Roth E, Zöch G, Schulz F et al 1985 Amino acid concentrations in plasma and skeletal muscle of patients with acute haemorrhagic necrotising pancreatitis. Clin Chem 31: 1305–1309
Rothe C F 1983 Reflex control of veins and vascular capacitance. Physiol Rev 63: 1281–342
Rowe J W 1980 Aging and renal function. Ann Rev Gerontol Geriatr 1: 161
Roza A M, Shizgal H M 1984 The Harris–Benedict equation reevaluated: Resting energy requirements and the body cell mass. Am J Clin Nutr 40: 168
Rudman D, Millikan W J, Richardson D et al 1975 Elemental balances during intravenous hyperalimentation of underweight adult subjects. J Clin Invest 55: 94–104
Russel D, Walker P M, Leiter L A et al 1984 Metabolic and structural changes in skeletal muscle during hypocaloric dieting. Am J Clin Nutr 39: 503–513
Rutherford R B, Balis J V, Trow R S et al 1976 Comparison of hemodynamic and regional blood flow changes at equivalent stages of endotoxin and hemorrhagic shock. J Trauma 16: 886–97
Ryan J A, Page C P, Babcock L 1981 Early postoperative jejunal feeding of elemental diet in gastrointestinal surgery. Am Surg 47: 393–403
Ryan J A, Adye B A, Weinstein A J 1986 Enteric fistulas. In: Rombeau J L, Caldwell M D (eds) Parenteral nutrition. W B Saunders, Philadelphia, ch 24: 434
Saar M G, Bulkley G B, Zuidema G D 1983 Preoperative recognition of intestinal strangulation obstruction. Am J Surg 145: 176–182
Sachar D B 1989 Cyclosporine treatment for inflammatory bowel disease. A step backward or a leap forward. N Engl J Med 321: 894–896
Sagar S, Harland P, Shields R 1979 Early postoperative feeding with elemental diet. Br Med J 1: 293–295
Sagawa T, Hitsumoto Y, Kanoh M et al 1990 Mechanisms of neutralization of endotoxin by monoclonal antibodies to O and R determinants of lipopolysaccharide. Adv Exp Med Biol 256: 341–344
Saito H, Trocki O, Alexander J W et al 1987 The effect of route of nutrient administration on the nutritional state, catabolic hormone secretion and gut mucosal integrity after burn injury. J Parenter Enter Nutr 11: 1–17
Salleh M, Ardawi M, Majzoub M F 1991 Glutamine metabolism in skeletal muscle of septic patients. Metabolism 40: 155–164
Salles M-F, Mandine E, Zalisz R et al 1989 Protective effects of murine monclonal antibodies in experimental septicaemia: *E. coli* antibodies protect against different serotypes of *E. coli*. J Infect Dis 159: 641–647
Sanstead H H, Henriksen L K, Greger J L et al 1982 Zinc nutrition in the elderly in relation to taste, acuity, immune response and wound healing. Am J Clin Nutr 36: 1046–1059
Sax H C, Warner B W, Talamini M A et al 1987 Early total parenteral nutrition in acute pancreatitis. Am J Surg 153: 117–124
Scheppach W, Burghardt W, Bartram P et al 1990 Addition of fibre to liquid formula diets: the pros and cons. J Parenter Enter Nutr 14: 204–209
Schoeller D A, van Santen E 1982 Measurement of energy expenditure in humans by double labelled water method. J Appl Physiol 53: 955–959
Schofield P F, Holden D, Carr N D 1983 Bowel disease after radiotherapy. J Roy Soc Med 76: 463–466
Schofield P F, Carr N D, Holden D 1986 Pathogenesis and treatment of radiation bowel disease: discussion paper. J Roy Soc Med 79: 30–32
Schroeder D S, Hill G L 1991 Postoperative fatigue: a prospective physiological study of patients undergoing major abdominal surgery. Aust NZ J Surg (in press)
Schroeder D S, Hill G L 1992 The importance of pre and immediate postoperative factors in the prediction of postoperative fatigue. World J Surg (in press)
Schroeder D S, Christie P M, Hill G L 1990 Bioelectric impedance analysis for body composition: clinical evaluation in general surgical patients. J Parenter Enter Nutr 14: 129–133
Schroeder D, Gillanders L, Mahr K, Hill G L 1991 Effects of immediate postoperative enteral nutrition on body composition, muscle function and wound healing. J Parenter Enter Nutr 15: 376–382
Scott N A, Leinhardt D J, O'Hanrahan T et al 1991 Spectrum of intestinal failure in a specialized unit. Lancet 337: 471–473
Shaw J H F, Humberstone D M 1988 Energy and protein metabolism in sarcoma patients. Ann Surg 207: 283–289
Shaw J H F, Wolfe R R 1986 Glucose fatty acid and urea kinetics in patients with severe pancreatitis — the response to substrate infusion and total parenteral nutrition. Ann Surg 204: 665–672
Shaw J H F, Wolfe R R 1987a Energy and protein metabolism in sepsis and trauma. Aust NZ J Surg 57: 41–47
Shaw J H F, Wolfe R R 1987b Free fatty acid and glycerol kinetics in severely septic patients and in patients with early and advanced gastroenterological cancer. Ann Surg 205: 368–376
Shaw J H F, Wolfe R R 1987c Glucose and urea kinetics in patients with early and advanced gastrointestinal cancer: the response to glucose infusion, parenteral feeding and surgical resection surgery 101: 181–191
Shaw J H F, Wolfe R R 1988a Metabolic intervention in surgical patients. An assessment of the effect of somatostatin, ranitidine, naloxone, diclophenac, dipyridamole or salbutamol infusions on energy and protein kinetics in surgical patients using stable and radio isotopes. Ann Surg 207: 274–282
Shaw J H F, Wolfe R R 1988b Whole body protein kinetics in patients with early and advanced gastrointestinal cancer: the response to glucose infusion and total parenteral nutrition. Surgery 103: 148–155
Shaw J H F, Wolfe R R 1989 An integrated analysis of glucose, fat and protein metabolism in severely traumatised patients. Studies in the basal state and the response to total parenteral nutrition. Ann Surg 209: 63–72
Shaw J H F, Wildbore M, Wolfe R R 1987 Whole body protein kinetics in severely septic patients Ann Surg 205: 288–294
Shields R 1965 The absorption and secretion of fluid and electrolytes by the obstructed bowel. Br J Surg 52: 774–779

Shimamoto Y, Chen R L, Bollon A et al 1988 Monoclonal antibodies against human recombinant tumor necrosis factor: prevention of endotoxic shock. Immunol Lett 17: 311–318

Shires G T, Canizaro P C 1977 Fluid and electrolyte management of the surgical patient. In: Sabiston D (ed) Davis-Christopher: Textbook of surgery. W B Saunders, Philadelphia, p 95–117

Shires G T, Cunningham J N, Backer C R F et al 1972 Alterations in cellular membrane function during haemorrhagic shock in primates. Ann Surg 176: 288–295

Shizgal H M 1991 Nutritional assessment with whole body biolelectric impedance. Am Society of Parenteral and Enteral Nutrition, Handbook of the 15th Clinical Congress, p 158–162

Silen W, Hein M F, Goldman G 1962 Strangulation, obstruction of the small intestine. Archives of Surgery 85: 121–129

Singleton A O, Redmond D C, McMurray J E 1964 Ileocaecal resection and small bowel transit and absorption. Ann Surg 159: 690–694

Sitzmann J V, Steinborn T A, Zinner M J et al 1989 Total parenteral nutrition and alternate energy substrates in treatment of severe acute pancreatitis. Surg Gynaec Obstet 168: 311–317

Skeie B, Askanazi J, Rothkopf M M et al 1988 Intravenous fat emulsions and lung function: a review. Crit Care Med 16: 183–194

Smiddy F G, Gregory S D, Smith I B et al 1960 Faecal loss of fluid, electrolytes and nitrogen in colitis before and after ileostomy. Lancet 1: 14–19

Smith C R 1991 Evidence supporting the efficacy of HA-1A in septic patients with gram negative bacteraemia. In: Duafala M E, Laden S K (eds) Immunotherapy with a human monoclonal antibody — a breakthrough in the management of gram negative sepsis. Scientific Therapeutics Information, Springfield

Smith R C, Hartemink R J, Hollinshead J W et al 1985 Fine bore jejunostomy feeding following major abdominal surgery: a controlled randomized clinical trial. Br J Surg 72: 458–61

Solomon S M, Kirby D F 1990 The refeeding syndrome: a review. J Parenter Enter Nutr 14: 90–97

Souba W N 1990 Proceedings of an international glutamine symposium — glutamine metabolism in health and disease: basic science and clinical aspects. J Parenter Enter Nutr 14: 39S–146S

Souba W W 1988 The gut as a nitrogen-processing organ in the metabolic response to critical illness. Nutr Supp Serv 8(5): 15–22

Stabile B E, Borzatta M, Stubbs R S 1984 Pancreatic secretory responses to intravenous hyperalimentation and intraduodenal elemental and full liquid diets. J Parenter Enter Nutr 8: 377–380

Stassen W N, McCulloch A J, Marshall J B, Eckhauser M L 1986 Percutaneous endoscopic gastrostomy: another case of benign pneumoperitoneum. Gastrointest Endosc 30:296

Steffe W P, Anderson C F 1984 Enteral nutrition and renal disease. In: Rombeau J L, Caldwell M D (eds) Clinical nutrition vol 1. Enteral and tube feeding. W B Saunders, Philadelphia p 362–375

Stokes M A 1991 The malnutrition of Crohn's disease. Ch M Thesis, University of Dublin

Stokes M A, Hill G L 1990a A new method for the measurement of total energy expenditure in surgical patients. Aust NZ J Surg 60: 715

Stokes M A, Hill G L 1990b The short gut. Current Practice in Surgery 2: 139–145

Stokes M A, Hill G L 1992 Effects of parenteral and enteral nutrition on physiological function. (Awaiting publication)

Stokes M A, Irving M H 1989 Mortality in patients on home parenteral nutrition. J Parenter Enter Nutr 13: 172–175

Stokes M A, Almond D J, Pettit S H et al 1988 Home parenteral nutrition: a review of 100 patient years of treatment in 76 consecutive cases. Br J Surg 75: 481–483

Stone H H, Fabian T C 1980 Peritoneal dialysis in the treatment of acute alcoholic peritonitis. Surg Gynaec Obstet 150: 878–882

Streat S J, Hill G L 1987 Nutrition in the management of critically ill patients in surgical intensive care. World J Surg 11: 194–201

Streat S J, Beddoe A H, Hill G L 1985a Measurement of body fat and hydration of the fat free body in health and disease. Metabolism 34: 509–518

Streat S J, Beddoe A H, Hill G L 1985b Measurement of body water in intensive care patients with fluid overload. Metabolism 34: 688–94

Streat S J, Beddoe A H, Hill G L 1986 Changes in body nitrogen — comparison of direct measurement with nitrogen balance. Aust NZ J Surg 56: 257–276

Streat S J, Beddoe A H, Hill G L 1987 Aggressive nutritional support does not prevent protein loss despite fat gain in intensive care patients. J Trauma 27: 262–266

Studley H O 1936 Percentage of weight loss: A basic indicator of surgical risk in patients with chronic peptic ulcer. JAMA 106: 458–460

Sturm J A, Wisner D H, Oestern H J et al 1986 Increased lung capillary permeability after trauma — a prospective clinical study. J Trauma 26: 409–418

Swaminathan R, Bradley J A, Hill G L et al 1980 The effect of varying amounts of intravenous glucose on the metabolism changes after surgery. Postgrad Med J 56: 652–655

Taggart D P, McMillan D C, Preston T et al 1991 Effects of cardiac surgery and intraoperative hypothermia on energy expenditure as measured by doubly labelled water. Br J Surg 78: 237–241

Tarzi R, Steiger E 1988 Enterocutaneous fistulas. In: Kinney J M, Jeejeebhoy K N, Hill G L, Owen O E (eds) Nutrition and metabolism in patient care. W B Saunders, Philadelphia, ch 13: 243–257

Theologides A 1979 Cancer cachexia. Cancer 43: 2004–2012

Thompsom J S, Rikkers L F 1987 Surgical alternatives for the short bowel syndrome. Am J Gastroent 82: 97–106

Thoren L, Wiklund L 1983 Intraoperative fluid therapy. World J Surg 7: 581–589

Tisi G M 1979 Preoperative evaluation of pulmonary function: validity, indications and benefits. Am Rev Respir Dis 119: 293–301

Tovey F I, Hall M L, Ell P J, Hobsley M 1991 Postgastrectomy osteoporosis. Br J Surg 78: 1335–1337

Tracey K J, Beutler B, Lowry S F et al 1986 Shock and tissue injury induced by recombinant human cachectin. Science 234: 470–474

Treves F 1924 Lectures on the anatomy of the intestinal canal and peritoneum in man. Br Med J 1: 415

Trunkey D 1991 Initial treatment of patients with

extensive trauma. N Engl J Med 324: 1259–1263
Twomey P, Ziegler D, Rombeau J 1982 Utility of skin testing in nutritional assessment: a critical review J Parenter Enter Nutr 6: 50–58
Twomey P L, Patching S C 1985 Cost effectiveness of nutritional support. J Parenter Enter Nutr 9: 3–10
Tzakis A, Todo S, Reyes J et al 1992 Clinical intestinal transplantation. Transplant Proc (in press)
Uehara A, Gottschall P E, Dahl R R et al 1987 Interleukin-1 stimulates ACTH release by an indirect action which requires endogenous corticotrophin releasing factor. Endocrinology 121: 1580–2
Ultman J S, Bursztein S 1981 Analysis of error in the determination of respiratory gas exchange at varying FO. J Appl Physiol Respirat Environ Exercise Physiol 50: 210
Unterman T G, Vazquez R M, Slas A J et al 1985 Nutrition and somatomedin XIII — usefulness of somatomedin-C in nutritional assessment. Am J Med 78: 228–234
Vaisman N, Pencharz P B, Koren et al 1987 Comparison of oral and intravenous administration of sodium bromide for extracellular water measurement. Am J Clin Nutr 46: 1–4
Van Buren C, Kulkarni A D, Schandle V B et al 1983 The influence of dietary nucleotides on cell mediated immunity. Transplantation 36: 350–352
Vincent J L 1991 Plugging the leaks? New insights into synthetic colloids. Crit Care Med 19: 316–317
Virgilio R W, Rice C L, Smith D E et al 1979 Crystalloid vs colloid resuscitation: is one better? A randomized clinical study. Surgery 85: 129–139
Viteri F E, Béhar M, Arroyave G, Scrimshaw N S 1964 In: Munro H N, Allison J B (eds) Mammalian protein metabolism. Academic Press, New York & London
Wahba W B 1983 Influence of ageing on lung function: clinical significance of changes from age twenty. Anaes Analg 62: 764–776
Wan J M, Haw M P, Blackburn G L 1989 Nutrition, immune function, and inflammation: an overview. Proceedings of the Nutrition Society 48: 315–335
Ward R A, Shirlow M J, Hayes J M et al 1979 Protein catabolism during haemodialysis. Am J Clin Nutr 32: 2443–2449
Warner M A, Hosking M P, Lobdell C M et al 1988 Surgical procedures among those greater than or equal to 90 years of age: a population based study in Olmstead County, Minnesota 1975–1978. Ann Surg 207: 380–386
Watters J M, Bessey P Q, Dinarello C A et al 1985 The induction of interleukin-1 in humans and its metabolic effects. Surgery 98: 298–306
Watters J M, Redmond M L, Desai D et al 1990 Effects of age and body composition on the metabolic response to elective colon resection. Ann Surg 212: 213–220
Watson M L, Lewis G P, Westwick J 1989 Increased vascular permeability and polymorphonuclear leucocyte accumulation in vivo in response to recombinant cytokines and supernatant from cultures of human synovial cells treated with interleukin-1. Br J Exp Pathol 70: 93–101
Webb A R, Moss R F et al 1991 Advantages of a narrow range, medium molecular weight hydroxyethyl starch for volume maintenance in a porcine model of fecal peritonitis. Crit Care Med 19: 409–416
Webb P 1984 Human calorimeters. Praeger, New York
Weinsier R L, Krumdieck C L 1981 Death resulting from overzealous total parenteral nutrition — the refeeding syndrome revisited. Am J Clin Nutr 34: 393–399
Welbourn R, Goldman G, Kobzik L et al 1990 Involvement of thromboxane and neutrophils in multiple-system organ edema with Interleukin-2. Ann Surg 212: 728–733
Wernerman J, Hammarqvist F, Vinnars E 1990 α-Ketoglutarate and postoperative muscle catabolism. Lancet 335: 701–703
Wilmore D W 1991 Catabolic illness-strategies for enhancing recovery. N Engl J Med 365: 695–702
Wilmore D W, Dudrick S J 1968 Growth and development of an infant receiving all nutrients exclusively by vein. JAMA 203: 860–864
Windmueller H G 1982 Glutamine utilization by the small intestine. Adv Enzymol 53: 201–237
Windsor J A 1989 Body protein loss in preoperative patients: the assessment of its impact on physiological function and surgical risk. MD Thesis, University of Auckland
Windsor J A, Hill G L 1988a Grip strength: a measure of the proportion of protein loss in surgical patients. Br J Surg 75: 880–882
Windsor J A, Hill G L 1988b Protein depletion and surgical risk. Aust NZ J Surg 58: 711–715
Windsor J A, Hill G L 1988c Risk factors for postoperative pneumonia: the importance of protein depletion. Ann Surg 208: 209–214
Windsor J A, Hill G L 1988d Weight loss with physiologic impairment — a basic indicator of surgical risk. Ann Surg 207: 290–296
Windsor J A, Knight G S, Hill G L 1988 Wound healing response in surgical patients: recent food intake is more important than nutritional status. Br J Surg 75: 135–137
Winkler M F, Gerrior S A, Pomp A et al 1989 Use of retinol-binding protein and prealbumin as indicators of the response to nutrition therapy. J Am Diet Assoc 89: 684–687
Wolfe R R, Allsop J R, Burke J F 1979 Glucose metabolism in man: responses to intravenous glucose infusion. Metabolism 28: 210–220
Wolfe R R 1984 Tracers in metabolic research: radio-isotope and stable isotope/mass spectrometry methods. Arliss, New York
Wolff S M 1991 Monoclonal antibodies and the treatment of gram negative bacteraemia and shock. N Engl J Med 324: 486–488
Wolfman E F, Trevino G, Heaps D R et al 1964 An operative technique for the management of acute and chronic lateral duodenal fistulas. Ann Surg 159: 563–569
Wolman S L, Anderson G H, Marliss E B et al 1979 Zinc in total parenteral nutrition: requirements and metabolic effects. Gastroenterology 76: 458–467
Woolf G M, Miller C, Kurian R et al 1983 Diet for patients with a short bowel. High fat or high carbohydrate? Gastroenterology 84: 823–828
Yamada N, Koyama H, Hioki K et al 1983 Effect of postoperative total parenteral nutrition (TPN) as an adjunct to gastrectomy for advanced gastric carcinoma. Br J Surg 70: 267–274
Yasumura S, Cohn S H, Ellis K J 1983 Measurement of extracellular space by total body neutron activation. Am J Physiol 244: R36–R40
Yeung C K, Smith R C, Hill G L 1979 Effect of an elemental diet on body composition — a comparison

with intravenous nutrition. Gastroenterology 77: 652–657

Yeung C K, Young G A, Hackett A F, Hill G L 1979 Fine needle catheter jejunostomy: an assessment of a new method of nutritional support after major gastrointestinal surgery. Br J Surg 66: 727–732

Young G A, Hill G L 1978 Assessment of protein-calorie malnutrition in surgical patients from plasma proteins and anthropometric measurements. Am J Clin Nutr 31: 429–435

Young G A, Hill G L 1980 A controlled study of protein sparing therapy after excision of the rectum. Effects of intravenous amino acids and hyperalimentation on body composition and plasma amino acids. Ann Surg 192: 183–191

Zager R, Venkatachalam M A 1983 Potentiation of ischemic renal injury by amino acid infusion. Kidney Int 24: 620–625

Zak J, Burns D, Lingenfelser T et al 1991 Dry beri beri: unusual complication of prolonged parenteral nutrition. J Parenter Enter Nutr 15: 200–201

Ziegler E J, Fisher C J, Sprung C L et al 1991 Treatment of gram-negative bacteraemia and septic shock with HA-1A human monoclonal antibody against endotoxin — a randomised, double blind, placebo-controlled diet. N Engl J Med 324: 429–436

Ziegler T R, Young L S, Ferrari-Baliviera E et al 1990 Use of growth hormone combined with nutritional support in a critical care unit. J Parenter Enter Nutr 14: 574–581

Index